Healthcare Management Dictionary

Annie Phillips
Independent Health Adviser
Management Consultant to General Practice

RADCLIFFE MEDICAL PRESS

Radcliffe Medical Press Ltd
18 Marcham Road
Abingdon
Oxon OX14 1AA
United Kingdom

www.radcliffe-oxford.com
The Radcliffe Medical Press electronic catalogue and online ordering facility.
Direct sales to anywhere in the world

British Library Cataloguing in Publication Data

A catalogue record for this book is available from the British Library.

ISBN 1 85775 802 1

Typeset by Advance Typesetting Ltd, Oxon
Printed and bound by TJ International Ltd, Padstow, Cornwall

Preface

The NHS has its own often bewildering array of management terms, acronyms, jargon and technical phrases. To anyone new to the NHS this can be confusing. Even experienced NHS clinicians or managers may be familiar with the jargon used in their own field, but may find that the terms used in different sectors sound like a foreign language. This dictionary provides plain English definitions of those hundreds of phrases that are commonly used within the NHS, with details of the websites where you can find more information.

This book aims to clarify the terminology and broaden the reader's understanding of healthcare. A mutual understanding of NHS terminology is also invaluable for multi-disciplinary teams, as it can assist communication between disciplines. It is aimed at all NHS workers, especially the new, inexperienced or overworked manager or clinician who has neither the time nor the energy to keep up to date with the new terminology as it emerges.

The main focus is on clinical management terms that are currently in use within primary care. Also included are terms more commonly used in secondary or social care, but which influence or impact on those working in primary care, and general management terms widely used in the private sector that may befuddle or bemuse managers and clinicians as they are imported into the NHS. It is particularly aimed at new or less senior managers who are aiming to take up the mantle of effective leadership and equip themselves with the skills required of them in the new NHS.

No single text can ever be fully comprehensive, and by its very nature some of the material in this book will date very quickly. Because of this, I also recommend the websites www.doh.gov.uk and www.guardiansociety.co.uk, both of which have alphabetical site indexes which are useful to visit in order to obtain information on current Government bodies, new legislation and reports.

I have endeavoured to select the terms that are likely to be most useful in current general practice. If I have not included something which you feel strongly should be included, or I have misinterpreted any material, please let me know so that any amendments can be included in future editions.

Annie Phillips
aphillips@cwcom.net or www.anniephillips.co.uk
May 2003

About the author

Annie Phillips has written professionally about health and health management since she qualified as a speech and language therapist in 1978. She has over 20 years of NHS experience in primary and secondary care as a clinician and manager.

Her 10 years practising as a speech and language therapist led to research on and publication of an international dysphasia/dementia screening test, presented at the 1986 British Aphasiology Conference. Annie has won various prizes and awards for her subsequent work, and in the 1990s she was a finalist in the Medeconomics Good Management Awards and a regional winner in a national British Institute of Management competition on change management.

She worked as a practice manager and fund manager for a five-partner training practice in central Brighton from 1989 to 1998. Since then she has returned to clinical work as a speech and language therapist and she also works as an independent health adviser, trainer and management consultant to general practice, health authorities, primary care groups and primary care trusts.

Throughout her career she has written extensively for the therapy, GP and management press. She currently writes on contemporary management issues for a range of publications, including *Health Service Journal*, *Community Care*, *Doctor*, *Practice Management* and Croner Publications, with a focus on healthcare politics and human resource management.

As a management consultant, her interest is in organisational analysis and the development of healthy organisations, with a focus on finding ways to manage stress and conflict, understanding and alleviating dysfunctional communication, and developing effective management strategies.

Annie can be contacted via aphillips@cwcom.net or www.anniephillips.co.uk.

A

ACAS

The Arbitration, Conciliation and Advisory Services. Founded in 1974, ACAS is considered to be the national employment relations expert. It is a public body funded by taxpayers and run by a council of members from business, unions and the independent sector. ACAS provides information and training for employers and employees on employment legislation, its core role being to prevent and resolve problems in the workplace.

www.acas.org.uk

Access

The extent to which service users are able to receive the care that they require. The issues involved in accessibility include travelling long distances, physical access (e.g. premises suitable for wheelchairs), communication (e.g. interpreters) and the availability of culturally appropriate services.

Access in healthcare is dominated by the focus on improving patient throughput. However, it is also about ensuring that patient care is:[1]

- accessible (no barriers, timely)

- appropriate (evidence based, meets the needs of the population)

- effective and efficient (best use of resources)

- equitable (respectful, provided on the basis of need)

- relevant (responsive and sufficient)

- acceptable (meets user expectations)

- knowledge based (sound information supports any decision making)

- accountable (principally and financially, outcome based)

- integrative (involves other agencies).

An accessible service ensures that all patient groups are catered for, regardless of their age, class or personal circumstances.

The Government introduced access targets in 2000, with the aim of increasing the proportion of patients who see a GP or health professional within 48 hours. Some GP practices improve their patient access by running *open-access* systems (surgeries with no appointments) or *mixed-access* systems (a mixture of booked and non-booked appointments). Although the *advanced-access* system takes more resources to set up, it is considered to be by far the most successful type, both by practices who use it and by the public.

Dr John Oldham's team at the *NHS Modernisation Agency* in Manchester disseminates information on how GPs can best improve their patient access arrangements by using an advanced-access system. This involves auditing consultation rates (telephone consultations, inappropriate follow-ups, etc.) and working out the best methods for resolving appointment problems (e.g. by having one doctor each morning devoted to seeing emergencies only, or using nurse triage).

The principle of advanced access can be summarised as follows.

1 Consultation data are produced by analysing how many patients the practice sees each day.

2 This demand is shaped as appropriate.

3 The demand is then matched to capacity.

4 A contingency plan for busy periods is put in place.

Assessment also takes into account the broader aspects of general practice work, such as the practice nurse/community nurse skill mix, the use of additional support services (e.g. optometry or pharmacy) or the use of NHS Direct, locum and deputising services. *See* **Quality team development**.

www.doh.gov.uk/scg/facs/index.htm

1 Maxwell R (1984) Quality assessment in health. *BMJ.* **288**: 1470.

Accountability
The duty to take responsibility for one's own actions, and to be able to give a full explanation of these actions to those who may request it (e.g. peers, or external agencies such as patients and policy makers).

Accreditation of healthcare
The formal recognition and achievement of a standard of quality attained by a healthcare unit. Accreditation agencies are usually independent of both the providers of care and those purchasing or commissioning it.

Practice accreditation schemes, originally developed by the Royal College of General Practitioners (RCGP), have been piloted and run by several primary care organisations throughout the country. Around 90% of practices in Scotland have now achieved accreditation. Accreditation requires practices to work within a specified quality framework; the RCGP scheme asks GPs to meet 46 essential criteria, based on what they are currently legally obliged to offer. GPs can then select 20 other 'good' or 'quality' criteria. An example of a 'good' criterion is an average length of booked appointments of not less than 7.5 minutes. An example of a 'quality' criterion is the team having a profile of patients' health needs and a strategy for tackling inequalities. *See* **Certification**.

Action-centred leadership

This approach is associated with the work of John Adair,[1] who noted that the effectiveness of the leader is dependent on meeting three areas of need within the work group, namely the need to achieve the common task, the need for team maintenance and the individual needs of the team members. Adair symbolises these needs by means of three overlapping circles. *See* **Leadership**.

1 Adair J (1979) *Action-Centred Leadership*. Gower, Aldershot.

Acute services

Medical and surgical treatment provided mainly in hospitals, but occasionally in satellite diagnostic and treatment centres. Acute trusts are management units in charge of hospitals that provide these services.

Additional clinical services

A group of services provided by the new GP contract. Most practices would be expected to provide these services, which would include vaccination and immunisation, contraception, child health surveillance, cervical cytology and chronic disease management. In exceptional circumstances it would be possible to opt out of providing one or more additional clinical services. Practices would have to give notice to the primary care organisation of their intention to opt out, so that alternative providers could be found for patients. *See* **GP contract**.

Administrator

Unlike managers, who oversee the planning and development of a piece of work, administrators administrate it. Administrators may plan work activities (e.g. meeting the month's production quotas), but they are rarely required to plan further ahead.

Algorithm

A procedure for problem solving, frequently used by NHS Direct and other computer users. It is a format often used to display clinical guidelines, showing the process of care diagrammatically as a series of branching 'if–then' or 'yes/no' statements. It usually consists of a series of boxed questions, the answers to which lead down to the next management step. *See* **Protocol**.

Allied health professional (AHP)

A professional healthcare worker who works alongside and supports medical personnel (also called a profession supplementary to medicine). Their training, roles and responsibilities vary widely, with some qualified to honours degree level, working autonomously as diagnosticians (e.g. speech and language therapists), and others working to a medical prescription (e.g. dietitians, radiographers). AHPs include art therapists, chiropodists, clinical scientists, dietitians, medical laboratory technicians, occupational, speech and language therapists, physiotherapists, orthoptists, paramedics, prosthetists, orthotists and radiographers. *See* **Health Professions Council**; **Professions supplementary to medicine**.

APD (Accredited Professional Development Scheme)

An initiative launched by the Royal College of General Practitioners (RCGP) in April 2002 to help doctors to meet revalidation requirements. A voluntary process undertaken over a five-year period, it requires GPs to prove ongoing competence in topics such as keeping up to date, improving care, referrals, prescribing and communication skills. GPs who are undertaking the programme require supervision from an RCGP-accredited facilitator; otherwise they complete the ADP pack alone following participation in an annual study day. *See* **Revalidation**.

www.rcgp.org.uk

Appraisal

The process by which an employee's performance is reviewed periodically against the various requirements of the job. Appraisals developed out of systems of 'merit rating' in the early 1900s. By the mid-1900s this had developed into a *management-by-objectives* approach, advocated by the management guru Peter Drucker, which deliberately excluded any attempt to give personality ratings. Between 1970 and 1990 *performance appraisal* schemes were introduced (which included an overall rating of performance and individual personality characteristics), which were closely linked to *performance-related pay* schemes. From 1990 to the present day, *performance management* has been conceived of as a normal and continuous process of management, rather than an annual ritual. It focuses on agreement and dialogue, and is concerned not only with outputs (results) but also with inputs (competencies).

The needs of the individual and the organisation within which they work do not always coincide, so appraisal is a means of exploring any conflict that exists. Modern appraisals are designed to be peer reviewed, fair, constructive, objective, positive, evidence based, unbiased and supportive, yet challenging. They form part of the *revalidation* system that is being set up for doctors.

There are various appraisal models, which may be one way (rated by the appraiser only), a joint process (self-rated and fed back by the appraiser) or 360 degree (where both appraisee and appraiser make a joint assessment). The *system* may be complex (with multiple-point self-assessment forms, peer reports and/or rating scales) or simple (with samples of notes and conversation). Supporting sources of evidence can be obtained from patients, superiors or peers. The system needs to be regularly evaluated in order to ensure that the process works effectively and efficiently.

The end result of the appraisal process is the individual's performance portfolio, which sits alongside and feeds into a *personal development plan*, which in turn feeds into the revalidation process, thus forming part of the *clinical governance* arrangements of the employing trust. Appraisal processes will differ between organisations, but appraisal should build on the strengths of both the organisation and the individuals who are working within it.

An appraisal is:

- a formal system for examining and building on strengths and minimising weaknesses
- a space for staff to assess their own needs and areas of difficulty
- an opportunity to discuss potential.

It is not

- subjective
- a disciplinary interview
- applied on the basis of insufficient, inadequate or irrelevant information
- presented as fact instead of opinion
- an opportunity to re-emphasise past problems.

During the appraisal interview, the objective is not to tell the individual what is going wrong, but to discuss their potential for development. Whoever appraises should use *assertive, counselling, problem-solving* and *facilitation* skills in order to be fair and unbiased, constructive and positive, objective and supportive, yet also challenging. Appraisals are not hierarchically based, but developmental. They focus on process, not outcomes. The appraisee should be given the opportunity to engage in the discussion, reflect on their own performance, state their needs and expectations and seek clarification. Meaningful (subjective and objective) targets should be set, and all judgements should be evidence based.

www.doh.gov.uk/gpappraisal
www.gmc-uk.org
www.appraisals.nhs.uk

Assertiveness

To be assertive is to communicate clearly, honestly and directly, without avoidance or resorting to manipulative or aggressive behaviour.

Assertiveness is regarded as an important component of cognitive–behavioural approaches to tackling anger, anxiety, depression and low self-esteem. The premise is that changing people's ideas will influence their behaviour, and likewise that changing their behaviour will lead to changes in their ideas.[1-3] Assertive techniques help people to communicate in constructive and satisfying ways and achieve workable results in difficult situations, and they assist in resolving conflicts without aggression. Some of the situations that can be helped with assertive behaviour include the following:

* time management
* identification of obstacles to career or personal development
* overcoming work and people demands
* making and refusing requests
* handling criticism or compliments
* coping with rejection
* building self-esteem
* giving constructive criticism
* staff appraisals and disciplinary procedures
* negotiating
* dealing effectively with conflict and violence
* goal setting.

Behaving assertively helps at both a professional and a personal level, as it can help to prevent aggressive or defensive behaviour. The assertive person takes charge and acts in ways that invite respect, accepting their own limitations and strengths. This in turn leads to clearer communication, as others understand clearly what their needs and desires are, and any potential confusion or discord is alleviated. Assertive skills enable people to cope more readily with feelings of frustration or inadequacy.

One of the first books to be published on assertiveness was written by Anne Dickson, an American psychologist.[4] Dickson's work is the source of much of the material that has subsequently been written on assertiveness in this country. She promoted assertiveness training as a popular method for self-development and for gaining self-confidence and control over one's life.

The assertive speaker:

* is specific
* negotiates

- repeats their message if it is misunderstood
- compromises if it is reasonable to do so
- listens
- self-discloses – expresses their feelings
- innovates – takes chances and risks
- accepts criticism where this is appropriate
- prompts others to express themselves honestly.

Assertive communication usually leaves both the speaker and the listener feeling more comfortable than do avoidance or confrontation. Assertiveness means communicating more honestly and directly. This leaves both parties feeling clearer and more at ease with the interaction. Assertiveness helps most in difficult or problematic situations – when dealing with critical comments or manipulative behaviour, when having to give criticism, or when negotiating.[5] *See* **Transactional analysis**.

www.anniephillips.co.uk

1 Grieger R and Boyd J (1980) *Rational–Emotive Therapy: a skills-based approach.* Van Nostrand Reinhold, New York.

2 Ellis A (1979) *RETR and Assertiveness Training* (audio cassette). Albert Ellis Institute for Rational–Emotive Behavior Therapy, New York.

3 Beck AT, Rush AJ, Shaw BF and Emery G (1979) *Cognitive Therapy of Depression.* Guildford, New York.

4 Dickson A (1982) *A Woman in Your Own Right.* Quartet Books, London.

5 Phillips A (2002) *Assertiveness and the Manager's Job.* Radcliffe Medical Press, Oxford.

Assertive outreach

An approach to working with severely mentally ill adults who do not engage effectively with traditional mental health services. Staff work with service users in their own environment (either at home or in another familiar environment, such as the park or the street), rather than through appointments at an office or hospital.

www.scmh.org.uk/

Assessment

The process of determining or measuring an individual's knowledge, skills or attitudes.[1] In healthcare, it is the term used for measurement of the performance, health or circumstances of an individual, family, group or community against one or more benchmarks in preparation for making a diagnosis or plan of action. *See* **Evaluation**; **Monitoring**.

1 Samuel O, Grant J and Irvine D (eds) (1994) *Quality and Audit in General Practice: meanings and definitions.* Royal College of General Practitioners, London.

Audit

Medical, clinical and *administrative audit* became popular in the early 1990s, as a risk management tool that was also useful for clinical and managerial purposes. Audit is an objective and systematic way of evaluating the quality of care or service delivery. It is a simple, effective and low-cost way of sifting and analysing data. It aims to promote higher standards of care, effectiveness and efficiency, and it helps to improve standards of care by highlighting discrepancies between perceived standards of practice and measured standards.

Audit is not a research tool. It does use some research methods (e.g. data collection, analysis), but it is not tied to research methodology. Scientific research methods are about proving facts in a way that can be replicated by other people using the same method. Audit is quite different. The aim of internal audit is to examine a particular practice and see whether it can be done better – no one else's practice is relevant. Audit does not require an hypothesis, a control group or a statistically significant sample.

Audit works best when a group of people decide on something to investigate and improve – ownership is important. Any system or method that requires improvement can be audited, whether it is a service, a building design, a way of working, a method of recording or a way of organising. Traditionally, management audit is concerned with two components, namely structure (which can include the environment) and process (which examines service delivery, for example). A classic GP practice audit is the examination and analysis of appointment availability.

- *Medical audit* concerns the performance and professional competence of doctors.

- *Clinical audit* evaluates an aspect of clinical care. Clinical audit is not exclusively medical – it may well involve all members of the healthcare team, patients and other care workers in looking at any aspect of clinical care.

- *Administrative audit* (or *internal audit*) is the audit of activities by non-medical staff, using criteria defined by the organisation itself.

- *External audit* is conducted by outsiders, using criteria defined by authorities outside the organisation.

- *Self-audit* is conducted by individuals or a group within the organisation.

- *Peer audit* is conducted by colleagues who combine resources to compare their audit findings.

Pre-audit involves meeting with all relevant personnel to define the problem, set standards and criteria and establish the required methodology. The audit itself involves collecting the data (*sampling*), analysing the data (comparing the observed practice with the standards set), presenting the findings, evaluating them, and finally implementing new standards, monitoring the change and ultimately reassessment (repeating the survey to test for evidence of effective change).

The audit cycle

Audit involves the following sequence of steps:

- observing the practice
- setting of standards
- gathering of data
- comparison of performance with standards
- implementing appropriate change
- monitoring the effects of the change – the *outcome*
- re-audit, in which the cycle is repeated.

Traditionally these steps are illustrated by a circular diagram, as a sequence that can be started at any point and taken in any order.

The focus in primary care is now moving away from medical audit towards multi-disciplinary or whole team audit activities, as it is thought improvement can only take place through changes to systems and organisation of care, rather than by changing individual working practice. The NHS Act 1999 recommends that audit should become a contractual activity for GPs. *See* **Criterion**; **Data**.

www.nice.org.uk
www.radcliffe-oxford.com

For further information on types of audit and how to audit, see the authors' book:

- Phillips A (2002) *The Business Planning Toolkit*. Radcliffe Medical Press, Oxford.

The National Institute for Clinical Excellence (NICE) and the Commission for Health Improvement (CHI) have launched a guide to clinical audit, *Principles and Best Practice in Clinical Audit*, which is available from the NICE website www.nice.org.uk or in print from Radcliffe Medical Press (www.radcliffe-oxford.com).

Audit assistant

The title for a member of staff who provides the technical support for medical audit.

Audit Commission

The Government quango responsible for ensuring that public money is well spent. The Audit Commission is in charge of local government's best value inspection regime, and is responsible for auditing the finances of councils and NHS organisations. *See* **Commission for Healthcare Audit and Inspection**.

www.audit-commission.gov.uk/home

Audit facilitator

A professional worker, usually employed by the Medical Audit Advisory Group within a primary care trust, whose role is to assist individual GP practices in implementing audit.

Autocratic leadership

An authoritarian style of management which is regarded as safe and paternalistic, and which carries a clear chain of command and authority. The divisions of work and hierarchy are fully understood by all, as it requires clear, detailed and achievable directives. The autocratic manager is usually an expert in their field, as they receive little or no information from others. This can be dangerous in today's work environment of technological and organisational complexity. Other weaknesses lie in the apparent efficiency of one-way communication – without feedback there are often misunderstandings, communication breakdowns and costly errors. However, the critical weakness of autocratic leadership is its effect on people – it is no longer acceptable for employees to accept and obey orders without question. Most people resent authoritarian rule and respond with resentment, resistance or sabotage. Authoritarian rulers cause low morale. *See* **Leadership**.

B

Balint group

Michael Balint, a Hungarian trained psychotherapist, has described a Balint group as a voluntary, self-selected group of people who meet to learn more about their own behaviour and emotions through reflection upon their work within the group.[1] Balint training for doctors uses group methods to look at the counter-transference process between doctor and patient, and the relationships between the group participants themselves and their leader. The aim is to assist each group member in evaluating his or her responses and recognising useful and difficult personality traits, thereby facilitating useful insight and change. *See* **T-group**.

www.balint.co.uk
www.familymed.musc.edu/balint/

1 Balint M (1964) *The Doctor, his Patient and the Illness.* Churchill Livingstone, Edinburgh.

Beacon services

A scheme that has been set up to identify and spread knowledge of examples of best practice in the NHS, highlighting innovative approaches to reduce health inequalities and improve service provision.

www.ohn.gov.uk
www.modern.nhs.uk/

Bedblocking

The phenomenon whereby older people are forced to stay in hospital beds because other forms of care (such as nursing homes or home care) are not available, thereby 'blocking' beds that could be used by other patients. *See* **Intermediate care**.

Belbin RM

Belbin is best known for the development of a *self-perception inventory* designed to provide members of a group with a simple means of assessing their best team roles.[1] Belbin researched and named the following different personality types found within groups: the Completer–Finisher, the Implementer, the Monitor–Evaluator, the Team-worker, the Resource Investigator, the Shaper and the Plant. *See* **Group**.

www.belbin.com/

1 Belbin RM (1991) *Management Teams: why they succeed or fail*. Heinemann, London.

Benchmarking

A method used by public sector organisations, charities and private companies for gauging their performance by comparing it with the performance of other similar-sized organisations. The Government encourages public sector bodies to compare their score on various published performance indicators as a way of improving services. Many organisations are now members of 'benchmarking clubs' in which they compare performance information (both published and unpublished).

www.ncvo-vol.org.uk/main/about/does/pdfs/QSTGbenchmarking.pdf

Bias

A predisposition or prejudice towards one particular viewpoint. In statistics, bias is a systematic distortion of a result, arising from a neglected factor.[1] When data are being collected, bias may arise from many causes, including the following:

• inappropriate selection of the population to be studied

• unsuitable measurement methods

• differences in interpretation.

Although attempts are made to avoid bias in research, if they occur they should be formally acknowledged.

1 Damuel O, Grant J and Irvine D (eds) (1994) *Quality and Audit in General Practice: meanings and definitions*. Royal College of General Practitioners, London.

Black bag

The doctor's bag. Traditionally a Gladstone bag made of soft black leather with a buckle fastening, it is now more likely to be a briefcase with foam inserts to separate the drugs and equipment inside. Ideally it should be coloured silver, not black, in order to keep the drugs cooler.[1]

• The bag must be lockable.

• It should never be left unattended on home visits (it contains drugs and blank scripts).

- It should be locked and kept out of sight in the boot of a car.

- It should be kept shut when not in use, as bright light may deactivate some of the drugs.

- The origin, expiry date and batch number of all drugs must be recorded.

- Out-of-date drugs should be regularly checked, replaced and disposed of.

It is useful for doctors to keep a second bag, which is more rarely used, for other equipment such as the following:

- peak flow meter

- specimen bottles

- venepuncture equipment, syringes and needles

- venflons and butterflies

- sterile gloves

- sharps box

- swabs

- disposable speculum

- equipment for giving saline infusion

- airways.

1 Rees (2001) The Doctor's Bag. *Doctor*. **27 September**: 63.

Booked admissions

The NHS national booked admissions scheme is an airline-style booking system that was introduced in pilot form in 1999. Originally devised by the National Booked Admissions Advisory Team (part of the Department of Health information technology proposals), it is planned that it will replace waiting-lists by 2005. Under the proposals, patients would be referred by their GPs, who would contact a central agency (NHS Bookings, possibly to be run by NHS Direct) by telephone, letter or email. The patient would then have the responsibility of directing any queries to the centre.

The system will be dependent on computerised links between primary and secondary care, enabling surgeries to book appointments electronically from the surgery as well as via the agency. Patients will be able to arrange outpatient and inpatient admission times at their own convenience, leading to fewer cancelled operations, less bureaucracy and more efficient use of NHS time and resources.

The Government estimates that 17% of GPs' patient contacts are related to referrals or hospital bookings, and the plan is that this telephone booking would free GPs from these patient-related queries.

www.poolehos.org/booked/home.htm
www.society.guardian.co.uk/nhsperformance/

Brainstorming

A method of finding creative solutions to longstanding problems. It starts with a group of people thinking up a list of solutions, including some ridiculous or impossible ones, and then involves sifting through them to see if there are any that, in retrospect, would seem to work.

British Association for Immediate Care (BASICS)

A charity formed in 1977 to foster education and the development of immediate care. Immediate care is defined as the provision of medical help at the scene of an emergency and during transit to definitive care in hospital. It also encompasses the sub-specialities of mass-gathering medicine and the medical management of major incidents and disaster.

www.basics.org.uk

British Medical Association (BMA)

An independent, member-only organisation that represents both primary and secondary medical members. The BMA works to represent and develop the careers, education and pay of its members.

www.bma.org.uk

British National Formulary (BNF)

A monthly publication published jointly by the British Medical Association and the Royal Pharmaceutical Society of Great Britain, available free to GPs. It provides information about drugs and their indications, interactions and cost. It is also available online.

www.bnf.org

Brown Bag review

The name given to repeat-prescribing projects which involve a method of reducing prescribing spend and improving clinical care in primary care by implementing tighter clinical and managerial controls. A full description of this method can be found in the author's book.[1] The steps involved can be summarised as follows:

- an audit of a sample of repeat prescriptions
- identification and analysis of prescribing type and spend (e.g. checking high-cost items and claims)
- a patient compliance check through patient recall or opportunistic consultation to establish use, polypharmacy, compliance, additional self-medication, contra-indications, pharmacokinetics or adverse reactions
- communicating with patients in order to explain, instruct and simplify the regime
- changing the computer recall and flagging system for repeat scripts
- instigating a patient review system for high-risk patient groups
- devising a mechanism for identifying and noting how prescribing is initiated or changed.

Given that two-thirds of all GP prescriptions are repeats, and that they represent 80% of total prescribing costs, such reviews can impact on patient care by considerably reducing risk, wastage and costs.

www.npc.co.uk
www.npc.ppa.nhs.uk

1 Phillips A (2002) *The Business Planning Toolkit*. Radcliffe Medical Press, Oxford.

Bureaucratic leadership

A leadership and management style that is commonly seen in public sector organisations where there is a demand for uniform treatment, regular procedures and accountability. This brings consistency, dependability and a sense of fairness and impartiality – people understand the rules and feel secure. Regularity of procedures helps to ensure essential values and ethics. However, bureaucracy has led to adherence to specified rules and procedures which can stifle flexibility, creativity and freedom. Although directives, policies and rules are essential in any business, there must be some flexibility. *See* **Leadership**.

Business ethics

This has been defined as the study of moral and ethical matters pertaining to business, institutions, practices and beliefs.[1] The following subjects fall within the domain of business ethics:[2,3]

- workers' rights

- consumer safety

- discrimination

- codes of conduct

- accounting practices

- energy utilisation

- company perks

- contracting

- relationships with trade unions

- whistleblowing

- computer data and privacy

- environmental protection

- research

- corrupt practices.

If dilemmas and disagreements are experienced at work due to a clash of values, this becomes an ethical issue. Some colleagues may be guided more than others by their principles or a sense of duty, their views being influenced by religious beliefs or moral values. Most people can agree on the importance of honesty, truthfulness and integrity, but this process may be assisted if healthcare organisations develop *codes of business ethics* so that individual members and stakeholders can be provided with clear guidance on the business stance. *See* **Sustainable development**.

www.defra.gov.uk/environment/greening/index.htm
www.nhsestates.gov.uk/
www.sustainable-energy.org.uk

1 Donaldson J (1989) *Key Issues in Business Ethics*. Academic Press, London.

2 De George R (1989) *Business Ethics* (3e). Macmillan, Basingstoke.

3 Webly S (1993) *Codes of Business Ethics: why companies should develop them – and how*. Institute of Business Ethics, London.

Business plan

A business plan covers all aspects of an organisation, including the service, finances, premises and team skills. The *process* of business planning enables the business to:[1]

- clarify some of the wider issues facing the business

- evaluate itself, detailing its strengths and weaknesses

- provide a statement of intent for interested stakeholders

- formulate goals and identify the action needed to achieve those goals

- identify resources required in terms of skills, activity and finance

- anticipate and plan for problems.

Business plans are usually issued to the business's professional advisers and sponsors – the bank manager and the accountant. Most practices keep information about practice income and expenditure private to the practice and its own business associates. Sharing the plan helps to firm up proposals so that everyone can ascertain whether or not the practice ideas are going to be viable. It is also useful to establish whether the practice aims and objectives coincide with those of the NHS as a whole.

The business plan provides details of the following:

- business aims and objectives

- staff/partnership structure

- current and future patient services

- the list or population size

- outside commitments

- capital resources – buildings and equipment

- clinical performance

- finance

- overall strengths and weaknesses

- external forces that may impact on the future of the organisation.

See **Planning cycle**.

www.anniephillips.co.uk

1 Phillips A (2002) *The Business Planning Toolkit*. Radcliffe Medical Press, Oxford.

Business process re-engineering (BPR)

A type of organisational analysis. It is defined as the fundamental and radical redesign of business processes, with the aim of achieving dramatic improvements in performance by critically measuring cost, quality, service and speed.[1] As with total quality management approaches, such exercises challenge the existing framework by questioning attitudes and behaviours, but unlike total quality management, business process re-engineering seeks major advances in performance, takes a strategic approach and is driven by top management. Total quality management requires a more supportive environment and aims for continuous (as opposed to 'one-off') improvement. *See* **Total quality management**.

1 Hammer M and Champy J (1993) *Re-Engineering the Corporation: a manifesto for business revolution.* Nicholas Brealey, London.

C

Caldicott

The work of Caldicott 'Guardians' within primary care organisations is to ensure that patient confidentiality issues are complied with and manual and IT systems are secure. Caldicott Guardians look at issues such as confidentiality and security, information, clarity, rights of access and documentation accuracy. Primary care organisations work with advice and guidance for protecting and using patient information through a programme of work recommended by Caldicott. *See* **Data Protection Act 1984 and 1998**.

www.doh.gov.uk/

CAMs

The term for therapists who practise *complementary and alternative medicine* (e.g. medical herbalism, aromatherapy, acupuncture). The tension between orthodox, allopathic medicine and the complementary therapies is easing as complementary therapies develop their evidence base and medicine becomes more open to the value of the CAM (complementary and alternative medicine) approach.

The NHS cannot recommend or purchase such care without evidence of the effectiveness of treatments, cost-effectiveness, professional regulation and local health needs assessment, so CAMs are encouraged and supported in research to help build the required evidence base. There are over 91 UK bodies representing 50 000 assorted CAM practitioners, and many more practitioners work without belonging to such a body.

Patients currently make 22 million visits each year to CAM practitioners – 34% to medical herbalists, 21% to aromatherapists, 17% to homeopaths, 14% to acupuncturists and 19% to other practitioners (massage, reflexologists, osteopaths, chiropractors). Osteopaths and chiropractors are now regulated (with aromatherapy, acupuncture and herbalism soon to follow). Around 40% of GPs provide some form of access to CAMs, and 68% refer at least monthly – most commonly to acupuncturists. They usually refer what they fail to manage, especially depression, sleep/eating problems and chronic illness.[1] A common request from GPs is that they need more information about what cases to refer and when. Most of them refer by personal recommendation.

www.ukcollege.com
www.harcourt-international.com

1 Fox M, CEO for the Foundation for Integrated Medicine, speaking at the Conference on Integrated Medicine in Primary Care, 6 October 2001, Brighton.

Capacity

The resources available to an organisation, including people, money, equipment, expertise and information.

www.doh.gov.uk/
www.local-regions.dtlr.gov.uk

Capital spending

Expenditure on new construction, land, improvements to existing property and the purchase of all other equipment and assets (e.g. computer hardware) that have an expected working life of more than one year. *See* **Care package**.

www.hmso.gov.uk/
www.dtlr.gov.uk/

Capitation fees

Part of the system of fees and allowances paid to General Medical Services GPs quarterly, pre the new GP contract. These payments are based on the number and age of people registered with a practice, with elderly patients attracting the highest fees. Additional payments are made each time a patient registers, and each time a doctor takes responsibility for child health surveillance, which includes those children who are on the at-risk register (i.e. at risk of physical, emotional or mental harm). *See* **Fees and allowances**; **New GP contract**.

Care management

This term, introduced in the NHS and Community Care Act 1990, refers to the management of the care of those in receipt of a care package. *See* **Care package**; **Care plan**.

Care package

A group of services brought together to achieve one or more objectives of a *care plan*. *See* **Care management**.

www.doh.gov.uk/

Care pathway

An approach to managing a specific disease or clinical condition that identifies what interventions are required, and which predicts the chronology of care and the expected outcome of the treatment. The approach is designed to ease the passage of the patient by co-ordinating care through the healthcare system from primary to secondary to tertiary care, and vice versa.

www.nelh.nhs.uk/carepathways.asp

Care plan

A plan (sometimes called a *collaborative care plan*) for providing care services to an individual or family. The plan should follow an assessment at a case conference or review and involve service users (patients/clients), carers and their families, as well as all relevant professionals. *See* **Care programme**.

Care programme

A detailed programme of care that contributes to one of the goals of a care plan. *See* **Care plan**.

Carer

A person who provides care on a regular basis, and who is not employed to do so by an agency or organisation. A carer is usually a friend or relative looking after someone who is frail or ill at home. The Government is introducing new legislation with the aim of assisting carers emotionally and financially, in recognition of the physical, emotional and financial savings that carers bring to the State.

Care trust

A local body that is responsible for delivering primary healthcare, community health services and social care for older people. Ministers believe that care trusts will facilitate and integrate joint working between health and social care. The first trusts, which were developed from existing primary care trusts, went live in April 2002.

www.doh.gov.uk/caretrusts/

Case mix

The mixture and severity of clinical conditions that are found in a particular healthcare setting. Healthcare commissioners often use their understanding of case mix to interpret clinical performance. Trusts use case mix crucially to defend their organisation's underperformance. For example, a specialist paediatric department might explain that it has higher than average postoperative disability rates on 'case-mix' grounds, because it has more complex and difficult cases than the norm.

Centralisation

Moving different parts of an organisation together in order to gain economic and administrative advantages. Centralisation makes it easier to implement common policies and develop consistent strategies, it is easier for management control and it leads to greater use of specialisation and improved decision making. It is more common in the public sector, where there is greater demand for accountability, regular procedures and uniform treatments. *See* **Decentralisation**.

Certification

Often used interchangeably with *accreditation*, this may be defined as the formal recognition of competence and performance.[1] The term is commonly used to describe the satisfactory completion of a period of training. Recertification describes the periodic revalidation of a doctor's certification status – a term that has now been superseded by revalidation. *See* **Accreditation of healthcare**; **Revalidation**.

www.rcgp.org.uk/

1 Samuel O, Grant J and Irvine D (eds) (1994) *Quality and Audit in General Practice: meanings and definitions.* Royal College of General Practitioners, London.

Chair

The person who is given responsibility for controlling a meeting by taking a leadership role and ensuring that the meeting keeps to time. He or she does this by discouraging side talking, allowing space for everyone to contribute, being aware that everyone has a different agenda, and encouraging participants to agree to abide by any decisions that are made.

Good chairing requires excellent interpersonal and communication skills. A chair's role will also be to elicit differing points of view. He or she requires knowledge of the subject under discussion, organisational skills, a broad understanding of group dynamics, and the ability to manage conflict. The chair encourages differing viewpoints while supporting the discussion, and ensures that everyone present sticks to the subject. They will do this by extracting ideas and summarising, thus helping the group to achieve a successful outcome. *See* **Facilitation**.

Change

Change is an inescapable part of working lives, yet most people resist change. There will always be powerful internal and external forces pushing for change, which will be viewed as positive by some in the organisation, and as negative by others. Change involves the whole team, and it is important to involve the whole organisation in any change, so that everyone is clear about the decisions. There is not necessarily ever a best or right way to change things – as this depends on the task and the state of the organisation at the time. *See* **Change management**; **Forcefield analysis**.

Change management

The process of managing change involves understanding the need to change, understanding the resistance to change, identifying the need for and planning for change. Successful change managers allow for a period of transition, seek commitment and support, problem solve, and use their supporters' energy, enthusiasm and lead. They involve staff and provide facts in order to avoid rumour and uncertainty, and finally they monitor and evaluate change.

Change management is particularly difficult for organisations that lead with an *autocratic* or *task-centred* leadership style, as this style of management is authoritarian and controlling, rather than *people centred*. Nor will change management be successful in organisations with *free-rein* leadership, where it is never clear who leads, and chaotic management results.

Good change management is *proactive* rather than *reactive*. Therefore successful organisations are those which actively prepare for change. Change is unsuccessful when it has been improvised and forced, rather than planned. There is no magic formula for change management, but there are some clear themes, which include the following:[1]

1 a clear sense of direction

2 good communication

3 strong feedback from service users

4 robust performance management systems.

The costs to organisations that resist expected change are dear, but the benefits to those that do not resist are fundamental, both financially (the organisation grows into the role expected of it) and personally (there is less stress and conflict for those working within it). *See* **Change**; **Forcefield analysis**; **Stakeholder analysis**.

1 Brindle D (2001) Clear sighted. *Guardian*. **11 July**: 12.

For more information on how to manage change successfully, see the following:

• Phillips A (2001) *The Business Planning Toolkit*. Radcliffe Medical Press, Oxford.

• Phillips A (2002) *Assertiveness and the Manager's Job*. Radcliffe Medical Press, Oxford.

Charges to patients

NHS GPs are permitted to charge their own patients for non-NHS-approved and private work. This includes certificates given with or without examination (e.g. sick notes, incapacity certificates for employers, insurance companies and sickness medicals), some travel vaccinations, and work done in the surgery on the patient's behalf (e.g. extracting and photocopying medical records for a solicitor's report).

Charismatic organisations

In one of the earliest studies of formal organisations, Weber[1] distinguished three types of authority relating to different types of organisations, namely traditional, bureaucratic and charismatic. Common to single-handed general practice, in charismatic organisations authority is legitimised by a belief in the personal qualities of the leader – the strength of their personality and inspiration. Charismatic organisations flourish only while the leader is established, and if routine procedures, systems and economic support are established in addition.

1 Weber M (1964) *The Theory of Social and Economic Organisation.* Collier Macmillan, London.

Charter mark

An award administered by the Cabinet Office for excellence in delivering a public service. It was launched as part of the Citizen's Charter scheme.

www.cabinet-office.gov.uk/servicefirst/index/markhome.htm

Chief executive bulletins

Circulars that are emailed from the Department of Health weekly to NHS and Council chief executives and directors of social services, and which are then placed on the Department of Health website. They replace the previously used HSC and LAC circulars, listings for which are set out in the bulletins, and are now used only for urgent and priority messages.

www.doh.gov.uk/cebulletin.htm

Child Protection Register

A confidential list, held by social services, of every child in a local authority with regard to whom there is serious concern about abuse or neglect. Registration aims to ensure that children and their families are receiving necessary help, but it does not affect a carer's legal responsibility towards their child. A case conference, usually attended by the family's GP, social worker and health visitor, can decide to place a child on the register. A child protection plan is put in place if there is concern about a child's physical and emotional well-being.

www.adss.org.uk
www.basw.co.uk/

Chi-squared test

A statistical technique that is used to test the frequency of a particular event (the number of times that it occurs). It thus tests the significance of proportions, or associations between categories used in an experiment.[1]

1 Robson C (1975) *Experiment, Design and Statistics in Psychology*. Penguin, Harmondsworth.

Clinical audit

See **Audit**.

Clinical Data Standards Board

The body that will provide the national standards to be used for data collection in any given clinical topic area. Clinical audit data sets developed to support National Service Frameworks, for example, will be scrutinised by the NHS National Information Authority's own data sets and, once ratified, will provide the national standard to be used for other data collection in the same topic area. Over time, this process of standards ratification will provide a library of accredited standards for use throughout the NHS. *See* **National Service Framework**; **NHS National Information Authority**.

www.doh.gov.uk/ipu/strategy/

Clinical governance

An umbrella term covering the implementation of evidence-based practice, supporting and developing the technological and clinical information infrastructure and ensuring that changing practice occurs in the light of *audit*, research and *risk management*.

Clinical governance is at its heart a quality improvement programme for healthcare. It is a concept which aims to bring together all of the components of good clinical practice and quality. It aims to improve patient care by achieving high standards, reflective practice and risk management as well as supporting personal and professional development.

The systems embraced by clinical governance include the following:

- clinical audit
- risk management
- revalidation
- evidence-based clinical practice (National Institute for Clinical Excellence, Commission for Health Improvement, protocols and local guidance)
- development of clinical leadership skills
- continuing education for all staff (personal development plan and practice professional development plan)

- audit of consumer feedback

- accreditation.

It has a strong resemblance to the concept of *total quality management (TQM)*, and involves the following:

1 co-operating and working with others

2 applying the principles locally

3 focusing on improving and maintaining high standards of care

4 helping to ensure good practice

5 setting clear service standards

6 performing clinical audit

7 ensuring that evidence-based practice is carried out

8 collecting records to help review performance and monitor patient care

9 implementing risk management plans

10 reporting adverse healthcare incidents

11 setting clear performance standards for all staff

12 promoting a learning environment

13 valuing openness

14 involving patients.

A good clinical governance programme would involve the application of good practice principles, such as the following:

1 the detection and investigation of *significant incidents* or adverse events

2 evidence-based clinical practice

3 the integration of clinical audit into the organisation

4 clinical risk reduction

5 the identification of and action against poor clinical performance

6 continuing professional development programmes in place for all staff.

This raises challenges for managers, who will have a role in assisting and encouraging the development of leadership skills and knowledge among clinicians, developing the appropriate accountability structures, and developing mechanisms to ensure that clinical audit is integrated into the organisation. *See* **Accreditation of healthcare;**

Commission for Health Improvement; Competence assessment schemes; National Institute for Clinical Excellence; Performance assessment framework; Performance indicator; Quality; Revalidation.

Clinical Governance Research and Development Unit (CGRDU)

The CGRDU was created in 1999 as a successor to the Eli Lilly National Clinical Audit Centre. Its main aim is research and development within the clinical governance field. The unit aims to support health service staff by providing information, guidance, training and publications on *clinical governance* and *audit* issues.

www.le.ac.uk/cgrdu

Clinical (practice) guidelines

Systematically developed statements (of principle) which assist in decision making about appropriate healthcare for specific conditions.[1] Clinical guidelines can also be used to define quality criteria in contract specifications. Guidelines are made up from collections of *criteria* which describe the nature and reflect the standard of care in precise terms. *See* **Protocol**.

1 Samuel O, Grant J and Irvine D (eds) (1994) *Quality and Audit in General Practice: meanings and definitions.* Royal College of General Practitioners, London.

Clinical supervision

A term used in the NHS to describe the offline management support of clinical staff. It is an opportunity to reflect on practice, to enhance skills and to clarify goals for professional development.[1] Staff who are counsellors, or who have some knowledge of counselling training, are often asked to act as clinical supervisors for other disciplines. *See* **Clinical supervision**; **Coaching**; **Mentoring**.

1 Kell C (2002) Can counsellors adequately supervise non-counsellors? *J Counsell Psychother.* **13**: 36–7.

Clinician

A health professional who is directly involved in the care and treatment of patients, for example a nurse, doctor, therapist or midwife.

Closing the loop

The term that is used for completing the audit cycle. It involves adjusting practice in the light of results and repeating the survey to test for evidence of effective change. *See* **Audit**.

Coaching

As part of the facilitation of learning, coaching is a 'process that enables learning and development to occur and thus performance to improve'.[1]

It is a term for bringing out the best in people and improving their skills by giving guidance, insight and encouragement during the learning process. The emphasis is on performance, success and developing one's full potential. A coach is usually someone who is not in their client's profession. MacLennan[2] has identified six main components of successful coaching:

1 first-hand experience and understanding of workplace achievement

2 a conceptual understanding of the process

3 performer-empowering attitudes and assumptions

4 skills in strong rapport creation and maintenance

5 excellent listening skills

6 sophisticated questioning skills.

Coaching is now divided into *executive coaching* and *life coaching*. The latter looks at all of the issues in a person's life, whereas the former is focused on life at work. It is widely accepted that coaching can have an important and revitalising effect on organisations. *Mentoring* requires a set of skills which include the role of a coach. *See* **Clinical supervision**; **Mentoring**.

1 Parsloe E (1999) The manager as a coach and mentor. *J Counsell Psychother*. **13**.

2 MacLennan N (1995) *Coaching and Mentoring*. Gower, Aldershot.

Code of conduct

See **Management code of conduct**.

Collaborative care

See **Care plan**.

Collaborative care planning

See **Care plan**.

Commission for Health Improvement (CHI)

A Government-sponsored inspection unit that seeks to ensure the quality of clinical practice while driving forward a concept of development, continued improvement, and encouraging and sharing best practice. The CHI aims to provide an accountability framework for NHS institutions and to improve public confidence in the NHS by addressing dangerous incidents and variations in performance. Like the National Service Frameworks and National Institute for Clinical Excellence guidelines, it aims to co-ordinate risk management, reinforce clinical audit and investigate adverse incidents. Its overall aims is to achieve a reduction in morbidity and mortality in the organisations that it inspects.

The principles of the CHI are:

- patient centred

- independent and fair

- developmental/involving active learning

- evidence-based

- open and approachable

- focused on patient care, not cost.

The CHI sees itself as having four roles, namely to investigate, review, evaluate and implement the following:

- clinical governance reviews

- National Service Framework studies

- National Institute for Clinical Excellence guidelines

- serious failures.

It aims to give advice and information to institutions that it inspects at corporate, patient, team and peer level.

The CHI aspires to provide a framework for NHS institutions to be accountable for their actions. *See* **Commission for Healthcare Audit and Inspection**.

www.nhs.uk
www.doh.gov.uk/
www.modern.nhs.uk/

Commission for Healthcare Audit and Inspection (CHAI)

A new independent body set up to regulate healthcare within the NHS. The Government announced its intention (in March 2003) to establish this new Commission which will bring together the health value-for-money work of the Audit Commission, the work of the Commission for Health Improvement and the private healthcare role of the National Care Standards Commission. This new single Commission will have responsibility for inspecting both the public and private healthcare sectors. Its principal roles will include:

- inspecting all NHS hospitals, with the ability to recommend special measures where there are persistent problems

- Licensing private healthcare provision

- Assessing the value-for-money of healthcare provision

- publishing reports on the performance of NHS organisations, including 'star ratings'

- publishing an annual report to Parliament on progress on healthcare delivery and the use of resources.

The intention is that CHAI becomes a powerful inspectorate and a force for improvement in the quality and equity of, and access to, NHS services.

www.doh.gov.uk/nhsacc/chai.htm

Commission for Patient and Public Involvement in Health (CPPIH)

An independent body charged with overseeing patient and public involvement in healthcare. This national commission was set up in 2002 as part of the Government plan to get more lay people involved in NHS decision making. Local networks began to be set up in 2003. The commission will oversee the Patient Advocacy and Liaison Service and patient forums that are set up in every acute and primary care trust, and the Independent Complaints Advocacy Service.

The CPPIH will also assist in the development of national patient surveys. *See* **Patient Advocacy and Liaison Service; Patients' forum**.

www.doh.gov.uk/involvingpatients
www.nhs.uk

Commissioning

The process by which the needs of the local population are identified, priorities are set, and appropriate services are then purchased and evaluated. Undertaken by the commissioning bodies such as primary care organisations and care trusts, it involves comparing waiting-list and league-table information provided by service providers such as trusts and special health authorities, and identifying variances in their costs and benefits. The consequences of these variances need to be established – a political and public debate is generated where funding judgements are made between services.

The information needs in commissioning healthcare are wide and complex. Commissioners obtain demographic facts about the numbers and health status of their population, and they try to identify an understanding of any *health outcomes* (any increased health benefits). Health gains may not always be clearly identifiable as clinical or financial, but may instead be physical, social, mental or emotional. Additional commissioning components include setting targets for health status, using information from existing services, and deciding on possible interventions from audits, research and opinion.

A picture of health is created by means of the following:

- epidemiology

- morbidity data

- mortality data

- locality analysis

- demographics

- auditing and evaluation of current and historical activity

- a review of current medical opinion and evaluation of clinical outcomes.

The *NHS Alliance*, which developed out of locality commissioning, has stated that commissioning should always include needs assessment, prioritisation and impact evaluation. It should be clinically driven, population specific, reflect patient experience rather than organisational boundaries, employ integrated care pathways, be sensitive to local need and have sophisticated service specifications with effective means of evaluating outcome. *See* **Health needs assessment/analysis**.

www.ohn.gov.uk/glossary/c.htm
www.doh.gov.uk/nhsfinancialreforms/
www.doh.gov.uk/finman.htm
www.nhsalliance.org

Communication

Communication may be defined as 'the exchange of information between a sender and receiver with the inference of meaning'. Around 85% of communication content is non-verbal – communicated in gestures, facial expression or tone of voice. Communication is complex, and involves the following:

- a message (statements, questions, commands or warnings)

- a language (words – written or spoken; symbols – music, art, body language and gestures)

- a system (listening, touch, silence, voice, gestures, writing).

The way in which something is communicated (its *delivery*) describes the content. A person's facial expressions, timing and speed, body language, voice tone and word choice will tell us whether the situation is public or private, doubtful or hopeful, formal or informal, serious or relaxed. These words and symbols have different meanings in different cultures.

Communication is multi-directional. It can be directional or one way, face to face, outward (towards the patient), 'up' from employee to employer, or lateral (when teambuilding, exercising leadership or motivating staff). Different communication styles are adopted for different functions (chairing, facilitating, presenting, instructing, etc.).

Personality, history, motivation and other less visible factors such as organisational structure, interpersonal relationships and the level of information also influence how and what we communicate.

Communication is a central organisational process. The exchange of information between different participants links the various subsystems and hierarchies within the organisation, and builds and reinforces interdependence between them. The larger and more specialised the work groups within the organisation, the greater the potential for misunderstanding. Differences in power, goals and expertise between departments may make communication difficult.

The relationship between the two people who are communicating also affects the accuracy with which messages are given and received – how much trust there is between the two, how much influence the sender has over the receiver, or expected standards of behaviour. All of these factors may limit the amount or type of information that people feel they can legitimately discuss. The amount of information that is held is also significant. If one is relying on only one source of information when judging performance, persistent biases are likely to occur.

Communication enables us to make discoveries about ourselves and others, to solve problems and develop new skills, to manage conflict, emotion and anger, and to question, adapt, change and grow. Some of the barriers to effective communication include the following:

- lack of feedback

- judging, controlling or evaluating behaviour

- internal or external 'noise' (interference)

- the use of language – misunderstandings can arise from the use of unfamiliar, abstract or technical terms

- the quality of listening by the receiver.[1]

The factors that most commonly affect clinical negligence claims are communication breakdown, poor systems and processes and human error.[2] Because of this, it is an important part of the job of any manager in healthcare to develop formal systems to manage administrative and clinical communication systems such as telephone protocols, tracer systems for records, systems for notifying patients of delays and results, and complaints procedures.

Good communication integrates quality through sharing good practice, listening and giving feedback. For communication to be successful, the following criteria have to be met.

- Both sides must be interested and involved.
- Both sides need to be willing to be open and honest.
- Both sides need to feel heard and understood.
- The atmosphere must be comfortable.
- Even if the talking is difficult, the important things need to be said.
- Conversations have to make a difference. Something useful or satisfying must happen as a result.

Good communicators 'read' the situation, engage people's attention, clarify meaning and check understanding. *See* **Listening skills**; **Non-verbal communication**.

1 Phillips A (2002) *Communication and the Manager's Job*. Radcliffe Medical Press, Oxford.

2 Wilson J (1995) General practice risk management. In: *News for Fundholders. Issue 4*. NHS Executive, London.

Community Health Councils
Locally elected bodies which were set up to independently assess local services and help patients to pursue formal complaints. They were replaced by the *Independent Complaints Advocacy Service*, set up as part of the Commission for Patient and Public Involvement in Health, in late 2003. *See* **Commission for Patient and Public Involvement in Health**.

www.btinternet.com/~cornwallchc/chc.htm

Community mental health team
A multidisciplinary team consisting of psychiatrists, social workers, community psychiatric nurses, psychologists and therapists who provide assessment and treatment outside hospitals for patients with severe and enduring mental health problems.

www.psychiatry.ox.ac.uk/
www.scmh.org.uk

Community/compulsory treatment order
Compulsory readmission to hospital of psychiatric patients in the community who fail to take their medication, a proposal introduced by the Government to reform

the 1983 Mental Health Act. Patients discharged from hospital would receive a compulsory care and treatment order specifying where they are permitted to live, as well as a care plan.

www.mind.org.uk/
www.smhc.org.uk

Competence assessment scheme

One of the measuring tools examined by the General Practitioners Council, General Medical Council and Royal College of General Practitioners is a competence assessment scheme, as it is recognised that doctors require not only academic competence but also operational competence.

Research[1] has identified several key competence criteria, which are those qualities most commonly mentioned by other GPs who are seeking medical care for their own family or friends. These criteria include the following:

- empathy and sensitivity

- team involvement

- personal organisation and administrative skills

- mechanisms for coping with stress

- communication skills

- legal, ethical and political awareness

- personal attributes

- professional integrity

- conceptual thinking

- job's relationship to society and family

- personal development

- clinical knowledge

- managing others

- learning and development.

See **Personal development plan**.

1 Ferguson E *et al.* (2000) A competency model for general practice: implications for selection, training and development. *Br J Gen Pract.* **50**.

Complaints

According to a General Medical Service report,[1] the most common complaints requiring resolution in general practice are the following:

- care management (35%)

- complaints associated with grief (20%)

- delayed or failed diagnosis (12.7%).

The recently bereaved are more likely both to attend the doctor for their own recent onset of illness, and to complain following the bereavement of a loved one. It is well documented that feelings such as fear, anxiety and loss of control greatly heighten physical and emotional pain and difficulties.

An effective *complaints procedure* would acknowledge these factors, and would be proactive in preventing complaints initially by supporting good practice. *See* **Complaints procedure**.

www.doh.gov.uk/complaints/index.htm

1 Green (2000) *Pulse*. **15 December**.

Complaints procedure

Primary care trusts require all primary care organisations to have complaints procedures. These procedures must be documented in waiting areas and patient literature, to make it easier for patients to make a complaint if they wish to do so.

Complaints procedures ideally include the auditing of any comments and complaints received, categorise the reason for the failure, are open about naming the person responsible, and encourage collective discussion and problem solving before implementing the solution. *Significant event analysis* can form part of this formal procedure. Here the evidence is presented back to the team so that it can inform future better practice.

If there has been cause for complaint, the complaints policy ideally outlines the best procedures to follow (e.g. a personal apology given over the telephone results in a higher level of complaints being resolved than an apology by letter; putting the problem right immediately causes the least anguish).

All NHS provider units, including GP practices, are required by their commissioning or employing trusts to have complaints procedures in place, so that patients are aware of how to make a complaint and the trust or practice understands the procedure to follow in the event of a complaint made against them. *See* **Complaints**.

Computing in healthcare

Visit www.phcsg.org.uk for the primary healthcare specialist group division of the British Computer Society medical group. Here you will find information on national user groups, discussion topics and *Informatics in Primary Care* (Radcliffe

Medical Press, Oxford, www.radcliffe-oxford.com/journals). *See* **Information technology accreditation**.

www.phcsg.org.uk

Confidentiality

The ethical duty of healthcare professionals to keep private any information which they have learned about their patients. According to the basic principles of confidentiality within the NHS, information may be passed to others if:

- the patient consents to this for a particular purpose, such as an insurance report
- it meets NHS purposes, including the effective management of healthcare
- it is a statutory requirement or in response to a court order
- it is in the public interest.

Healthcare workers must not disclose or use any confidential information obtained in the course of their work, other than for the clinical care of the patient to whom that information relates. The legal and medical exceptions include exceptional circumstances such as disclosure in the patient's own interest, that required by law, any overriding duty to society because of national security or public health concerns, teaching and research or the storage and transmission of records and information. Others may be engaged to handle confidential information, but only to meet management needs.

All health service workers sign up to an ethical obligation to keep information about patients private and confidential. Any staff member who handles patient data has a duty not to disclose learned sensitive information to any third party. In 1993 the General Medical Council allowed that information may be disclosed with the explicit consent of the patient. However, in the case of audit, the general rule is that anonymised data should be used wherever possible. If at any stage a disclosure would enable an individual patient to be identified, that person must be informed and advised of their right to withhold consent to disclosure. In order to ensure patient confidentiality, NHS workers are advised to:

- obtain prior consent from patients
- anonymise patient information
- avoid codes that could identify patients or doctors
- destroy audits when these are complete
- register with the Data Protection Act.

See **Data Protection Act 1984 and 1998**.

Confidential enquiry

An anonymised, often national, survey or data collection of identified adverse events and their related circumstances.[1] See **Significant event analysis**.

1 Samuel O, Grant J and Irvine D (eds) (1994) *Quality and Audit in General Practice: meetings and definitions*. Royal College of General Practitioners, London.

Conflict management

Conflict management means to actively seek out the sources of stress within an organisation, either in individuals or in groups, and to devise ways either to accept and manage the difficulties, or to change the situation.[1] See **Change management**.

1 Phillips A (2002) *Assertiveness and the Manager's Job*. Radcliffe Medical Press, Oxford.

Constructive criticism

This is criticism given wisely, the only aim being that the person being criticised should learn in a positive manner from the experience. It is specific, avoids attack or blame, and does not give unsolicited or unwanted advice. It is given without judgement, and avoids global or generalised statements about behaviour, as these can be construed as an attack on an individual's personality. Those giving constructive criticism do not assume that they know what motivates other people, for they may be mistaken. Constructive criticism spells out the consequences of changed behaviour, while acknowledging that people may not be able to change. Constructive criticism views others as equals. See **Appraisal**; **Assertiveness**; **Disciplinary interview**.

Continuing professional development (CPD)

A process of planned, continuing development of individuals throughout their career. Sometimes termed lifelong learning, it is regarded as the systematic maintenance, improvement and extension of professional knowledge and skills, and the development of the personal qualities necessary to execute the job. An important part of any job is self-development. CPD is designed so that individuals will derive personal satisfaction from their work and contribute fully to the success of their organisation. Management organisations such as the Institute of Health Service Managers (IHSM) are now investigating how to incorporate CPD into the manager's job in healthcare.

CPD was set up by the Government to encompass the entire workforce.[1] It encourages rigorous self-regulation, continued implementation of recertification or revalidation, and acceptance of professional accountability. It requires the development of appraisal systems, learning organisations, revalidation and regulation.

Clinical training is planned for and supported nationally. GPs are now required to keep records of their ongoing clinical development in *personal development plans*.

Nurses have requirements to keep up to date built into their contracts. Other clinical support services (e.g. therapists) have revalidation or registration requirements which ensure that they are kept up to date professionally. It is expected that the Government and primary care trusts will support all NHS professionals (support and ancillary staff), who do not currently have the backing of professional bodies to guide and inform their practice, in CPD.

1 Department of Health (1998) *A First-Class Service: quality in the new NHS*. The Stationery Office, London.

Continuity of care

If a patient or client undergoes a smooth passage through the health and social care system, despite the involvement of many different disciplines in their care, they are said to have received continuity of care. This is often facilitated by the patient being given a named person, or *key worker*, who co-ordinates the episode of care. *See* **Care pathway**.

Contract: GP

Strictly speaking, there is no single GP contract – the term is used in the wider sense, referring to the regulatory framework which governs how GPs work within the NHS (the *Red Book*, terms of service, the legislation and regulations). Negotiations to produce new national (General Medical Service) and local (Personal Medical Service) contracts are currently under way. The Government priorities are for local pay, a fixed budget, quality-driven, quicker and better patient access, skill mix within practices, and developing specialist GP services.

A potted history of general practice shows how this contract has developed.

1 In the nineteenth century, doctors were paid on the basis of the amount that patients paid into sick clubs and friendly societies – this was known as *capitation*.

2 In 1911, the National Insurance Act created a framework of GPs as independent contractors. The 'pool' system of payments was introduced, with the total amount for GPs decided centrally.

3 In 1948, Aneurin Bevin set up the NHS. GPs were persuaded to become employees, but preserved their self-employed status.

4 In 1966, the Government conceded to GP demands for substantial contract changes, including pensions and Government-funded premises and staff.

5 In 1990, health secretary Kenneth Clark imposed a new contract on GPs with higher capitation-based payments, fundholding and an extension of GP services such as health promotion.

6 In 1992, GPs began to express an interest in the salaried option.

7 In 1998, the NHS Primary Care Act introduced the idea of *personal medical service* (PMS) pilots.

8 In 2000, the NHS Plan resolved to expand the local PMS system, and looked to build in national arrangements so that both would operate within a single contractual framework by 2002.

9 GPs voted in early 2003 on whether to accept a new GP contract. *See* **New GP contract**.

www.rcgp.org.uk/

Control

A *control experiment* is an experiment performed to provide a standard of comparison for other experiments. A *control group* is a group of subjects that provides such a standard of comparison.

Managerially, the type and amount of control that is exercised in an organisation has an effect on employee performance.[1] Organisational leaders are aware of the forces in themselves, in the people whom they manage, and in the situation that is being managed.

Control also implies something about the individual's standing within the organisation. It provides either a safe or constraining boundary, and it either restricts or gives freedom of choice. In general, people feel good and powerful when they exercise control, and they may be more willing to conform in these circumstances. Control seems to help individuals to identify with their workplace, but there will always be resistance to control among people with low self-esteem and less belief in authority.

1 Tannenbaum R and Schmidt WH (1973) How to choose a leadership pattern. *Harvard Bus Rev.* **May–June**: 162–75, 178–80.

Controls assurance

A systematic self-assessment procedure for identifying and managing clinical risk. *See* **Clinical governance**; **Health and safety**; **Risk assessment/management**.

Core value system

This represents the key values that are important to people. Common examples of such values include security, respect, money, achievement, health, success, ambition, freedom, integrity, compassion, independence, family, children, travel and trust. When we live in conflict with our own inner values, this can lead to unhappiness, frustration and blocks. Becoming aware of our values, and prioritising them, helps us to reassess our goals. If freedom, independence and achievement are high on our list, we will need to be in a job that can give free rein to these qualities.

Correlation

A statistical term that is used to describe the relationship between one variable and another.[1]

1 Robson C (1975) *Experiment, Design and Statistics in Psychology*. Penguin, Harmondsworth.

Cost rent scheme

A scheme in which GPs pay a notional rent for premises rented from private developers. Primary care organisations are now less likely to use these, preferring *private finance initiative* schemes. *See* **Local Improvement Finance Trusts**; **Premises improvements**.

Council for the Regulation of Healthcare Professionals (CRHP)

Shaped by the Kennedy Report,[1] a body that was established to strengthen the framework of professional self-regulation and to ensure greater consistency between the nine health profession regulatory bodies covering doctors, dentists, nurses, midwives, health visitors, opticians, pharmacists, osteopaths and chiropractors. The Council has now been replaced by the Health Professions Council.

The functions of the CRHP include the following:

- protecting and promoting the interests of service users and the public

- managing a framework for self-regulation

- comparing and reporting on the regulator's performance to promote continuous improvement

- promoting co-operation and the sharing of good practice.

The CRHP was set up as a key part of the Government's drive towards greater co-ordination and accountability in professional self-regulation. Professional regulation in healthcare provides independent standards of training, conduct and competence for each profession in order to protect the public and guide workers and employers. *See* **Health Professions Council**; **Regulation**; **Self-regulation**.

www.hp-uk.org/

1 Kennedy I (2000) *The Report of the Public Inquiry into Children's Heart Surgery at the Bristol Royal Infirmary.* The Stationery Office, London.

Counselling skills

Interpersonal communication skills developed by counsellors but also used by any good communicators. They include effective listening, active questioning, summarising, problem-solving, diagnosing, evaluating and reflecting skills, and accepting behaviour patterns.

Managers may be required to listen to and give advice on problems that may directly or indirectly affect their staff's work. Here person-centred and first-line counselling skills should ideally be used. They include the following:[1]

- empathy

- non-intrusive support

- listening

- open questions
- reflective questions
- observational skills
- accepting and non-judgemental comments
- summarising.

The interviewer will direct or guide the interviewee, with the aim not of telling them what to do, but rather of helping the interviewee to solve or come to terms with the problems him- or herself. In humanistic counselling practice the counsellor adapts their way of working to suit or 'fit' the individual. The interviewee in this instance acts to provide a sense of:

- choice
- safety
- positive self-regard
- focus of evaluation
- congruence
- open presence
- encouragement
- ongoing commitment to the interviewee.

The interviewee, if given adequate time and space in which to explore their problem, will know when the work begins and ends, but the interviewer provides a safe boundary.

For more information on interviewing and counselling skills, see the author's book.[2] *See* **Interpersonal communication skills**.

1 Rogers C (1967) *On Becoming a Person*. Constable, London.

2 Phillips A (2002) *Communication and the Manager's Job*. Radcliffe Medical Press, Oxford.

Crisis resolution

A service, led by a mental health team of nurses and support workers, designed to provide a 24-hour time-limited service for adults over 18 years of age who have a mental health problem and who have been seen by a GP within the last 24 hours. *See* **Intermediate care**.

Criterion

A standard or benchmark by which something can be judged or decided. Criteria are set as part of the audit cycle. A criterion has been defined by Donabedian as 'a set of discrete, clearly definable and measurable phenomena that are (in some way) relevant to the definition of quality'.[1] A criterion may be defined as an ideal standard that is as clear and specific as possible, and that may be measured both qualitatively and quantitatively. A practice example would be 'a 25% reduction in complaints by X, or X number of telephone calls to be answered within X minutes'.

An *explicit criterion* is one that is declared and written down. An *implicit criterion* is one that uses personal experience and knowledge, that may assess attitudes or subtle variations in care, or that uses values which may be spoken but not written.

Criteria may be *external* (chosen by those outside the audit, e.g. professional colleagues, societies, etc.) or *internal* (external standards that have been readjusted to suit the audit team). Internal criteria are the most successful type, as they meet the particular needs of the individuals in the organisation undertaking the audit. *See* **Audit; Standards**.

1 Donabedian A (1982) Explorations in quality assessment and monitoring. In: *The Criteria and Standards of Quality. Volume 2*. Health Administration Press, Ann Arbor, MI.

Critical incident technique

A procedure in which episodes which reflect both good and poor practice are collected in order to develop criteria for rating professional behaviour. Developed by psychologists in the 1950s,[1,2] it is now used extensively in clinical medicine, in hospitals and in other care settings. *See* **Confidential enquiry; Significant event analysis**.

1 Flanagan W (1954) The critical incident technique. *Psychol Bull*. **51**: 327–58.

2 Samuel O, Grant J and Irvine D (eds) (1994) *Quality and Audit in General Practice: meanings and definitions*. Royal College of General Practitioners, London.

D

Data

A collection of facts, observations or measurements. In *data collection*, particular attention is paid to make certain that the facts are representative, complete and relevant. In *data handling*, the data are stored, protected, manipulated, analysed or presented. In *prospective data collection*, data are collected over a defined period of time or for a predetermined number of cases. Retrospective data collection involves reviewing records in order to gather facts about past performance.[1] *See* **Audit**.

1 Samuel O, Grant J and Irvine D (eds) (1994) *Quality and Audit in General Practice: meanings and definitions.* Royal College of General Practitioners, London.

Data Protection Act (DPA) 1984 and 1998

This was set up in order to protect individuals and organisations from problems relating to confidentiality of data.

The 1984 Act gave individuals extensive rights to examine personal information held on computers, and the 1998 Act strengthens this right by extending the right of access to manual records. The legislation is complex, and some measures may not be in place until as late as 2007.

The Data Protection Acts and the Caldicott Review alert all healthcare providers to the need to improve their computer security and risk management systems, and to be aware of the legal implications of allowing third-party sources access to confidential patient data. The DPA specifies that any individual or organisation that holds third-party information of any kind, either as manual records or on computer, must ensure that they do not disclose this to any third party without the necessary data protection notifications, even if they have the explicit agreement of the individual whose details are being held.

If patient data are made available to external sources such as pharmaceutical companies, in order to improve clinical management, the DPA advises on methods to improve computer security and risk management systems. Data protection notification must cover all of the potential disclosures to third-party organisations. The DPA also makes organisations aware of their responsibilities and liabilities in the event of a complaint.

For further information on patient access to computerised records, or the code of practice on data registration for GPs, contact the Data Protection Registrar, Wycliffe

House, Water Lane, Wilmslow, Cheshire SK9 5AF. Tel: 01625 535777 or 545700. *See* **Confidentiality**.

www.dataprotection.gov.uk/
www.bma.org.uk

Day care

Also known as day services, this is daytime care provided in a centre away from a service user's home. Day care covers a wide range of services, from training, therapy and personal care to social, recreational and educational activities.

www.doh.gov.uk/ncsc/

Day case surgery

Clinical interventions that involve the patient being admitted for planned (*elective*) surgery, treated and discharged all on the same day. It is estimated by the Royal College of Surgeons that almost 50% of all elective surgical interventions can be performed on a day case basis. Both commissioners and the public prefer day case surgery; it is cheaper and more efficient than inpatient care, and the clinical outcomes are just as good.

Day centre

A centre for the provision of day care or day services. *See* **National Care Standards Commission**.

Day rehabilitation

A short-term programme of therapeutic support, provided as one of the intermediate care models at a day hospital or day centre. *See* **Intermediate care**.

Decentralisation

A process of separation of different parts of an organisation, or the extension of activities or services to remote areas once an organisation has become too large to be functional. The advantages are as follows.

- Decisions can be made closer to the actual operating levels of work.

- There is increased responsiveness to local circumstances.

- Support services are more likely to be effective.

- It has an encouraging effect on staff morale and motivation.

However, decentralisation can lead to a loss of control and increased lack of dependence on the main power base, leading to mutual lack of respect and cultural misunderstandings. *See* **Centralisation**.

Delegation

The process by which work is passed on to someone who can do it better, quicker or more cheaply than, or instead of, the delegator, so the latter can concentrate on those tasks that only they are equipped (and paid) to do. It is the process by which someone permits the transfer of authority to another to operate within prescribed limits. Whoever delegates is entrusting responsibility and authority to others (not necessarily subordinates), who then become responsible to the delegator for results. The delegator remains accountable for the performance of the delegatee. What is delegated is essentially the right to make decisions – a person cannot be responsible for a task if authority to act is not given.

In general, the subordinate should tackle predictable tasks, while the more experienced worker should handle exceptional ones. Confidential matters, legally or contractually restricted jobs and ultimate accountability can never be delegated. Delegation is not abdication.

The following factors militate against delegation:

- poor time management

- unclear remits and responsibilities

- underestimatation of a subordinate's competence

- the senior worker feeling insecure with regard to his or her job and work relationships

- fear of criticism.

During the process of delegation the delegator clarifies objectives, agrees the terms of reference, authority and responsibility, gives guidance, support and training, and agrees monitoring and review periods.

Delegation has the advantages that it gives the senior worker more time for thinking and planning, it encourages initiative, and it equips people to solve their own problems.

- Phillips A (2002) *Communication and the Manager's Job*. Radcliffe Medical Press, Oxford.

Department of Health, Social Services and Public Safety (DHSSPS)

The department responsible for promoting and providing integrated health and social care services in Northern Ireland. It sets the overall strategy and is responsible for health and social services policy and legislation.

www.dhsspsni.gov.uk

Deprivation allowance

A series of payments made to General Medical Service GPs, based on an index of deprivation devised by Professor Jarman, and paid on an enumeration per district basis. The payments are banded – one for England and Wales and one for Scotland. *See* **Fees and allowances**.

Desktop review

A form of inspection in which the performance of an organisation is assessed by submitted statistics rather than by a visit from an inspector.

Developmental assessment

An assessment of a child's language, cognitive (intellectual) and physical development that 'screens' for any difficulties. It is usually undertaken by the health visitor, doctor or another paediatric specialist worker (e.g. speech and language therapist or child psychologist). Normal developmental assessments are made as follows:

- developmental assessment at 11–14 days
- developmental assessment at 6–8 weeks
- developmental assessment at 7–9 months
- developmental assessment at 18 months
- developmental assessment at 2½ years
- eye test at 3 years
- developmental assessment at 4 years.

The assessment will provide comprehensive information about the child's development and attainment targets.

www.wellclosesquare.co.uk/protocol/pae/pdevass.htm

Diagnostic and treatment centres

Centres that focus on routine elective operations. *The NHS Plan* announced that more than 20 diagnostic and treatment centres will be developed by 2004, of which eight will be operational. Some of these will be built and managed by the private sector in order to increase the number of elective operations. The Government wishes to support the development of these centres, as they operate at the patient's convenience, away from the interruptions and pressures of general hospital emergency work. *See* **Elective operation**.

Did not attend (DNA)

A term that refers to patients who fail to turn up for their appointments for whatever reason (usually without advance warning), or those who arrive late and cannot be seen. They are recorded in the patient notes as DNAs. A major NHS goal is to improve and simplify its waiting-list procedures so as to minimise the number of DNAs, which cost the health service around £280 million a year.

www.nelh.nhs.uk/management/

Diplomatic leadership

A leadership and management style where the manager has no real line of authority and is dependent on the skills of persuasion for obtaining the co-operation that he or she requires. This approach has advantages in that people work more enthusiastically if they are given reasons for doing a task, and they feel respected. The manager is rewarded by co-operation. However, staff often interpret the attempts to persuade rather than to order as a sign of weakness. The manager has lost out by not having a clear-cut line of authority – and any attempt to revert to a frank autocratic order will have obvious and disastrous effects, while the manager in turn loses the respect of his or her colleagues. *See* **Leadership**.

Directorate of Counter Fraud

An NHS directorate that was established in 1999 to investigate fraudulent activity in every sector of the NHS. *See* **Fraud**.

www.doh.gov.uk/dcfs/index.htm

Disability Discrimination Act 1995 (DDA)

An Act which sets minimum standards demanding that public buildings and private companies which provide a public service make their service accessible to disabled people. It was recently updated to include educational establishments. The DDA requires all organisations to audit their premises and take reasonable measures to ensure that they are accessible to all employees and customers. The DDA also contains legislation to prevent discrimination against job candidates on the basis of their disability. *See* **Employments Rights Act 1996**.

www.disability.gov.uk/

Disability Rights Commission (DRC)

An independent body set up by the Government to help secure civil rights for disabled people. The DRC advises the Government as well as campaigning to encourage good practice, eliminate discrimination and promote equality.

www.drc-gb.org/drc

Disability team

A team consisting of social work managers and occupational therapist care managers who work with older people and those with physical disabilities.

www.dlf.org.uk/

Disciplinary interview

An interview whose aim is to inform an employee of and correct mistakes or unwanted behaviour by helping the employee to improve, thus preventing the situation from arising again. It is not used as a means of imposing sanctions, but with the objective of improving performance in the future. The interview should have a problem-solving style that involves obtaining the facts, exchanging opinions and deciding upon appropriate action. The focus is on performance, not on personalities.

During a disciplinary interview the interviewee does much of the talking, thus allowing the interviewer to obtain the facts. The aim is to reach agreement on the problem and the action decided. Having investigated the facts thoroughly and allowed the employee to put their case, the manager will be expected to clarify expected standards of performance or organisational policy.

Disciplinary interviews may form part of a dismissal procedure, so staff have the right to be accompanied by another individual if they so wish. Each disciplinary interview should be approached according to the stage of the procedure that has been reached. During the initial stages, an informal problem-solving approach may be best, and considerate handling at this stage may prevent the matter from going any further.

Before embarking on a disciplinary procedure, all training options should be taken into consideration before considering dismissal. See **Constructive criticism**.

- Phillips A (2002) *Dealing with Conflict and Criticism. Assertiveness and the manager's job.* Radcliffe Medical Press, Oxford.

Discrimination

Discrimination occurs when individuals or organisations treat other people unequally or unfairly. Discrimination is usually shown against people who are perceived to be in the minority by the more powerful majority (in a patriarchal society, usually white, non-working-class, able-bodied men). People who have made different lifestyle choices (e.g. those who are gay) are frequently discriminated against, as is anyone who is perceived to have less money and therefore less power (e.g. women, the elderly, the working classes).

Discriminatory practice often occurs in organisations or institutions where there are long-held power imbalances, and where these power inequalities are considered to be natural, necessary and beneficial. If there is an hierarchical and patriarchal management style, self-interest prevents any real change.

Anti-discriminatory training recognises the need both to be honest in the face of a natural resistance to losing that power, and to cultivate awareness of cultural advantages. Training aims to raise awareness of oppressive practices and encourage participants to become aware of their own prejudices and responses. The objective is to raise awareness and thereby change attitudes. *See* **Equal opportunities; Institutional racism**.

- Phillips A (2002) *The Business Planning Toolkit*. Radcliffe Medical Press, Oxford.

Disease registers
Computerised information systems that are set up as a way of managing patients with chronic, long-term diseases such as asthma, diabetes, hypertension or cardio-vascular disease. They include diagnostic and prescribing details as well as consultation and morbidity data, and they incorporate systems for calling and recalling patients.

Dispensing doctors
Doctors who both prescribe and dispense medication to their patients. The General Practitioners Council and the NHS Confederation are currently working on a reform of the mechanism for payments to dispensing doctors under the new GP contract umbrella. The intention is that rural practices should not have to rely on dispensing for their economic viability, and that payment for dispensing should be separate from the allocation formula used to calculate the global sum. The aim is for Government, managers and patients to feel confident that dispensing by doctors is both clinically effective and ethical, and for doctors to feel that the work involved is appropriately rewarded.

District audit
The arm of the Audit Commission that is responsible for ensuring that local government and the health service spend its budget wisely. *See* **Audit Commission**.

www.district-audit.gov.uk

Doctor–patient partnership (DPP)
An organisation that is developing initiatives which empower and involve patients in managing their own chronic, long-term illnesses. The DPP sets up and evaluates projects which seek to involve people other than doctors (e.g. nurses and pharmacists) more in the long-term clinical management of patients with chronic illness.

Research shows that a self-management approach in patients with chronic diseases gives rise to improvements in health outcomes, such as improved psychological adjustment, reduced severity of symptoms, a significant decrease in pain, improved life control and activity and increased life satisfaction, with a consequent reduction in demands on the health service. *See* **Expert Patient Project; Patient empowerment**.

Drug action team (DAT)

A multi-agency partnership that operates the Government's drugs strategy at a local level. The team usually includes police, social services, health authority and voluntary sector groups.

www.drugscope.org.uk/dat/home.asp

Drug companies

Pharmaceutical companies involve themselves in general practice in many ways. Practices will be familiar with their representatives calling for appointments to discuss new products or services. Drug companies support general practice by sponsoring product changes and clinical meetings.

E

Effectiveness

A measure of success in achieving a clearly stated objective.[1] *See* **Audit**; **Quality**.

1 McCormick JS (1981) Effectiveness and efficiency. *J R Coll Gen Pract*. **31**: 299–302.

Efficacy

The term for the maximum potential benefit that can be expected from the use of an intervention. In medicine, this refers to the ability of a medical or surgical intervention to produce the desired outcome in a defined population under ideal circumstances.[1]

1 Hopkins A and Costain D (1990) *Measuring the Outcomes of Medical Care*. Papers based on a conference held in September 1989, organised by the Royal College of Physicians and the King's Fund Centre for Health Services Development. Royal College of Physicians, London.

Efficiency

The effectiveness of an intervention relative to the resources (one of which may be money) required to achieve it.

Elective operation

Non-emergency operations (also known as routine operations, planned or 'cold' surgery) such as hernias, cataract removal, hysterectomy or hip replacements. *See* **Day case surgery**.

Electronic medical record (EPR)

A record, held on a computer database, which contains a patient's personal details (name, date of birth, etc.), their diagnosis or condition, and details of the treatment/ assessments undertaken by a clinician. It typically covers the episodic care provided mainly by one institution, but the aim is to make clinical details available across the full spectrum of care.

Electronic medical records (EPRs) have different characteristics to their paper-based equivalent. For example, they can be accessed simultaneously by different people, audits are easier and alert warnings are improved. However, they do also have disadvantages. When individual trusts and practices have different electronic inter-faces, data transfer is problematic. Systems need to be adapted to accept remote data entry from other sources. There are high training, staff and infrastructure costs. Furthermore, legal and security characteristics have to be considered, such as medical confidentiality, access to records, and coding and linking problems. Accurate codes need to be devised, used and understood by every user of the system. Appropriate links (e.g. between drugs and diagnoses) also need to be devised. There may be prob-lems in retaining coherence in coding over time (e.g. when a diagnosed condition develops or changes).[1]

The Government's IT targets are stringent, but in recognition of the difficulties involved, the NHS National Information Authority in charge of IT within the NHS has set up a funded, centralised programme. Work has begun on the *health records infra-structure (HRI)*, with the aim of achieving full electronic medical records (EPRs) in trusts by 2008. *See* **Electronic record development and implementation programme**; **NHS National Information Authority**; **Paperless practice**.

www.doh.gov.uk/ipu/whatnew/itevent/tables/epr.htm

1 NHS Executive (2000) *Electronic Patient Medical Records in Primary Care (changes to the GP terms of service)*. Ref: PC – 01/10/00 and Good Practice Guidelines for General Practice Electronic Patient Records. Prepared by the Joint Computing Group of the General Practitioners Committee and the Royal College of General Practitioners, 31 August 2000, version 2.6.

Electronic record development and implementation programme (ERDIP)

A national scheme to promote best practice in electronic record-keeping. *See* **Electronic medical record**.

www.nhsia.nhs.uk/erdip/

Electronic staff record (ESR)

A major initiative of the National Shared Service Authority, this is a national integrated human resources and payroll system. It is planned that it will be delivered across the entire NHS by 2012. *See* **National Shared Service Authority**.

Emergency capacity management system (ECMS)

A system which co-ordinates GP emergency admissions to acute trusts, currently being piloted locally, with national roll-out planned in 2003. The electronic booking system aims to equalise workloads in Accident and Emergency departments.

Emotional intelligence (EQ)

The understanding of emotion; the ability to perceive, integrate, understand and effectively manage one's own and other people's feelings.

The following five domains of EQ have been identified:

- knowing one's emotions
- managing one's emotions
- motivating oneself
- recognising emotions in others
- handling relationships.

The concept of emotional intelligence recognises qualities such as self-control, persistence, resilience, and sensitivity to others' feelings. Clinicians can hone their emotional intelligence by discussing difficult consultations with peers in small groups, or by video analysis, shared surgeries or problem case reviews. Personal and professional success correlates with high IQ and EQ scores.

Employee volunteering
The encouragement and support of their staff by employers in giving their time to volunteer in the local community. The employer supports their employees practically by giving them time off, matching their funding or allowing them to use office equipment.

www.volunteering.org.uk

Employers' liability insurance
Insurance that covers employers against a claim for compensation that is made by a worker injured at work. The certificate of insurance must be displayed in the workplace. If the organisation has not complied with health and safety regulations, the insurer may sue to reclaim any compensation paid out.

Employers' organisation
A body that

- represents local government bosses in national pay negotiations
- supports councils in their human resources role
- provides expert advice and information on people management and development.

www.lg-employers.gov.uk/

Employment law

Employment law is formulated by either statute law (Acts of Parliament), case law (tribunals), European Community directives and court decisions or common law. The legislation covers employment rights for all contracted staff, including bank staff, locum and casual workers. The most relevant acts of employment law to NHS managers are the following:

- Equal Pay Act 1970

- Rehabilitation of Offenders Act 1974

- Race Relations Act 1976

- Employment Rights Act 1993

- Employment Relations Act 1999

- Sex Discrimination Act 1975 and 1986

- Human Rights Act 1998

- Disability Discrimination Act 1995

- National Minimum Wage Act 1988

- Public Interest Disclosure Act 1998

- Working Time Regulations 1998

- Health and Safety at Work Regulations 1992

- Health and Safety at Work Act 1974

- Employment Relations Act 1999.

Careful employers keep within the law by keeping ahead of policy changes and checking that they give all of their employees all of the job opportunities that are offered within the organisation. They keep the necessary paperwork and document all decision making.

Further information on employment regulations for new employers can be obtained from the following sources:

- The Employers Orderline (Inland Revenue). Tel: 0845 764 6646.

- The Inland Revenue helpline. Tel: 0845 607 0143.

- The Department of Trade and Industry (DTI) publications orderline. Tel: 0870 150 2500.

- Arbitration, Conciliation and Advisory Services (ACAS) Reader Ltd. Tel: 01455 852225.

See **Employment Rights Act 1996**.

www.dti.gov.uk
www.acas.org.uk
www.croner.co.uk

Employment Rights Act 1996

The main statutory employment rights are consolidated into this Act and the Industrial Tribunal Act 1996. In addition, there is a considerable amount of anti-discrimination legislation that affects employment, namely the Equal Pay Act 1970 as amended, the Sex Discrimination Act 1975 as amended, the Race Relations Act 1976 and the Disability Discrimination Act 1995. *See* **Employment law**.

www.acas.co.uk

Empowerment

The process of assisting people to enable them to take responsibility for themselves and to make decisions about their own lives.

Enhanced clinical services

See **GP contract; Local enhanced service; National enhanced services**.

Enhanced records

Elaborated clinical records which allow consistent comparison and effective future prospective audit. *See* **Retrospective audit**.

Epidemiology

The branch of medical science that is concerned with the occurrence, distribution and control of diseases in populations. Epidemiologists usually work within public health departments or academia. They collect and examine medical data and identify health trends in order to establish which diseases are on the increase and where, and which treatments are effective and which are not.

www.pho.org.uk/
www.ije.oupjournals.org

Equality awards

The Government, with an eye on the litigation league-tables, recognises the importance of promoting good practice within the NHS, and has therefore set up this award to encourage the NHS to improve equality of provision.

www.doh.gov.uk/nhsequality

Equal opportunities

The Equal Opportunities Commission was set up under the 1975 Sex Discrimination Act to work towards eliminating discrimination in the workplace on the grounds of sex or marital status, while promoting equal opportunities for both men and women. It continues to campaign to close the pay differentials between the sexes, and to eliminate sexual harassment in the workplace.

An equal opportunities employer provides equal opportunities for every individual in their organisation by treating everyone with whom they have contact (patients, staff, representatives of external organisations) equally and fairly. The Human Rights Act 1998, the Sex Discrimination Act 1975 and 1986, the Race Relations Act 1976 and the Employment Relations Act 1999 cover several aspects of increased protection for workers, and demonstrate good models for anti-discriminatory practice. For example, under the Human Rights and Sex Discrimination Acts, the right to equal treatment opens up the risk of employment claims from women who allege discrimination on the grounds of sex.

Equal opportunities employers are aware of the broader issues and barriers that face those who try to access the services to which they are entitled. These may be attitudinal or environmental barriers (e.g. limited transport, poor lighting, cluttered corridors, complicated forms) or institutional/organisational barriers (e.g. queue management systems).

Equal opportunities employers:

- make efforts to understand the complexities and culture of their organisation

- regularly examine any areas of vulnerability

- conform to all relevant employment law

- anticipate the impact of new legislation

- train in disability awareness and equal opportunities

- counsel staff as a first-line management approach to poor performance

- examine reports on complaints, consultation and referral rates

- ask service users what they want

- instigate and develop appraisal systems for clinicians.

Equal opportunities policies outline any necessary disciplinary and grievance procedures. They apply to all procedures and individuals across the organisation, and they aim to offer equity of access, ensuring that services are delivered sensitively and recognising linguistic and cultural barriers. *See* **Discrimination**; **Equality awards**; **Institutional racism**.

- Phillips A (2002) *The Business Planning Toolkit*. Radcliffe Medical Press, Oxford.

www.eoc.org.uk/

Equal Pay Act 1990

Anti-discrimination legislation to promote equal work. Equal pay law is meant to help ensure women and men in the same employment are treated equally in pay and other contractual terms and conditions of employment. 'Pay' has a wide definition and includes basic salary and other pay benefits, such as occupational pensions, holiday pay, sick pay and shift pay.

Equal pay law in Britain is set out in the Equal Pay Act (EPA) 1970 as amended. European Union law also covers equal pay. Article 141 of the Treaty of Amsterdam requires that women and men should receive equal pay for equal work. Under the EPA employees may claim equal pay with colleagues of the opposite sex where they are in the same employment and are doing:

- work which is the same or broadly similar (known as 'like work')

- work rated as equivalent under an analytical job evaluation scheme

- work which is different but which is of equal value in terms of the demands of the jobs.

Equal pay law covers a broad range of workers regardless of their length of service and whether on full-time, part-time, casual or temporary contracts.

The EOC Code of Practice on Equal Pay recommends that employers should adopt and implement an equal pay policy and carry out a review of the pay system. An equal pay policy should include a statement of commitment to providing equal pay by adopting a transparent and objective pay system. It should also indicate that action in the form of a pay review will be undertaken in order to implement the policy and a system set up to monitor effectiveness. *See* **Discrimination**; **Equal opportunities**; **Pay-and-reward system**; **Pay review**.

www.acas.co.uk
www.eoc.org.uk/

Essential clinical services

The first group of services to be offered within the new GP contract, these are services that will be provided by every practice. They include services initiated by patients who are ill, or who believe themselves to be ill, with conditions from which they are expected to recover. Essential clinical services also cover the general management of terminally ill patients. Other essential clinical services include patients who present with new symptoms such as chest pain, upper respiratory tract infections, fever and other health problems for the first time. *See* **GP contract**.

Evaluation

The gathering of information about an event or process so that judgements may be made about the merit or acceptability of that event or process. *See* **Assessment**; **Monitoring**.

Evidence-based medicine

The systematic analysis of data in order to assess the clinical efficacy and cost-effectiveness of treatments. First described in the *British Medical Journal* in 1996 as 'the conscientious, explicit and judicious use of current best evidence in making decisions about the care of individual patients', it is a discipline that aims to invalidate previously accepted diagnostic tests and therapies and replace them with new ones that are more powerful, accurate, efficacious and safe.

The practice of evidence-based medicine means integrating individual clinical expertise with the best available external clinical evidence from systematic research.[1] This process underpins, for example, the work of the National Institute for Clinical Excellence (NICE), which decides the technologies and treatments that should be made available on the NHS. The aim of NICE is for the responsibility for decision making to be being taken away from doctors and given instead to multi-disciplinary teams of academics, statisticians, health economists and health practitioners working alongside service users and carers to negotiate the available evidence and disseminate the results to clinicians. The aim is not to dictate or explain, but rather to present clear evidence both to doctors and to the public.

The Department of Health, in their *NHS Psychotherapy Services in England Review of Strategic Policy*,[2] adapted some principles applied to psychotherapy research and produced a four-step model for improved patient care. This model can be used reliably for any service provision:

- to commission systematic research reviews

- to secure professional consensus

- to implement evidence-based practice

- to benchmark service outcomes

- to provide improved patient care.[3]

See **National Institute for Clinical Excellence**.

www.jr2.ox.ac.uk/bandolier
www.nhsdirect.nhs.uk
www.nelh.nhs.uk
www.harcourt-international.com/journals/ebhc
www.sheffield.ac.uk/

1 Sackett DL, Rosenberg WH, Gray J *et al.* (1996) Evidence-based medicine: what it is and what it isn't. *BMJ.* **312:** 71–2.

2 Department of Health (1996) *NHS Psychotherapy Services in England Review of Strategic Policy.* HMSO, London.

3 Roth A and Fonagy P (1996) *What Works for Whom. A critical review of psychotherapy research.* Guildford Press, New York.

Publications on evidence-based practice include the following:

- *Effective Healthcare Bulletins*: available from NHS Centre for Reviews and Dissemination, University of York, York YO1 5DD; subscriptions are available from Royal Society of Medicine Press, PO Box 9002, London W1A 0ZA.

- *Bandolier*: a monthly newsletter on healthcare effectiveness, available from *Bandolier*, Oxford Pain Relief Trust, Oxford, www.jr2.ox.ac.uk/bandolier/

- *Health Updates*: available from the Health Development Agency, www.hda-online.org.uk/

Executive summary

Written by the most senior member of an organisation (the executive partner, chief executive or manager), this is a summary of a document. In a business plan, it identifies the key issues to be considered following a business evaluation. It overviews the organisational strengths and weaknesses, representing the collective view of the whole team, and it summarises the main aims and objectives for the year ahead. Key recommendations are given at the end of the summary.

Experiment

An experiment is a controlled observation in which the relationship between two variables is investigated by deliberately producing a change in one of them and observing the change in the other. It differs from a survey, case study or natural observation in which no outside manipulation occurs. By deliberately manipulating one variable, the experiment aims to control all other variables so that they do not affect the outcome.

Designs for experiments may be complex, and can involve any of the following:

- *independent subjects*, where a sample of people is obtained with individuals allocated randomly to one or other of the experimental conditions

- *matched subjects*, often used in twin studies, where subjects are matched in pairs and each is allocated randomly to each experimental condition

- *repeated-measures design*, where a single subject appears under both of the experimental conditions

- *single-subject design*, where only one subject is used for the experiment.[1]

See **Audit**; **Research**; **Survey**; **Variables**; **Write-up**.

1 Robson C (1975) *Experimental Design and Statistics in Psychology*. Penguin, Harmondsworth.

Expert Patient Project

A pilot project which supports volunteers running groups with the aim of educating, informing and encouraging patients with chronic diseases to self-manage. Research has demonstrated that this approach can lead to improvements in health outcomes, with a consequent reduction in demand on the health service. It has been demonstrated to be clinically effective in leading to improved psychological adjustment and fewer visits to GPs. Empowering patients with chronic illnesses to undertake increased monitoring of their condition has been shown to lead to reduced severity of symptoms, a significant decrease in pain, improved life control and activity and increased life satisfaction. *See* **Doctor–patient partnership**; **Patient empowerment**.

www.ohn.gov.uk/

F

Facilitation

A facilitator is someone who leads or presents formal or informal group meetings. Their role may be to encourage decision making or to elicit differing points of view, depending on the function of the meeting or training day. A facilitator requires experience, knowledge, organisational skills, a broad understanding of group dynamics, chairing and counselling skills, and the ability to build teams and manage conflict.

The role of the facilitator is to encourage differing viewpoints while supporting the discussion, to keep time and to ensure that everyone present sticks to the subject. They will do this by:

- extracting feelings and ideas from the audience

- summarising the content of the meeting

- helping to pull the ideas of a group together

- enabling the group to move forward

- helping the group to achieve a successful outcome.

A facilitator co-ordinates the group activities, following and accompanying the group rather than leading them. They seek ways of reinforcing positive behaviour and challenging negative behaviour. Facilitators address and balance conflict and are able to tolerate criticism. Overall, their role is to involve everyone, and to allow useful debate while keeping to the agenda and time. Good facilitation requires excellent interpersonal and communication skills. *See* **Group**; **Team**.

- Phillips A (2002) *Communication and the Manager's Job*. Radcliffe Medical Press, Oxford.

Feedback

The reporting of the results of a survey, audit or process.

Fees and allowances

These General Medical Service allowances are the backbone of GP pay. Detailed in the *Red Book*, and updated annually in the medical press, they are paid quarterly in arrears. They include a set of basic practice allowances (area, initial practice, associate, assistant and seniority allowances), training grants, deprivation payments, capitation fees and payments for reaching certain clinical targets (immunisation, pre-school booster and cytology). Other item-of-service (IOS) payments include those made for immvacs (vaccinations and immunisations), and fees for providing contraceptive and maternity and chronic disease management services. Additional payments cover consultation or telephone treatments for temporary residents, emergency care (including arrest of dental haemorrhage) and miscellaneous allowances for provision of maternity services, health promotion work, minor surgery sessions, night visits and locum/maternity/paternity cover. *See* **General Medical Service allowances**.

Flexible pay enhancements

These may include long service awards, help with childcare, accelerated access to medical services, achievement awards, the availability of job shares, or flexible working schemes such as part-time, term-time only, evening/weekend work, homework or annual hours contracts. Other awards could include the development of profit share/bonus rewards schemes, employee-led roistering, career breaks or flexible retirement.

Flexible pay enhancements work outside the constraints of common pay scales. They are based on identified service needs and reflect the local position. Schemes that do not 'cost' can be developed, such as job enlargements (which increase the scope and range of tasks), job rotations (which decrease boredom and increase variety) and job enrichments (which permit workers greater autonomy and freedom). Such enrichments may involve giving staff more challenging tasks, changing the timing, sequence or pace of the task, or giving them with responsibility for outcomes.

Flexible working has developed across industry as it is recognised that it increases efficiency, meets customer demands, and assists employees in balancing work and personal commitments. *See* **Improving Working Lives standard**; **Pay-and-reward system**.

Floor targets

Targets that have been set by the Government to cover five areas, namely unemployment, crime, education, health and the environment. They are intended to be minimum standards for improvements in deprived areas, set to test the Government's neighbourhood renewal policy.

www.neighbourhood.dtlr.gov.uk/

Forcefield analysis

A system for analysing the support for and resistance to change, usually illustrated by drawing arrows between the (opposing) groups that are driving and resisting change. A forcefield analysis can help to ensure that people move beyond the status quo either by reducing the impact of some of the driving forces (thereby enabling the resisters to move forwards), or by influencing those who are resisting so that they themselves come to realise the need for change.

The following example shows the opposing weights of groups of people (the stakeholders) who stake an interest in general practice:

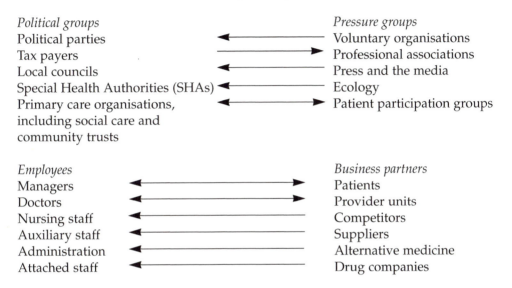

Political groups
Political parties
Tax payers
Local councils
Special Health Authorities (SHAs)
Primary care organisations,
including social care and
community trusts

Pressure groups
Voluntary organisations
Professional associations
Press and the media
Ecology
Patient participation groups

Employees
Managers
Doctors
Nursing staff
Auxiliary staff
Administration
Attached staff

Business partners
Patients
Provider units
Competitors
Suppliers
Alternative medicine
Drug companies

The analysis will help to identify who drives the change and who has the greatest influence. *See* **Change management**; **Stakeholder analysis**.

Foundation hospitals

From 2003, the Government will permit these high-performing hospitals to run independently, freed from Department of Health controls, as a reward for running high-quality services to audited and regulated standards. The aim is to provide a new model of working with ownership devolved to local communities. Critics, however, see this as one step towards privatisation of the NHS.

Franchising

NHS franchising involves identifying the top NHS managers and appointing them to what are seen as the greatest challenges, which could be either failing trusts, key modernisation initiatives or strategic health authorities. The 'franchise' bid for a top job will involve the management team producing a business plan and operational strategies and appointing its own top team. The bidding team may be from the private, voluntary or public sector.

www.doh.gov.uk/

Fraud

Fraud happens every day across the whole NHS. In primary care, fraudulent activity is commonly found in the areas of false reimbursement claims, false invoices or quotes. Bribery, stealing and corruption are also not uncommon. Good organisation and tight management, including the following, can help to prevent fraud:

- evidence-based practice
- use of policies, especially whistleblowing policies
- double-accounting systems
- risk management
- systematic monitoring
- high-quality healthcare delivery
- teamwork
- scrutiny by an informed public
- Staff training
- Practice performance indicators
- Systems and structures.

See **Directorate of Counter Fraud**.

www.doh.gov.uk/dcfs/index.htm

Free-rein leadership

A particular style of leadership in which the manager uses delegation to optimise full use of time and resources. The freedom given motivates people to make a full effort. However, there is a high degree of risk with very little managerial control. If this style of leadership is used, the manager needs to have a very good knowledge of the competence and integrity of their team and the ability of that team to handle high levels of freedom. Free-reign management is usually only given to senior managers in an organisation. If misused, it can create chaos within the organisation. *See* **Leadership**.

G

Gap funding

A regeneration initiative that was developed in order to attract private investment in potentially risky projects. The idea was to make up the cash difference between the extra cost of developing difficult sites and the possible market values if the project failed. In 1999, the European Commission claimed that the scheme breached its State aid rules. Alternatives have now been approved by the Commission. *See* **Local Improvement Finance Trusts; Private finance initiative**.

General Medical Council (GMC)

A professional regulatory body that licenses doctors to practise medicine in the UK. All working doctors have to be registered with the General Medical Council. The role of the latter includes keeping a register of qualified doctors and disciplining those whose conduct fails to meet professional standards. If a doctor is removed from the register, they may no longer practise medicine in the UK.

The GMC is a charity whose purpose is the protection, promotion and maintenance of the health and safety of the community. It has strong and effective legal powers designed to maintain the standards the public expect of doctors. Their self-declared job is not to protect the medical profession but patients. Hence, if any doctor fails to meet set standards, their right to practise medicine is removed.

The GMC consists of some 104 members: elected doctors, members of the public and doctors appointed by educational bodies – the universities, medical Royal Colleges and faculties.

www.gmc-uk.org

General Medical Service allowances

The services that GPs are currently contracted to provide under national contract standards, for which they are paid a standard set of quarterly fees and allowances. The details and funding of General Medical Services are described in the *Red Book* (Statements of Fees and Allowances), and include a set of basic practice allowances based on practice locality or seniority, as well as training grants, deprivation payments, capitation fees and payments for reaching certain clinical targets. Other payments include those made for vaccinations and immunisations, fees for providing contraceptive and maternity services, and payments covering treatments for temporary patients, emergency care or out-of-hours visits. Personal Medical Services (PMS) GPs have a different, locally negotiated contract for their work, which will usually include modified GMS services, unless a specialist scheme is run.

www.gmc-org.uk/

General Medical Services cash-limited budget (GMSCL)

Budgets held by primary care organisations which cover most of the cost of GP practice staff, including nurses, premises improvements and information technology.

General Practitioners Council (GPC)

The committee of the British Medical Association that negotiates pay and conditions for GPs.

Glass ceiling

A metaphorical, discriminatory barrier that prevents professionals from reaching senior positions in an organisation, even though no formal barriers to advancement exist. Glass ceilings are usually encountered by women and other oppressed groups.

Goal setting

Goals tell us where we want to go, and *objectives* tell us how to get there. Goals provide the basis for objectives, and they assist in planning and control and help to focus direction.

Goals need to be:

- specific, precise

- measurable (in terms of cost, quality, quantity and timeliness)

- achievable within the available time scale

- realistic (but provide a challenge and stretch the employee)

- jointly established, not imposed

- broken down into objectives

- planned – indicate priorities (must do, could do), subject to a deadline

- continually updated

- checked for success.

A commonly used acronym is SMART: **s**pecific, **m**easurable, **a**chievable, **r**ealistic, **t**argetted.

Goal setting involves planning ahead, addressing the major strategic issues and not simply concentrating on the operational management issues. Goal setting requires clarity, realistic time estimates, patience and the ability to distinguish between 'urgent' and 'important'.

Goal setters map the environment and paint a vision of the future. If personal and organisational goals are met and integrated, a stronger sense of identity and value will result. The art of good management lies in identifying which goals are important, and in achieving them using the minimum possible resources and without unnecessary stress. *See* **Change management**; **Planning cycle**.

- Phillips A (2002) *The Business Planning Toolkit*. Radcliffe Medical Press, Oxford.

- Phillips A (2002) *Assertiveness and the Manager's Job*. Radcliffe Medical Press, Oxford.

Golden handcuff

Incentive payment for GPs who continue working past 60 years, payable pro rata for every year that GPs work between 60 and 65 years of age. Eligible GPs have to be working at least 25% of full time, and the scheme only covers principals, not locums. *See* **Incentive payments**.

Golden hello

Government-funded payments to doctors who choose general practice, with additional sums for those doctors who join general practice in an under-doctored area. *See* **Incentive payments**.

Good medical practice

The General Medical Council is seeking to raise the level of GP professionalism. The changes proposed in the 2001 guidance[1] give GPs responsibility for managing themselves and their business more professionally.

1 If doctors have good reason to think that their ability to treat patients is seriously compromised by a lack of resources, they should either put the matter right, or alert their employing/contracting body to their concerns. They should also record these, and the steps taken to resolve them.

2 All doctors are required to make clear, accurate, legible and contemporaneous notes.

3 Doctors must now inform patients, either orally or in writing, why they are being removed from their list. GPs should not end relationships with patients because of a complaint or for financial reasons.

4 GPs are required to encourage and value their teams and to support, monitor and review teamwork. Team leaders will be expected to communicate well and deal openly and supportively with problems concerning the performance, conduct or health of their team members.

5 If there are serious concerns about a colleague's performance, health or conduct, steps must be taken immediately to investigate concerns, protect patients and report concerns to the appropriate body. *See* **Management code of conduct; Professionalism: a code of practice for doctors; Professionalism: a code of practice for managers; Whistleblowing**.

www.gmc-org.uk

1 Lee M (2001) *Pulse*. **13 October**: 29.

GP contract

The Government recognises that GP contracts are outdated and limiting. The way in which family doctors have been rewarded has remained largely unchanged since 1948. The fees and allowances given relate to the number of patients registered and, the Government considers, insufficiently to the services provided and the quality of those services. By 2004, both local Personal Medical Services and national arrangements are set to operate within a single contractual framework, namely the *new GP contract*, which aims to completely amend the current *Red Book* contract. Salaried GPs will become more common, and there will be an inbuilt expectation that GPs will accept and adhere to certain common quality standards.

The new GP contract has been set to meet the objective of allowing GPs to control and manage their workload. It is designed to achieve this by the following means.

- It will make available resources that will take into account the needs of the practice population.

- New work will attract new resources.

- Practices will be allowed to opt out of providing some services.

- Practices will be able to choose the level of quality of service that they provide, by selecting one of five levels to which to adhere.

- Primary care organisations will assume responsibility for the provision of out-of-hours services.

- The current arrangements for patient allocation will be changed.

- Demand management initiatives will be introduced.

The new contract framework delivers a wider range of contractual options, including salaried service. It allows more flexible ways of working, is more family-friendly and encourages career development. It is practice based rather than partner based, which encourages the development of skill mix within the practice.

The aim is to incorporate the best features and the flexibility of the Personal Medical Services contract, but with the security of national negotiation and pricing, and with a greater opportunity to control GP workload. It has been developed as the vehicle for achieving the Government's objective of a single contractual framework for GPs.

The proposed categorisation divides the medical work in general practice into three groups:

1 essential clinical services

2 additional clinical services

3 enhanced clinical services (national and local).

It will be possible for clinical services to move from one group to another.

The new GP contract will be priced ready for the profession to vote on it by April 2003, with implementation planned for 2004. *See* **Access**; **Salaried GPs**; **Short-term contracts**.

www.rcgp.org.uk/

GP retainer
A GP who is temporarily absent from work while on leave, usually for pressing or family reasons such as maternity, paternity, adoptive or parental leave, or for sickness, annual or family emergency leave. A retainer fee is paid to the practice while the retainee is absent, to enable them to employ cover for him or her.

Green Paper
A consultation document formed by the Government that sets out their views and invites discussion on a particular policy area, such as planning or the NHS. It is the first step in a policy-making process that usually leads to legislation (White Paper). *See* **White Paper**.

www.explore.parliament.uk/

Grievance procedure and interview
A procedure for staff to object either to an order from a senior, or to any work problem that they believe to be illegal, unethical or counterproductive.

The objective of a grievance interview is to enable an individual to air a complaint, to discover the causes of dissatisfaction and, if possible, to remove them. Organisational policy should clarify the organisation's grievance procedure, which may involve investigating the facts and clarifying possible causes of action. *See* **Counselling skills**; **Whistleblowing**.

www.pcat.co.uk
www.acas.co.uk

- Phillips A (2002) *Communication and the Manager's Job*. Radcliffe Medical Press, Oxford.

Group
A number of people who share the same task. Combinations of different motivations and personalities within groups can be difficult, but groups usually work to find common ground so that they can work together comfortably. As the group forms, it will unconsciously start to develop shared patterns of perceiving, thinking and communicating to counteract any feelings of individual isolation. Group members

converge towards overt or covert 'norms', and anyone who does not conform to those norms will be under pressure from the rest of the group to do so.

Achieving groups support and reward team members, have a mission, co-operate and work to maintain good interpersonal relationships. They are active, and the individuals within them are clear about their own and others' roles and competencies. They use these different team roles to contribute to the overall aims and to develop the capacity to meet new challenges and demands. The team scans and responds to the environment in order to identify trends, ideas and opportunities and actively promote its mission. If they are to be successful, groups must have autonomy, accountability, authority, responsibility and a remit.

Researchers have shown that groups go through certain processes during their development. Tuckman[1] noted that groups pass through different stages in their development, and classically demonstrate *forming, storming, norming, performing* and *deforming* behaviour. The stages are not linear – a group may regress back to an earlier stage if it is under pressure or stress. In the first stage, known as *dependency*, group members will expect to be told what to do, and they may be defensive and not take any risks. In the second stage, known as *conflict*, the group may begin to feel more confident and therefore become more competitive and challenging. Subgroups and hidden agendas will emerge. In the third stage, known as *togetherness*, individuals begin to feel good about being members of the group, and this leads to a productive phase of group life. As *interdependency* is reached in the fourth stage, groups perform optimally and good interpersonal relationships are evident. The level of commitment to the team is high, and there is flexibility of working practices towards individuals, subgroups or the whole team. During the last stage, known as *loss and grieving*, members may feel threatened or saddened by the ending of the group, and therefore resist the ending.

Some rules of group dynamics can be summarised as follows.[2]

- A group leader will emerge if unelected.
- Working groups should be kept small. In a group of 8 people, there are 8 different agendas but potentially 28 different relationships going on.
- There will be a tendency for men to interrupt women or to dominate the space.
- Oppression will rule – the 'experts' and higher social classes will dominate.

Belbin[3] researched and named the following different personality types that are found within groups: the Completer–Finisher, the Implementer, the Monitor–Evaluator, the Teamworker, the Resource Investigator, the Shaper and the Plant.

1 Tuckman BW (1965) Developmental sequences in small groups. *Psychol Bull.* **63**: 384–99.

2 Middleton J (2000) *The Team Guide to Communication.* Radcliffe Medical Press, Oxford.

3 Belbin RM (1991) *Management Teams: why they succeed or fail.* Heinemann, London.

For more information on teams and groups, see the following:

- Mullins LJ (1999) *Management and Organisational Behaviour* (5e). Financial Times/Pitman Publishing, London.

Guideline
See **Algorithm**; **Protocol**.

H

Halo effect

The process by which the perception of a person is formulated on the basis of (usually unconscious) impressions, which may be a favourable or unfavourable trait or impression. Interviewers in particular must be aware of their tendency to appoint or not on the basis of the halo effect, as it tends to shut out other relevant characteristics of the person under consideration. The danger is that the perceiver/interviewer may or may not remember or be aware of whom the interviewee reminds him or her. When such quick judgements are made, the interviewer may ignore subsequent stimuli that vary from the original perception, and only (subconsciously) note those characteristics which support the original judgement.

Health Action Zone

A partnership that is set up between the NHS, local authorities, community groups and the voluntary and business sectors in areas of high deprivation. Its aim is to tackle health inequalities and poor health.

www.ohn.gov.uk
www.haznet.org.uk

Health and safety

In 1974 the first Health and Safety at Work Act (HASAWA) created a broad base of duties set up to ensure that employers identified workplace risks and took steps to prevent accidents and ensure the good health of their employees. Subsequent EEC directives have been issued which make employers' requirements more explicit. Employers can be criminally prosecuted for any health and safety breaches. The legal requirements are as follows:

1 to own a written safety policy

2 to have a health and safety law poster or leaflet visible

3 to consult with employees

4 to have employers liability insurance

5 to record and notify accidents

6 to have clear first-aid arrangements

7 to identify those responsible for each procedure.[1]

A health and safety *risk assessment* provides a structured method aimed at protecting individuals, leading to effective action to control the major causes of harm. This involves controlling the risks – that is, identifying and assessing the hazards, establishing whether the existing precautions are adequate, and devising plans to meet any short-comings. Legislation requires that the assessment must be recorded for employers with five or more employees.

The commonest health and safety risks in general practice relate to people, procedures and the working environment. Health and safety legislation is aimed at protecting patients and staff from dangerous hazards or procedures at work. The clinical and organisational risks inherent in running health services are mul-tiple, covering anything from managing the risks of stress in staff, to the risk of fire, or clinical risk such as infection from spillage, clinical waste or needlestick injury.

Health and safety legislation requires that organisations audit regularly – that is, assess potential hazards, take action to control the situation, and then monitor it.

All employers have a duty of care to their staff under the Health and Safety at Work Act 1974. Further regulations (*The Management of Health and Safety at Work Regulations 1992*) require 'health surveillance', which involves detailed risk assess-ment for employees. Under the regulations, organisations need to protect their staff from and manage the risks of the impacts of stress at work. Employers are legally bound to provide a safe system of work, and are required to make regular assessments of the potential risk to staff of bullying, harassment or excessive workload. *See* **Controls assurance**.

www.hda-online.org.uk/
www.hse.gov.uk
www.hsebooks.co.uk/

1 *The Management of Health and Safety at Work Regulations 1992. Approved code of practice.* Available from Health & Safety Executive, Tel: 08701 545500 or 01787 881165.

For literature and more information about health and safety, see the following:

• Scriptographic Publications Ltd, Channing House, Butts Road, Alton, Hampshire GU34 1ND. Tel: 01420 541738.

• Moore R and Moore S (1995) *Health and Safety at Work: guidance for general practitioners*. Practice Organ-isation Series 1. RCGP Publications Unit, London.

• Business and Legal Reports Inc., 6 Redwood, Burnham, Buckinghamshire SL1 8JN. Tel: 01628 666166. Fax: 01628 668522.

• Health and safety: HSE Books, PO Box 1999, Sudbury, Suffolk CO10 2WA. Tel: 01787 881165. HSE Infoline: 0870 154 2200.

For a further discussion of health and safety and risk assessment, see the following:

- Phillips A (2002) *The Business Planning Toolkit.* Radcliffe Medical Press, Oxford.

Health and social services boards (HSSB)

The Northern Ireland health and social services boards that plan, commission and monitor the health and social services for people in their areas. Four boards cover the country – northern, southern, eastern and western.

www.n-i.nhs.uk

Health and social services councils (HSSC)

In Northern Ireland, each of these councils monitors the operation of the health and personal social services in its board area. It provides advice to the public about services, recommends how services might be improved and advises boards in order to ensure that the whole community's needs are met.

www.nhscc.org

Health and social services trusts (HSST)

In Northern Ireland, the 19 trusts that are responsible for managing hospital and community staff and services under agreements with health and social services boards and GP fundholders. They are managerially independent of health and social services boards and directly accountable to the Department of Health. *See* **Health and social services boards**.

Health authority

Now termed strategic health authorities, these bodies will have strategic responsibilities for healthcare within their regions. They will no longer hold commissioning budgets, as primary care organisations have developed their commissioning role, but will set and oversee standards for the health and social care trusts within their region.

www.nhs.uk/

Healthcare resource group tarrif (HRG)

Developed as a commissioning tool, this classifies healthcare services into different categories based on the type of clinical care offered and the amount of resources being used. The HRG system replaces the 'consultant episode of care' system that commissioners used in the past with one that buys the entire care pathway. Initially there will be 15 HRGs covering six surgical specialities, and these will expand to encompass all specialities by 2006.

The Government has introduced this new tool as part of their NHS financial reforms[1] which cover payments by result, nationally agreed prices for procedures and episodes of care, and commissioning based on case-mix-specific volumes (i.e. volumes which are adjusted according to the case mix). *See* **Commissioning**; **Service level agreement**.

www.doh.gov.uk/nhsfinancialreforms/

1 *Reforming NHS Financial Flows. Introducing payment by results: 2002 consultation document.* www.nhs.uk/.

Health Development Agency (HDA)

Established in 2000, this agency is part of the NHS and is funded mainly by the Department of Health. It was set up to tackle inequalities and improve the community's health. The HDA has a public health role and is a national organisation. It also assists primary care trusts in supporting practices with their own health needs assessments.

The HDA has developed policies and guidance for local health planners to access, and it uses examples from health improvement and modernisation plans and Health Action Zones to bring together the theory and practice of reducing health inequalities. The planners whom it is targeting are those agencies which are working to improve the well-being of their population, namely local government, primary care trusts and strategic health authorities.

Evidence and guidance are available from the HDA for all of the following Health of the Nation targets:

- reducing accidents

- teenage pregnancy

- drugs and alcohol

- mental health, diet, nutrition and obesity

- housing and transport

- neighbourhood renewal

- sexually transmitted diseases

- smoking.

To order HDA publications, contact the HDA distributor. Tel: 0870 121 4194. Email: onlinecommunications@HDA-online.org.uk *See* **Health gain**; **Health needs assessment/analysis**.

www.hawnhs.hda-online.org.uk

Health gain

This is a step beyond health promotion. Improving health gain and reducing health inequalities involve identifying high-risk groups of patients and developing educative approaches to modify risky or unhealthy lifestyle behaviour. Organisations that sign up to health needs analysis are automatically assuming health gain as an outcome. Any primary care organisation that incorporates National Service Frameworks into practice working, and which works to improve access to services for high-risk patients, is supporting the Government plans for overall health gain. The Government health objectives which support health gain are to develop NHS partnerships with social care, to confront the causes of ill health (poverty, deprivation and social exclusion), and to respond more positively to patient need.

The NHS Act 1999 has set standards and targets to improve health and reduce inequality, such as the following:

- the reduction of social exclusion, poverty, discrimination and unemployment

- the reduction of teenage conceptions

- the development of a National Health Poverty Index

- improving service access

- a 10-year programme to reduce heart disease

- 1000 new graduate mental health workers in primary care

- early intervention with regard to psychosis, and assertive outreach

- breast, cervical, colorectal and prostate screening programmes to be set up

- for the elderly, a single assessment process to be shared with social care

- a new sexual health and HIV strategy

- new prescribing regimes.

See **Health needs assessment/analysis; Health promotion**.

www.ohn.gov.uk/
www.modern.nhs.uk/

For further details, see the following:

- Department of Health (2000) *The NHS Plan: a plan for investment, a plan for reform.* The Stationery Office, London.

Health Improvement Programme (HimP)

A local plan drawn up by primary care professionals to improve health and health-care. The primary care organisation works in conjunction with other agencies, such as local authorities and the voluntary sector.

www.doh.gov.uk/himp/

Health inequality

The gap in health status, and in access to health services, between different social classes and ethnic groups, and between populations in different geographical areas.

www.doh.gov.uk/healthinequalities/index.htm

Health needs assessment/analysis

An overview of patient health needs that also summarises recommendations for action. The analysis calculates and compares local/national consultation and morbidity/mortality rates for all targeted clinical areas of concern (e.g. cancer, mental health, teenage pregnancy). A profile is presented showing current service activity and the aims and objectives for the target group stated. The current management and clinical roles and responsibilities and any resource implications would be documented, together with current and future audit activity. The analysis would also review any clinical training needs, assess the skills required, and describe any interventions planned.

Needs assessment is growing increasingly complex, and the aid of public health workers and epidemiologists is becoming essential. However, it is possible for even a small health organisation such as a general practice to make a start in understanding their patient profiles, provided that the problems of data comparison and small sample sizes are addressed.

The following information is needed for health needs analysis:

- demographic data (age/sex/census data)

- birth and death information

- morbidity data on illness and disability

- services used.

Health needs assessment can equip an organisation with working models that may help both to provide the evidence required to re-evaluate their work, and to provide information to enable them to prioritise the service that they provide.

The methods of analysis vary according to the circumstances, and include the following:

- collecting evidence

- defining measurable outcomes

- judging the effectiveness of interventions

- reviewing and comparing data

- keeping abreast of external influences and the local factors that impact on health in the organisation (e.g. socio-psychological forces, legal and political influences, economic trends).

See **Health gain**; **Health promotion**.

For more information on how to conduct a health needs analysis at GP practice level, see the following:

- Phillips A (2002) *The Business Planning Toolkit.* Radcliffe Medical Press, Oxford.

Health outcomes

One way of measuring the success of clinical or management interventions on patients. Health outcomes can be assessed by using specific tools that measure a process, an outcome or a structure.

- *Measuring the process.* If there are too many variables in your clinical population, a process measurement could look at the success of an intervention by, for example, noting the use of a new service by your client group compared with that by the general population.

- *Measuring the outcome.* If you are looking at changes in mortality rates, this measurement may take many years. It may be more appropriate to look at 'surrogate' indicators such as the reduction of risk (e.g. the number of smokers in the population who have stopped smoking).

- *Measuring the structure.* When attempting to change patterns of behaviour, there are many factors beyond the experiment's control. For example, if one is aiming to reduce the number of teenage pregnancies, it would be essential to record the number of pregnancies. For a more robust indicator, it may be better to measure the number of teenagers who are contacted, counselled and advised. *See* **Health gain**; **Health promotion**.

Health Professions Council (HPC)

This body came into being on 1 April 2002, replacing the Council for Professions Supplementary to Medicine (CPSM) and all of the 12 uniprofessional boards. Now the sole regulatory body for the 12 allied health professions that were previously covered by the CPSM, it will operate under the Professions Supplementary to Medicines Act 1960 until May 2003.

All allied health professionals working within the NHS must be state registered by the Health Professions Council, so that their qualifications, registration address and professional standing can then be made available for public scrutiny. *See* **Allied health professional**; **Council for the Regulation of Healthcare Professionals**; **Professions supplementary to medicine**; **Regulation**.

www.hpc-uk.org

Health promotion

All NHS agencies can contribute to promoting the nation's health if they have adequate funding, are able to make long-term plans, and are willing to co-ordinate services and recognise the barriers to health promotion. GPs in particular can play a key role in patient education, and are also well positioned to research, evaluate and monitor patient health.

Services committed to health promotion define health broadly and holistically as a sense of physical, mental, emotional, social and environmental well-being. They see themselves as instrumental in shaping the future health of their patients, and would ideally demonstrate good, equal relationships with local stakeholders and communicate well with those sections of the community who experience the greatest disadvantage. The services offered would strive to be efficient, economical, effective, appropriate, accessible and equitable. *See* **Health Development Agency; Health gain; Health needs assessment/analysis**.

Health Protection Agency

An independent body established by the Government to improve the provision of health and emergency planning.

Health service ombudsman

There are health service ombudsmen for England, Scotland and Wales. The position of ombudsman was established under the 1973 Health Service Commissioners Act. Accountable directly to Parliament, not to Government, the ombudsman has the power to launch independent investigations into complaints from the public that hardship or injustice has been caused by any of the following:

- the failure of the NHS to provide a service or access to information

- failure of a service

- maladministration (e.g. failure to respond to complaints).

The ombudsman's brief was extended into primary care in the 1990s. A request to have a complaint taken to the ombudsman is the penultimate part of the practice complaints procedure, to be undertaken if a complainant is not happy with the practice, primary care organisation and local independent review panel responses.

The cases that the ombudsman deals with are sensitive and complex, and the majority of those involving GPs focus on service inflexibility, poor complaints handling and badly managed removals from a GP list.

If the ombudsman upholds a complaint, they can demand an apology or seek changes in practice from the offending service provider.

www.health.ombudsman.org.uk/

Health status

In medicine, health status may be measured in many different ways, including the following:

- biomedical control

- symptom level

- functional status

- psychosocial status

- patient satisfaction

- increased knowledge

- behaviour changes.

See **Audit**; **Outcome**.

Healthy living centres

A network of centres set up from 1999 across the UK in areas of rural or urban deprivation. Their aim is to promote health and healthy lifestyles and to tackle social exclusion among the most disadvantaged members of those communities. Each centre may be a physical building, or alternatively a form of outreach. Services that may be provided by healthy living centres include Well Man and Well Woman clinics, sexual health or dietary advice, physical exercise facilities and English language classes.

www.ohn.gov.uk/ohn/partnerships/hlc.htm

Heartsink patient

An anecdotal term used by doctors to refer to one of those patients who induce feelings of mental fatigue, hopelessness, despair and frustration in their doctor. In psychological terms, such counter-transference is the doctor's emotional response to the patient. Any patient who attends frequently, worried that they are ill when no cause can be found, is at risk of being labelled a 'heartsink'. The term can be inappropriate and derogatory, as some of these patients have complex emotional problems which can affect the way that they feel physically, and which may lead to illness (somatisation). Dr James Groves[1] divided heartsink patients into the following four categories:

- dependent clingers

- entitled demanders

- manipulative health-rejectors

- self-destructive deniers.

These features may defeat and stress their carers. Some doctors now consider that their own behaviour and responses may be part of the problem – a failure to come to some shared understanding at the end of a consultation, and a failure of mainstream medicine to recognise adequately the complex psychological, social and emotional aspects of illness.[2] It has been suggested that if clinicians do not deal with patient ideas, concerns and expectations (ICE), patients are more likely to return or complain.[3]

1 Groves J (1978) Heartsink patients. *New Engl J Med.* **298**: 883–7.

2 O'Dowd T (1988) Five years of heartsink patients in general practice. *BMJ.* Mentioned in S Saini (ed.) (2002) Everything you wanted to know about heartsinks. *Doctor (Registrar).* **14 Feb**: 55–7.

3 Jamil T (2003) Coping with patients' unreasonable demands. *Registrar Pulse.* **24 March**: 71.

Hepatitis B vaccine
It is a statutory requirement that anyone working in close contact with body fluids must be vaccinated against hepatitis B. Registered patients and the GP's own employees are exempt from any fee for this, unless it is prescribed as a travel vaccine. A fee for both the vaccine and the administration may be charged to unregistered patients, but it is usual for occupational health departments for NHS or private health and social care organisations to provide this to their own at-risk employees free of charge. If patients require an occupational health service, it is reasonable to refer them to a GP who has no responsibility for them under the terms of service.

Histogram
A pictorial or graphical view of the distribution of a set of scores.

Horizon scanning
A term used in NHS planning for identifying the potential costs of and demands for new clinical developments in the NHS. It describes the identification at an early stage of new drugs, devices and medical procedures that are likely to emerge in the future and have an impact on the NHS in terms of cost and demand.

www.publichealth.bham.ac.uk/horizon/

Hospital-acquired infection (HAI)
Antibiotic-resistant infections or diseases that are on the increase in hospitals. Methicillin-resistant *Staphylococcus aureus* (MRSA) is a common example.

Hospital at home
Intensive support in the patient's own home, including investigations and active treat-ment of a limited number of conditions that would otherwise require acute hospital

inpatient care, for a limited period. The treatment is above the level of care normally provided by primary care, but does not necessarily require the resources of an acute hospital stay.

Hospital at home can be used as a way of avoiding an acute admission, or to enable earlier discharge from hospital.

This scheme is popular with patients but not with carers. The idea originated in France and has since spread to other countries, where it is undertaken in different ways. In the UK it aims to be a personal, nurse-led service, whereas in the USA the focus is more 'hi-tech'. The primary aims of the scheme are to cut costs and reduce the duration of care, although research suggests that the scheme achieves neither of these objectives for medical patients, nor does it improve health outcomes overall.[1]
See **Intermediate care**.

1 Shepperd S and Liffe S (2001) *Hospital at Home Versus Inpatient Hospital Care (Cochrane Review)*. The Cochrane Library. Issue 4. Update Software, Oxford.

House officer

A doctor in training who has successfully completed five years at medical school and is learning general medicine in a hospital in preparation for becoming a registrar, and eventually a GP or consultant. House officers are also called junior doctors.

www.bma.org.uk

Hub and spoke

A technical term for concentrating specialists in the centre and having small outreach services for minor forms of the speciality on the outskirts. This approach is considered to be one answer to growing recruitment problems in small specialist services.

Human resource management (HR management)

Human resource managers take personnel management a step further and work with an underlying understanding of the subtext, context and complexities of their organisation. They manage not only operationally but also strategically, and they have in place strategies for managing the risks of staff failing to perform. This understanding embraces the following theories:

- workplace motivation

- organisational communication

- organisational structure and design

- leadership

- group processes

- learning

- personality

- culture, conflict and change

- management control and power.

Human resource management refers to strategic and long-term people management, whereas *Personnel management* deals with the short-term, operational level of people management. Human resource management looks beyond people management, policies and laws to whole system management, where managers work on cultural issues and the organisation moves beyond only directing and controlling people. People management then becomes a key element in the strategic planning of a business.

Where people management policies demonstrate significant concern for employee welfare, and organisations pay more than lip service to investing in their staff, a human resource model is adopted. This ensures that staff are well trained and competent, there is a good skill mix, the working environment is safe and comfortable, and working practices are cost-effective. *See* **Improving Working Lives standard**; **Personnel management**.

Human Rights Act 1998

This European directive was passed in 1998, and it is significant that case law is still being made on the basis of the Act. It primarily gives the right to equal treatment to everyone regardless of age, sex, class, culture or ability. It legislates for personal human rights that can be defended in court, including the right to life, the right to liberty, freedom from inhuman treatment and the right to a family. It has been used by individuals to claim services and benefits that have been denied, and by charities to mount campaigns for changes to Government policies. The Human Rights Act, which was made law in 2001 in the UK, requires public services to respect human rights.

www.hmso.gov.uk

Hypothecated tax

A tax that is raised for spending on a specific purpose (e.g. going to war or improving health services) rather than for general spending by the chancellor. Politicians in the UK rarely rely on this type of taxation.

Hypothesis

A supposition or proposition that is assumed for the sake of argument; a theory to be proved or disproved by reference to facts; a provisional explanation.[1] *See* **Experiment**; **Research**.

1 *Chambers English Dictionary* (1988) Cambridge University Press, Cambridge, p. 702.

I

Iatrogenic

Relating to illness, death or infection caused by doctors. This usually occurs through ignorance, as when drugs prescribed in a good cause interact negatively with each other, or it may be a result of simple random human error. Systems of clinical governance (health and safety, risk management, protocols and clinical guidelines) are put in place to help to reduce this margin of error.

Ideal

The best standard obtained in the best conditions.

Improving Working Lives standard (IWL)

This new standard, set by the NHS Act 1999, means that every member of staff working within the NHS is entitled to belong to an organisation which can prove that it is investing in training and development.

The NHS Plan[1] states that by April 2003 all NHS employers are expected to be accredited as putting IWL standards into practice. These standards, which are part of a set of core performance measurements, will demonstrate that staff are treated well, and this will be linked to the financial resources that the organisation receives. One of the key objectives is for organisations to conduct annual attitude surveys, which involve asking their staff relevant questions and acting on the key messages received.

IWL standards will be conferred on organisations that:

- invest in the training and development of staff

- tackle discrimination and harassment

- improve diversity

- apply an attitude of zero tolerance towards violence against staff

- reduce workplace accidents

- provide occupational health and counselling services

- conduct annual attitude surveys

- ask staff relevant questions and act on the key messages received

- provide access to learning for all NHS staff without a professional qualification

- commit to providing flexible working conditions

- Involve staff in the design and development of better working practices.

Other supporting measures are being developed by the NHS Executive, including a Performance Framework for Human Resources, an Occupational Health Service for all NHS employees, and Employee Accreditation Standards.

www.doh.gov.uk/iwl

1 Department of Health (2000) *The NHS Plan: a plan for investment, a plan for reform: investing in NHS staff.* The Stationery Office, London.

Incentive payments
Part of a scheme to improve recruitment and retention, these payments are Government-funded sums of money given to doctors who choose to work in or remain in general practice. *See* **Golden handcuff; Golden hello.**

Independent Complaints Advocacy Service
A service that was set up as part of the Commission for Patient and Public Involvement in Health to help patients to pursue formal complaints through the complaints procedures. It is planned that it will replace Community Health Councils. *See* **Commission for Patient and Public Involvement in Health; Patient Advocacy and Liaison Service.**
   Details of the plans are available at www.nhs.uk

Index of deprivation
An official measure used by the Government to target regeneration policies to the most deprived areas.

www.regeneration.dtlr.gov.uk/

Indicator of care
An element of care which is definable, measurable or amenable to change.[1] *See* **Criterion**.

1 Samuel O, Grant J and Irvine D (eds) (1994) *Quality and Audit in General Practice: meanings and definitions.* Royal College of General Practitioners, London.

Industrial tribunal

Industrial tribunals are independent employment tribunals that assess employee claims for unfair dismissal or discrimination using the Sex Discrimination or Disability Discrimination Acts. Staff who are claiming for unfair dismissal can also seek arbitration through the Advisory, Conciliation and Arbitration Service (ACAS). The main statutory employment rights are consolidated into the Employments Rights Act 1996 and the Industrial Tribunal Act 1996.

www.bbc.co.uk/business/work/issues/articles/

Infection control

The process of managing the risk of inadvertently reinfecting oneself or others when working with or handling infectious material. For example, during minor surgery sessions, blood, body fluids, sharps (needles, scalpels, stitch cutters) and laboratory specimens should be handled and disposed of correctly, and needlestick injuries reported correctly and appropriate action taken. The simplest and most important measure is to ensure that hands are washed before and after procedures. *See* **Health and safety**.

www.medical-devices.gov.uk

Information for Health strategy

The NHS Information Strategy introduces information about the use of and plans for IT in the NHS. Strategic health authorities have a duty to implement its recommendations locally. As an example of the type of strategies produced by the NHS Information Strategy, one aim is to develop information strategies to support each National Service Framework, including information for patients and the public:

- to support patient and social care

- to support the quality agenda (clinical audit data and access to evidence)

- to support health improvement (e.g. through disease registers)

- to support management needs.

The strategies are being developed in partnership with all stakeholders, including NHS professions and other care and patient organisations. Related security, confidentiality and data protection issues will be addressed in each case. Each information strategy will cover the following:

- the development of information for patients and the public

- national clinical and clinical audit data sets

- input to the national information infrastructure, such as the National Electronic Library for Health

- input to generic information programmes (e.g. to support, rapid referral).

The contents of the strategies will need to conform to national data standards. Over time, this process of standards ratification will provide a library of accredited standards for use throughout the NHS. *See* **Information technology accreditation**; **National Electronic Library for Health**; **National Service Framework**; **NHS National Information Authority**.

www.doh.gov.uk/ipu/strategy/
www.nhsia.nhs.uk

Information technology accreditation

Accredited IT systems are those that have been approved by the Government and IT industry meeting expected standards. The Government aim is to have compatible systems in place throughout general practice by 2010, so that common data can be easily transferred to central, primary care trust-held servers. The Government recognises the need for the NHS to establish a reliable and coherent information base of patient-related data. This information base, together with the analytical tools required to make use of the data, provides the necessary information to manage the many and various Government-supported schemes, such as Health Improvement Programmes and National Service Frameworks.

At present, accredited systems must:

- be compliant with a nationally recognised coding system

- have data that can be easily extracted and manipulated and easily expanded

- be able to be networked

- be Windows based.

Primary care organisations currently only credit systems that have:

1 user interfaces

2 patient reminder or recall displays

3 appointment books

4 a sound medical diagnostic and drug coding base

5 item-of-service links

6 pathology links modules

7 dispensing modules with drug formularies

8 portable protocol builders

9 anatomical dictionaries

10 NHSnet communications for email, Web browsing and structured messaging

11 bulletin boards to manage emails

12 a facility for collecting immunisation and screening histories.

www.doh.gov.uk/ipu/strategy/

Informed consent

The requirement for patients to understand the care to which they are consenting. In order to prevent adverse patient complaints, patients must consent to their own or their relatives' treatment. This covers all patient groups. Organisational policies must make the route to this explicit, and ensure that everyone understands both the concept and what consent they are giving to the intervention (investigations, research or treatment). Such a policy may include, for example, the way in which patients confirm their agreement to intimate examinations, an explanation of false-negative and false-positive results, or an outline of the limitations of screening. *See* **Data Protection Act 1984 and 1998**.

Inpatient

A patient who has been admitted to hospital for treatment and who is occupying a hospital bed.

www.doh.gov.uk/waitingtimes

Institute of Health Service Management (IHSM)

The largest UK professional body for managers working in healthcare and health services, the IHSM acts as a leading provider of education, training courses, seminars and events, and as a publisher of material on healthcare policy issues. It aims to improve health, medical and healthcare services across the UK by providing information on policy, resources and employment support.

www.ihm.org.uk

Institutional racism

Sir William McPherson first coined the term *institutional racism*, which was used during the Stephen Lawrence Inquiry.[1] The definition refers to 'the collective failure of an organisation to provide an appropriate and professional service to people because of their colour, culture or ethnic origin. It can be seen or detected in processes, attitudes and behaviour which amount to discrimination through unwitting prejudice, ignorance, thoughtlessness and stereotyping which disadvantage minority ethnic people'.

This definition could usefully be broadened to incorporate all dimensions of discrimination on the grounds of gender, age, sexuality, class, disability or lifestyle choice. In most organisations, negative attitudes prevail with regard to diversity and difference; these are often not publicly expressed, but they are frequently expressed internally. *See* **Discrimination; Equal opportunities**.

1 McPherson W, Sir (1999) Institutional racism at work. *The Independent*. **25 February**.

Intelligence

This has been defined as mental agility, *fluid intelligence* being a type of abstract reasoning that is free of cultural influence, and *crystallised intelligence* being dependent on learning and experience. It is now accepted that there are multiple intelligences – verbal, mathematical, special capacity, kinaesthetic, musical and emotional. More questions than answers are raised about the nature of intelligence (e.g. whether it is inherited, constant, dependent on life experience, culture or education, and whether it can be measured or not).[1] Binet and Simon were the first psychologists to measure intelligence in a structured and systematic way. From this work the Stanford Binet test was developed for measuring intelligence quotient (IQ).[2]

1 Binet A and Simon Th (1905) Methodes nouvelles pour le diagnostic du niveau intellectual des anormaux. *Ann Psychologique*. **11**: 191–244.

2 Terman LM (1916) *The Measurement of Intelligence*. Houghton Mifflin, Boston, MA. Cited in LJ Mullins (1999) *Management and Organisational Behaviour* (5e). Pitman Publishing, London.

Intermediate care

Nursing home, rehabilitation or home care services provided to ease the transition of the patient from hospital to home and from medical dependence to functional independence. One of the crucial elements of *The NHS Plan*, intermediate care is an umbrella term used to describe a range of services that incorporate a multi-disciplinary approach, and which are designed to promote independence in line with the 'care closer to home' principle.

The Department of Health has marked intermediate care services with the following standard definitions.

- They are targeted at people who would otherwise face unnecessary or prolonged secondary or long-term residential care.

- They have a planned outcome of maximising independence.

- They are time limited, the average care package running from 1 to 6 weeks.

- They involve cross-professional working, a single assessment framework and records and shared protocols.

There are various models of care services for people with physical, mental and social needs (see above). However, older people are given special focus because of their much higher rate of growth in numbers of acute admissions and use of nursing and residential home care placements.

Intermediate care packages are clinical support packages developed in collaboration with community and secondary care staff, with the aim of supporting patients in need during their transition between hospital and home. Future schemes that are being piloted in some parts of the country train their intermediate care workers as specialised workers who have been taught to take on several health and social care roles, so that patients can be attended by a single care worker rather than the three or four who were previously used.

The current expansion of intermediate care reflects the outcome of the National Beds Inquiry consultation, which demonstrated overwhelming support for 'care closer to home'.

As part of their modernisation agenda, the Government sees GPs as playing a large part in supporting the wider healthcare of their community, and wants them to be more involved with this type of development. It sees general practice as having the necessary technical and interpersonal attributes to provide primary healthcare as well as personal, co-ordinated continuity of care for its patients.

The GP vision of intermediate care is to develop early discharge protocols, and to have nurse-managed beds with GP input and expertise to call upon. It is seen as a transient stage, and not as a cheap alternative to acute or long-term care – although it is more costly than other services, it is patient friendly.

GPs can access support and assistance via the primary care organisation's intermediate care co-ordinator, who has responsibility for securing the development of care pathways and access to service protocols, and for ensuring that intermediate care is integrated across all health and social care communities, including housing and the independent sector.

Government Public Private Partnership (PPP) monies can be used to help to fund these schemes.

See the BMA website www.bma.org.uk/public for more details. Information on intermediate care and specialist GPs can be found on www.bma.org.uk or the Royal College of General Practitioners website at www.rcgp.org.uk. *See* **Crisis resolution; Day rehabilitation; Hospital at home; Rapid response; Residential rehabilitation; Supported discharge**.

Interpersonal communication skills

Communication skills that are widely based, functional or process orientated. They include such skills as the following:

- motivating

- leading

- listening

- instructing

- organising

- writing

- presenting

- chairing

- counselling

- facilitating

- supervising

- delegating

- interviewing

- appraising.

See **Communication**.

Investors in People (IiP)

IiP was launched in 1991 by the Department of Employment as a standard for training and development of individuals within an organisation. The organisation was taken over by a private company in 1993. It is a Government-sponsored initiative, based on a commitment to the benefits that organisations can gain from a rigorous approach to the development of their human resources. The aim is to develop a more highly skilled and flexible workforce, and to reward organisations that achieve the prescribed training standards with a Kitemark logo.

The IiP initiative provides a national framework for maintaining and increasing the UK's competitive position in world markets. The standard provides a framework for improving business performance and competitiveness through a planned approach to setting and communicating business objectives and developing people to meet those objectives. The standard is held for three years, after which the organisation must apply for reassessment in order to retain it.

The standard is a cyclical process based on four key principles:

1 a public commitment from the top to invest in and develop people in order to achieve business goals

2 planning how individuals and teams are to be developed in order to meet those goals

3 taking the relevant action to achieve this

4 evaluating the outcomes as a basis for continual improvement.

Organisational success is dependent on the effective development of human resources. IiP is recognised as one of the most successful quality awards ever to be introduced. It can be viewed as part of a wider quality management process with natural progression towards total quality management. *See* **Total quality management**.

www.smartman.co.uk
www.artetch.co.uk

Item of service (IOS)

Payment made to GPs following submission of evidence of provision (via an IOS link to the payment section of the primary care organisation). These include payments made for vaccinations and immunisations, and for providing contraceptive, maternity and chronic disease management services. Additional payments cover consultation or telephone treatments for temporary residents, emergency care and miscellaneous allowances for provision of health promotion work, minor surgery sessions and night visits. These payments were phased out for Personal Medical Services GPs, and will also be phased out under the terms of the 2002 New National Contract. *See* **Fees and allowances**.

J

Job analysis

A managerial task which identifies whether there is a job to be done. This occurs prior to selection and will involve the following steps:

1 reviewing the job description and job specification

2 speaking to the new appointee's manager and subordinate in order to establish what is needed and who would fit in

3 ascertaining whether some of the tasks can be delegated to staff who are already in post

4 listing the pressing reasons for employing a new member of staff

5 looking at the anticipated pros and cons of having the post filled

6 consider the implications for the organisation and related services (e.g. other surgeries, hospitals, health authority) if the post were not filled.

Salary costs are identified, using the mid-point of the incremental scale, to include the following:

1 potential training costs

2 associated capital costs (e.g. new equipment)

3 the overall plans for the organisation in terms of staffing levels and developments (e.g. if you are considering computerising in the near future, you may be able to afford to cut clerical time but increase VDU operation time).

See **Job description; Job specification; Staff profile.**

Job description

The job description should contain the following information:

1 job title

2 grade

3 hours worked

4 Main job purpose (key role(s) and result areas)

5 duties and responsibilities

6 specific limitations of authority

7 areas of responsibility

8 working relationships (reporting and accountability arrangements)

9 any personal competencies required

10 signature of manager

11 date prepared.

Good job descriptions paint an accurate picture of the job. They are clear about any difficulties (any aspects of the job that are particularly demanding or difficult to perform) and tedious or unpleasant aspects.[1] The emphasis should be on purpose and accountability rather than on tasks and responsibility (a cleaner may well vacuum floors, but that is not the purpose of the post – the purpose of such a job is to keep the floors free from dirt). *See* **Job analysis**; **Job specification**; **Staff profile**.

1 Roger A and Cavanagh P (1967) Personnel selection and vocational guidance. In: AT Welford *et al.* (eds) *Society: problems and methods of study*. Routledge, London.

Job enlargement
Increasing the scope of a job and the range of tasks that the worker usually carries out. It is regarded as horizontal job design, as it makes the job structurally larger. However, it may do little to improve staff motivation or performance, as it may simply increase the number and type of tasks that the worker has to complete. *See* **Job enrichment**.

Job enrichment
An extension of the more basic job rotation and enlargement methods, this involves vertical job enlargement. It aims to give the worker more control and greater authority over the planning and execution of their work. It increases the complexity of the work, and should provide a more challenging opportunity for psychological growth. It aims to give workers, especially those higher up in the hierarchy, greater freedom and responsibility. *See* **Job enlargement**.

Job redesign
Restructuring either the nature of a work task or a method of working. *See* **Job enlargement**; **Job enrichment**; **Job rotation**.

Job rotation

The basic form of job redesign, which involves moving staff from one job to another in an attempt to train them, prevent boredom and add variety. Neither the nature of the task nor the method of working is restructured. Job rotation can help to give staff a better understanding of the purpose of the organisation's work. *See* **Job enlargement**; **Job enrichment**; **Job redesign**.

Job specification

More detailed description of the skills required of the employee, identifying the task(s), knowledge and specialist skills required for the job that is being advertised. Also known as a *person specification* or *candidate profile*, it looks at the essential and desirable qualifications and personal competencies required for the job. If selection is matched to this, it considerably reduces interviewer bias. A job specification helps to eliminate the contravention of any equal opportunities laws. It determines the primary skills in the job description and stipulates the essential and desirable qualifications and/or experience. For example:

- *skill*: typing medical letters

- *desirable qualification*: Medical Secretary Grade

- *essential minimum*: 50 wpm audio typing, shorthand typing

- *experience*: able to describe a significant period of employment as a medical secretary

- *personal competences*: to set and prioritise work and objectives, to report personal learning and development needs to manager, to be able to influence, build and maintain a network of relevant contacts.

See **Job analysis**; **Job description**; **Staff profile**.

Joined up working

The working together of organisations such as councils, hospitals and schools to identify and solve local problems. Joined up working is commonly found in primary care organisations where managers work on issues of joint interest with others in social services, local government or the voluntary sector. The Government has pushed this idea as a means of closing the gaps between public services and improving overall performance. *See* **Joint funding**.

Joint Committee for Postgraduate Training for General Practice (JCPTGP)

The Medical Education Standards Board will shortly take over the role of the JCPTGP and the specialist training authority. *See* **Medical Education Standards Board**.

Joint funding

The agreement of two or more agencies to share the cost of running a project or service. *See* **Joined up working**.

www.doh.gov.uk/jointunit/partnership/htm

Joint investment (and implementation) plan (JIP)

Plans, produced by health authorities and local authorities, that form part of *local action plans (LAPs)* for purchasing care services jointly. JIPs identify workforce plans for the development of intermediate care by identifying key issues (e.g. existing investment, number of beds available and occupied) and detailing the expected benefits of service change for users and carers. JIPs are commonly developed across social care, education and housing sectors, as well as other key agencies such as the voluntary and charity sector and other representatives of service users and carers. *See* **Joint funding**.

K

Key role development

Section 9.5 of the NHS Plan[1] itemises how NHS employers will be required to empower appropriately qualified nurses, midwives and therapists to undertake a wider range of clinical tasks. The expectation is that nurses and the professions supplementary to medicine will be trained to take a broader role in assessment and diagnosis so that they will be able to:

- order pathology and X-rays

- refer directly to allied professionals

- identify areas/specialities where nurses can admit and discharge patients

- manage more chronic disease caseloads

- prescribe limited medicines

- undertake resuscitation training (including defibrillation)

- run minor surgery clinics

- undertake IT triage.

www.modern.nhs.uk

1 Department of Health (2000) *The NHS Plan: a plan for investment, a plan for reform.* The Stationery Office, London.

Key workers

Public sector staff, such as nurses, police officers and teachers, who are crucial to the economy and vital for better public services, but who are relatively poorly paid. The term is often used in relation to the lack of affordable housing for such people in areas with high house prices. The definition is now being broadened to include almost all poorly paid workers. Key workers are sometimes referred to as *named workers*.

www.london.gov.uk/

King's Fund

A charitable foundation whose goal is to improve health, especially in London. The King's Fund audits, assesses and makes recommendations to improve healthcare, with a focus on the following:

- tackling health inequalities and social injustice

- enabling health and social care staff and organisations to work in partnership across traditional boundaries

- promoting cultural diversity in healthcare

- encouraging patient and wider public involvement in health and healthcare.

www.kingsfund.org.uk/

Knowledge workers

Employees who apply their theoretical and practical understanding of a specific area of knowledge in order to produce outcomes of commercial, social or personal value. Their performance is very much judged both on their cleverness and creativity and on the commercial value of their applied knowledge. Knowledge workers are increasingly being employed in the consultancy, telecommunications, scientific and technical fields.

L

Laissez-faire leadership
A particular style of leadership in which the manager withdraws leadership if it is observed that team members are working well together – with the proviso that help is on hand if it is required. *See* **Leadership**.

Leadership
Leadership may be hierarchical, top driven, autocratic or bureaucratic. Leadership skills can be learned and developed, but there is no single style of leadership that is appropriate to all situations – different styles are appropriate for different stages of the business.[1]

Common leadership patterns include the following:[2]

- high level of concern for production and low level of concern for people

- low level of concern for production and high level of concern for people

- high level of concern for people and production

- a maternalistic or paternalistic management style in which reward and approval are shown to those who are loyal and obedient to the organisation

- approval of aims to keep people happy

- avoidance of conflict

- risk-taking and innovative behaviour

- high levels of control, with reward and punishment systems

- opportunist behaviour – adapting situations and adapting to people in order to gain the maximum advantage

- a willingness to explore options and alternatives openly and flexibly

- a willingness to change

- manipulation, coercion and changeability

- unfair authority.

Best practice shows us organisations where the decision making is devolved downwards, and ideas are fed upwards. Significant employee involvement is recommended in the 'excellence' literature.[3] People are encouraged by being involved and directing the agenda for change. If the power base is held by expert teams rather than by individuals, people work collectively on clearly defined subject areas. This promotes innovation and creativity, and demonstrates respect for employees.

Leadership styles give a clue to the type of culture within the organisation, and each has its own strengths and weaknesses. Managers have their own individual way of leading. Most adopt a style with which they feel comfortable, that matches the expectations of the people for whom they work and the situation facing them. For example, it is necessary to be autocratic at times of rapid and imposed change or crisis – someone has to make decisions fast. Managers can afford to adopt a more diplomatic stance when there is time to consult and debate.

The leader is not necessarily the manager – the leader visions and the manager controls. A *supportive* style of leadership is related to lower turnover and grievance rates and higher levels of subordinate satisfaction, and results in less inter-group conflict. This is the preferred (and expected) style of leadership in today's work culture.

Directive leadership can increase productivity – but only if the task is routine. Some people prefer a structured style, so that they are being led. This is often the most productive style to use when managing a crisis. *See* **Autocratic leadership; Bureaucratic leadership; Diplomatic leadership; Participative management; Free-rein leadership.**

1 Mintzberg H (1973) *The Nature of Managerial Work.* Harper and Row, New York.

2 Blake RR and Adams McCanse A (1991) *Leadership Dilemmas: grid solutions.* Gulf Publishing Company, Houston, TX.

3 Peters TJ and Waterman RH (1982) *In Search of Excellence.* Harper and Row, London.

Learning difficulty

The condition which affects people who experience more problems than the general population with activities that involve thinking and understanding. *See* **Learning disability.**

www.doh.gov.uk/learningdisabilities

Learning disability

The condition which affects people who need additional help and support with their everyday lives, because they find activities that involve thinking and understanding difficult. Some people with a learning disability may also have an additional impairment, such as a sensory impairment or a physical disability. *See* **Learning difficulty.**

Learning needs

As part of the revalidation and appraisal process, GPs and all NHS staff are required to demonstrate that they understand and can prioritise their own learning or training needs. These can be ascertained formally (e.g. by objective testing, audit or research, peer assessment, educational appraisal or mentoring schemes) or informally (e.g. by self-appraisal, reading and reflection, case review or video-tape consultations). In order to identify their own need to learn, clinical staff (and others, where appropriate) need to:

- be open to new ideas
- undergo continual professional development
- have an intimate knowledge of their role
- learn from experience
- listen actively
- respond fairly to assessments of practice
- learn on the job
- keep up to date
- be willing to make suggestions for improvement in their practice.

The Government is keen to apply personal development plans for all professional workers within the NHS. A range of methods is used to identify learning needs, including the following:

- obtaining feedback from colleagues
- self-appraisal (of individual attitudes, knowledge, awareness of health politics, skills)
- conducting audit or research
- comparing one's performance with that of others
- observing work role and environment
- reading and reflecting
- taking part in educational appraisal or mentoring schemes
- analysing patient/staff contacts by case review
- video-taping consultations
- analysing practice activity data
- undergoing objective testing
- attending educational meetings or training programmes.

See **Learning plan; Patient unmet needs; Personal development plan; Practice professional development plan; Revalidation.**

Learning organisation

An organisation that facilitates learning by all of its members and which continually transforms itself.[1] Learning organisations are said to adapt particularly well to change as they reposition *human resource management* centrally and view employees as key stakeholders. This facilitates an increase in teamwork and employee involvement.

1 Burgoyne J (1995) Feeding minds to grow the business. *People Management*. **21 September**: 22–5.

Learning plan

This documents individual or organisational learning priorities and training needs, and notes where any information that is needed can be obtained. It requires an honest analysis of the present position and how that position was reached, identifies the progress required, and analyses what must be achieved in order to achieve that progress. The contents of a learning plan can be summarised as follows:

• what has been achieved to date

• current knowledge, abilities and opportunities

• future career and life goals

• outcome measurements.

See **Learning needs; Personal development plan.**

Learning sets

A method of *self-managed learning* in which a group of colleagues meet, and each participant is given equal time within the group. The person who is the focus of attention learns and evaluates for him- or herself. There is a shift in his or her ideas in relation to the issue under consideration. The process can be supportive and empowering but challenging, as each person takes personal responsibility for their own learning.
  In learning sets:

• more innovative solutions to problems emerge

• learning is disseminated more widely

• the organisation as a whole often develops a learning approach to problem solving

• participants find other people whom they can rely on to continue to support them through change

- participants learn to support and challenge behaviour appropriately, to listen actively and to be honest and open, and they take these skills back to their organisations

- the facilitation skills can be learned and extended to others

- progress may be made in resolving problems to which there may have been no clear solutions before

- effort and resources are not wasted on inappropriate learning

- participants are more open to further self-development

- the focus is on approaching and dealing with practical problems, not on theory

- risk is soon regarded as a developmental and acceptable tool

- individuals adapt the process to suit their own needs

- real issues are addressed, and there is practical, immediate application of the learning

- individuals identify their own needs and arrive at their own solutions.

Learning styles

Researchers have identified several different types of learner:[1]

- the activist who learns by doing

- the pragmatist who learns best when the practical application is obvious

- the theorist who needs to understand the fundamental principles

- the reflector who learns by thinking about things.

Everyone has a different learning style, and these can be recognised along with a broad understanding of group process and behaviour and some of the obstacles to learning (an unwillingness to learn about difference, a fear of change and development). Learning will be more complete, and is more likely to persist, if the learner is empowered to construct their own learning and therefore actively participate in the process. The teacher's role here is to facilitate or mentor, not to impart knowledge.

1 Honey P (1994) Styles of learning. In: A Mumford (ed.) *Handbook of Management Development* (4e). Gower, Aldershot.

Listening skills

Active listening requires the receiver to listen for the total meaning that a person is conveying, in order to try to determine both the content of the message and the feelings underlying it. Active listening also involves noting all of the cues, both verbal and non-verbal, in communication.

We listen and process information faster than we can speak. Good listeners:

- eliminate distractions
- stop talking
- stop interrupting
- relax, and do not rush
- are alert to non-verbal cues
- empathise
- demonstrate understanding – paraphase/summarise frequently
- use open-ended questions to clarify and understand
- use silence
- are not afraid of tension
- allow for reflection.

See **Counselling skills**.

Lloyd George wallets

Buff-coloured A3-sized medical record wallets in use in GP practices which have not yet become paperless. The wallets and their contents are owned by the State.

Local action plan (LAP)

These are used to define healthcare plans developed by primary care trusts in collaboration with local healthcare planning agencies such as social care, housing, education and the independent sector. The plans commonly cover particular groups of people with special care problems, such as services for older people or those with specific physical, mental or social needs. LAPs identify workforce plans for the development of intermediate care covering the NHS, social care and the independent sector. *See* **Joint investment plans**.

Local delivery plan (LDP)

A new system of three-year planning and capital allocations undertaken by trusts. It was set up in response to the Government's *Investment, Expansion and Reform Paper* to replace the Service and Financial Framework.

www.doh.gov.uk/planning2003-2006/index.htm

Local enhanced services

Unlike the other categories of clinical services provided under the GP contract, these will be subject to local discretion and will be locally commissioned. Like national enhanced services, they will be agreed locally between practices wishing to offer them and the primary care organisation, with, if desired, the involvement of the Local Medical Committee. Unlike national enhanced services, they will not be nationally priced. The category could include pilot schemes for innovative services, or provision for a specific local need (e.g. an influx of asylum seekers). *See* **GP contract**.

Local Government Association

A body that represents local authorities in England and Wales, working with central government with the aim of promoting better local government and service working, one approach being to assist joint working with health and social services.

www.lga.gov.uk/

Local implementation strategy (LIS)

A document that has to be produced by special health authorities to describe how they intend to implement *Information for Health* and other local strategies.

Local Improvement Finance Trusts (LIFT)

NHS LIFT is a private limited company set up by the NHS and private sector property developers under the public–private partnership initiative in order to fund, replace and refurbish primary care premises in England. LIFT was developed by the Department of Health and Partnerships UK plc (PUK). Originally a commercial company, it is now a limited company owned by the Department of Health and the private sector. It is regarded as a single corporate entity with a focus on one objective, namely building primary care facilities, and it will take slightly greater risks than other property developers. LIFT will own and lease premises, and it will supplement rather than replace current premises investments. It will build new premises or refurbish old ones for lease. At a local level, a LIFT venture has its funding split 50:50 between the private and public sectors, and its management board consists of NHS managers, GPs and private sector partners, all of whom work together to develop and agree investment locally.

The NHS Plan committed the NHS to entering into a new public–private partnership within a new equity stake company to improve primary care premises in England. This is now being taken forward through Partnerships for Health, a 50:50 joint venture between the Department of Health and Partnerships UK plc (PUK). *See* **Premises improvements**.

www.doh.gov.uk/pfi/nhslift.htm

Local Medical Committee (LMC)

A statutory body consisting of groups of locally elected GPs representing a particular locality who have the power and authority to make comments and recommendations to their local primary care organisations on issues of interest and concern. NHS authorities must consult the Local Medical Committee on issues ranging from GP terms of service to investigations into professional conduct.

www.bma.org.uk/

Local Negotiating Committee (LNC)

Any of the bodies that have been set up in some areas of the country in response to the growing number of GPs contracted for salaried services to primary care trusts. These committees draw up local generic contracts and job descriptions, and also represent other staff-grade doctors and dentists. Representatives from the British Medical Association and Local Medical Committee are included on the committees, which are seen as a particularly effective way of representing GP interests. Contracts are based around a national core service framework with locally negotiated elements, rather like the current Personal Medical Services contract and the proposed new General Medical Services contract. *See* **Salaried GPs**.

www.bma.org.uk/

Locum

A self-employed doctor who is paid to provide cover for absent GP colleagues. Locums are expected to cover surgeries, and also to be proactive and constantly strive to improve their competencies by analysing complaints and compliments, changes in patient care and unexpected outcomes, and requesting feedback from referrals or investigations. Locum workers now have to sign up to clinical governance demands, and also demonstrate reflective learning as part of their continuing professional competence to practise. Thus they may ask practices for feedback on interesting or significant patient outcomes.

Long-stay mental hospital

A hospital that provides long-term care for patients with a mental health problem or a learning disability. Most of these hospitals evolved out of nineteenth-century asylums and were the main form of residential care for these patients until the development of community care in the 1980s.

www.rcpsych.ac.uk/

Looked-after children

Children who are either in care (subject to a care order) or accommodated by a local authority. Children become looked after if, for example, they have been neglected or abused, or their birth parents are temporarily unable to care for them. Social services and voluntary agencies arrange alternative care arrangements either within the children's birth family or in a foster family or a residential children's home. The majority (70%) of looked-after children return to their birth families within one year. The remaining 30% continue to be 'looked after' by the local authority, usually in residential accommodation. The Government has set stringent educational targets to be met by this group.

www.baaf.org.uk

M

Management code of conduct

A locally managed code of conduct, developed by the NHS Confederation, the Institute of Health Service Management and the Financial Management Association, that requires those who agree to its terms to adhere to strict criteria (e.g. with regard to honesty, openness and probity) while holding senior management positions within the NHS. Other requirements are to be open to continuing professional development, to keep informed of developments both within and external to the profession, to monitor medical and management trends, and to develop a positive relationship with the consumer. The code is regarded as a public affirmation of continued commitment and high values.

The three groups that developed the code hope that it will be incorporated into staff contracts so that managers can be judged by clear and achievable targets, and that breaches of the code will be handled effectively and consistently. Breaking the code could bring serious penalties, including dismissal and a bar on re-employment within the NHS. The code covers the rights as well as the responsibilities of managers. *See* **Professionalism: a code of practice for managers**.

www.doh.gov.uk/managingforexcellence
www.ihm.org.uk

Management role

The manager has a variety of roles within an organisation:

- commercial (buying, selling)
- financial (obtaining capital and making optimal use of funds)
- security
- accounting (stocktaking, balancing accounts, costing, analysis)
- administrative.

The managerial role will include, among other things, planning, problem solving, networking, co-ordinating, organising, supervising, controlling, measuring, motivating, managing conflict, and developing and disciplining staff. *See* **Middle management**.

Manual handling

The Manual Handling Regulations 1992 require employers to make a 'suitable and sufficient' assessment of the risks to health incurred by moving and handling objects at work, taking into account the individual's ability, the load and the working environment. If hazardous handling cannot be avoided, the regulations require the task to be either redesigned ergonomically or automated. *See* **Health and safety**.

Mean

The statistical term for the mathematical average; an intermediate value between two extremes.

Median

The statistical term for the middle value in a series of numerical values arranged in order of magnitude.

Medical Abbreviations

A website designed to help patients, medical secretaries and others to understand some of the abbreviations used by medical personnel.

www.rcgp.org.uk/rcgp/corporate/patients/abbreviations.asp

Medical Defence Union (MDU)

The most well-known medical defence organisation in the UK. It acts to support its doctor and dentist members' medico-legal needs and professional reputations. The MDU acts as a mutual organisation and offers its members indemnity services as well as advising on medico-legal matters. In addition, it offers surgery premises insurance and insurance against clinical/medical negligence, and advises on issues such as risk management. It also supports nurses and practice managers.

www.the-mdu.com

Medical Devices Agency (MDA)

An executive agency of the Department of Health. Its role is to safeguard public health by working with users, manufacturers and law makers to ensure that medical devices meet appropriate standards of safety, quality and performance, and that they comply with the relevant Directives of the European Union.

In order to achieve its objectives, the MDA investigates adverse incidents relating to medical devices, offers advice and practical guides for health and social care professionals involved in primary care, and contributes to the establishment of safety standards and protocols.

www.medical-devices.gov.uk/

Medical Education Standards Board (MESB)

The Government is setting this up as a single supervisory body to replace the Joint Committee on Postgraduate Training for General Practice and the Specialist Training Authority (which supervises training for secondary care doctors). Accountable to the Health Secretary, it will ensure that medical training meets UK requirements, it will issue GP certificates, it will control entry to the new GP register, and it has the power to suspend doctors. The 25-strong board will consist of lay representatives and medical members. The registers will be available to the public. The MESB will maintain links with the General Medical Council on issues such as revalidation.

The aim is to provide a coherent, robust and accountable approach to postgraduate medical education.

Medical model

A model or philosophy of health that works on the premise that all illness has a biological/physiological cause, and can therefore be cured by medical/biochemical intervention (drugs, surgery, etc.). *See* **Social model**.

Medical negligence

A legal term used to describe an error or 'a breach in the duty of care' by a clinician who has caused a medical injury, complicated an existing medical problem or caused the death of a patient. It is also known as clinical negligence. The patient or their dependants can sue the clinician for compensation.

www.the-mdu.com

Medical Protection Society

A mutual association of doctors and other professionals that offers its members professional indemnity cover and advice on risk management.

www.mps.org.uk

Medicines Control Agency (MCA)

An executive agency of the Department of Health whose primary objective is to safeguard public health by ensuring that all medicines on the UK market meet appropriate standards of safety, quality and efficacy. Safety aspects cover potential or actual harmful effects, quality relates to development and manufacture, and efficacy is a measure of the beneficial effect of the medicine on patients.

The MCA aims to achieve its objective by means of the following:

- a system of licensing before the marketing of medicines

- monitoring of medicines after they have been placed on the market
- checking standards of pharmaceutical manufacture and wholesaling
- enforcement of requirements
- responsibility for medicines control policy
- representing UK pharmaceutical regulatory interests internationally
- publishing quality standards for drug substances through the *British Pharmacopoeia*.

The MCA works with governing bodies of medical professions to assess the theoretical and practical aspects that underpin prescribing practice. *See* **National Prescribing Centre**.

www.mca.gov.uk/

Meetings

Good meetings are short and constructive, allowing ideas to be presented and actioned with minimal debate. The format for successful meetings is as follows.

- Circulate an agenda.
- Record apologies of the current meeting.
- Approve the minutes of the last meeting.
- Deal with matters arising.
- Identify and discuss regular issues.
- Identify and discuss specific issues.
- Note any other business (AOB).

Mental Health Act Commission

This watchdog is a special health authority that is fully independent of mental health service providers. It consists of more than 170 members from the medical, nursing, psychology, social work and legal professions. Its main function is to review the operation of the Mental Health Act 1983 in relation to detained patients.

www.mhac.trent.nhs.uk/

Mentoring

This has been defined as 'off-line help by one person to another in making significant transitions in knowledge, work or thinking'.[1] Traditionally it is a master–pupil relationship offered by someone more experienced in a profession, who passes on their wisdom and experience in order to give the novice a helping hand. Mentoring usually occurs by means of a series of supportive and educational meetings for a defined period.

Mentoring is one of the principles of ongoing learning. It is based on the relationship with an experienced organisation member who can share, guide and provide feedback to the employee. The mentor should provide a structured opportunity for the employee to review and discuss their career plans. Researchers suggest that organisations need to be fully committed to the idea of mentoring and ensure that individuals are adequately prepared for the programme.[2] Benefits include managerial effectiveness, communication improvements, the promotion of equal opportunities and self-learning. *See* **Clinical supervision**; **Coaching**.

1 Clutterbuck D and Megginson D (1999) *Mentoring Executives and Directors*. Butterworth-Heinemann, Oxford.

2 Clutterbuck D and Wynne B (1994) Mentoring and coaching. In: A Mumford (ed.) *Handbook of Management Development* (4e). Gower, Aldershot.

Middle management
Management that concentrates on tactics (i.e. how the overall strategies are to be achieved). This often involves devising and operating short-term plans (from 6 months to 2 years ahead). Senior managers operate more strategically than middle managers (i.e. looking ahead by up to 5 years).

MIQUEST (Morbidity Query and Export System)
This software, commissioned by the NHS National Information Authority, allows extracted data to be standardised and pooled from a variety of proprietary GP systems. All GP systems currently need to be MIQUEST compliant in order to achieve official computer accreditation.

The Primary Care Data Quality project provides a mechanism for capturing the quality data that are required to support clinical governance and National Service Frameworks. Using a set of queries written by this system, and following a data collection plan, GP practices build their own disease registers. The MIQUEST package includes support on installation, training, data extraction and interpretation. It interrogates GP systems to look for clinical data, clinical values or measurements (e.g. minimum or maximum, particular records and criteria). MIQUEST is run with the assumption that improved data quality does ultimately lead to improved patient care.

For more information on MIQUEST, contact any of the following:

1 The General Practice Section, St George's Hospital Medical School, London SW17 ORE. Tel: 020 8725 5661. Email: buckwell@Drs.desk.sthames.NHS.uk

2 The Primary Care Data Quality project. Website: www.drsdesk.sghms.ac.uk\pcdq\pcdq.htm

3 NHSnet. Website: http://www.nelh-pc.mhs.uk

See **NHS National Information Authority**; **PRIMIS**.

www.nhsia.nhs.uk

Mission statement

A statement that encapsulates the vision of the organisation studied – that is, its goals, aims and objectives. It is used to give a flavour of the organisation, by detailing the values and commitments that will be reflected in the organisation's management, policies and organisational literature.

An example of a mission statement is given below.

Practice mission statement

This practice strives for public accountability. We want to maintain a responsive and better-quality service for our patients, sharpened and more flexible clinical practice, and see an improvement in communications with our stakeholders. We want to continue to achieve the recent clinical improvements in patient care, delivered with sensitivity at a practice level. To this end we will continue to strive for an improved, efficient and cost-effective service.

Mixed health economy (see LIFT)

The type of economy that is said to be developing where the private sector invests in public sector projects.

Mode

The statistical term for the most frequently occurring item or number in a series. It also refers to the peak(s) in a frequency curve. *See* **Mean; Median.**

Modernisation Agency (NHS)

A national body created by the Government in 2000 to help local clinicians and managers to redesign services so as to make them more patient friendly, quick and efficient, and to secure continuous service improvements across the entire NHS.

The agency co-ordinates management and leadership development in order to foster leadership talent at all levels within the health service. It thus has responsibility for the NHS Leadership Centre and the NHS Beacon Services Programme.

www.modern.nhs.uk/

Monitoring

Making pre-specified, objective observations about the characteristics of an event or process using standard forms of data collection. Monitoring is usually done by means of checklists or questionnaires. It should be undertaken against known standards. *See* **Assessment; Evaluation.**

Motivation

Motivation to work, job satisfaction and performance are determined by a variety of factors, including economic rewards, social relationships, personal attitudes and values, the nature of the work, leadership styles and the satisfaction derived from the work itself. Employees have an interest in work beyond the actual mechanics of the task in hand – people also need recognition, intellectual stimulation and socialisation. Different people are motivated by different things. The employer's role is to ensure that the motivational needs of their staff are met, that these are taken into account when managing pay-and-reward systems, and that the organisation's aims and values are addressed.

Multi-agency

Referring to the working together of differently funded bodies to share funds and projects so as to achieve the best care for a common client group (health working with social care, the voluntary sector, local authorities, etc.). *See* **Care plan**; **Team**.

Multidisciplinary team

A team or group consisting of representatives from several different professional backgrounds who all have different areas of expertise (e.g. a community mental health team). *See* **Care pathway**; **Intermediate care**.

Myers–Briggs Type Indicator (MBTI)

A form of personality testing[1,2] developed by psychologists from Carl Jung's work on personality attitudes and functions. Jung defined the basic extrovert/introvert personality types, and also postulated that personality differences would be manifested by different cognitive functions of feeling, sensation and intuition. The MBTI is based on these theoretical constructs, with some additional dimensions reflecting the particular personality styles of individuals. The MBTI is usually presented as a table showing characteristics frequently associated with particular personality types – for example, shy and sensitive (prefers ideas to people) versus enthusiastic and high-spirited (but may be too quick). Thus each personality 'type' has both positive and negative characteristics.

www.discoveryourpersonality.com
www.opp.co.uk
www.skepdic.com/myersb.html

1 Briggs Myers I (1987) *Introduction to Type*. Oxford Psychologists Press, Oxford.

2 Hirsch SK and Kummerow J (1990) *Introduction to Type in Organisations*. Oxford Psychologists Press, Oxford.

N

National Association of Primary Care (NAPC)

A professional body open to those who work in primary care. It was set up to represent the interests of all primary care professionals and to negotiate primary care organisations' interests with central government and other political parties.

www.primarycare.co.uk

National Audit Office (NAO)

An independent body that scrutinises public spending on behalf of Parliament. The NAO audits the accounts of all Government departments and agencies as well as a wide range of other public bodies, and it reports to Parliament on the economy, efficiency and effectiveness with which Government bodies have used public money.

www.nao.gov.uk/

National Beds Inquiry (NBI)

Established within the Department of Health in 1998, its roles are:

- to review assumptions about growth in the volume of general and acute hospital services and the implications for services and bed numbers in the future

- to review the service implications of current mental health policies

- to assess the 'appropriate' use of acute beds by older people and to consider scope for alternative care models, including the further development of intermediate care and community services.

See **Intermediate care**.

National Booked Admissions Programme

A programme set up by the Government to achieve the NHS target plan of replacing waiting-lists with booking systems by 2005. The aim is to allow GPs or their patients to book their own healthcare appointments online. The National Patient Access Team (NPAT) is charged with achieving this target. *See* **National Patient Access Team**.

www.doh.gov.uk/waitingtimes
www.npat.org.uk/

National Care Standards Commission (NCSC)

A non-departmental public body, responsible to the Secretary of State for Health, that sets, monitors and improves standards of care for vulnerable adults and children in the field of health and social care. It is to take on the regulation of social care and private and voluntary healthcare in England. The NCSC is the independent regulatory body that has been responsible for inspecting and regulating almost all forms of residential care and other voluntary and private care services in England from April 2002. It can order the withdrawal of a care home's licence and the exclusion of individuals from the residential care sector.

The NCSC will regulate the following services:

- care homes

- children's homes

- domiciliary care agencies

- residential family centres

- voluntary adoption agencies

- independent fostering agencies

- private and voluntary hospitals and clinics

- nurses' agencies

- day centres.

See **Commission for Healthcare Audit and Inspection**.

www.doh.gov.uk/ncsc/
www.centrepointgroup.co.uk

National Clinical Assessment Authority (NCAA)

A special health authority set up in April 2001 to provide rapid and objective expert assessment of a doctor's performance, where concerns about that doctor have been raised locally. It produces a report to the referring employer recommending a course of action to address those concerns.

The NCAA also offers support and advice to doctors who are directly referred by their employers for irregular behaviour. It has a complementary function to the General Medical Council, which is the first point of referral in situations of more serious professional misconduct. Primary care organisations, the Commission for Health Improvement and the NCAA have signed a memorandum of understanding to ensure that doctors are not passed between organisations unnecessarily. GPs in difficulty can self-refer. Not all doctors who are referred will be assessed, but those who are can expect assessment to take between five and six months. This assessment may include psychometric tests to investigate the doctor's attitudes and personality traits. The aim is to identify the doctor's areas of strength as well as their deficiencies. The NCAA will draw up a confidential report and action plan, including recommendations, which is sent both to the doctor and to the referring organisation. The NCAA expects around 100 assessments a year to take place. Cases of poor conduct or performance are dealt with by the General Medical Council, so the NCAA should not pose a threat to self-regulation.[1]

www.ncaa.nhs.uk/

1 Comerford C (2001) Irvine dismisses NCAA threat to self-regulation. *Doctor.* **11 October**: 11.

National Council for Voluntary Organisations (NCVO)
An umbrella body for voluntary organisations and charities in England. The NCVO represents more than 1000 organisations. It negotiates with the Government over service levels, charity law and consultation, and it also provides support and services to organisations.

www.ncvo-vol.org.uk/

National Electronic Library for Health (NELH)
An electronic accredited NHS library of health information, which enables clinicians to access information on the latest treatments and best practice. This primary care library aims to:

- rate the information sources to which it has links

- apply strict criteria of evidence base

- be relevant to primary care

- provide the right volume of information

- use accredited sources only.

It is hoped that the NELH will discourage clinicians from accessing unauthorised, unstandardised and poor-quality material now available on the Internet by using only approved (accredited) material. *See* **NHS National Information Authority**.

www.nelh.nhs.uk

National enhanced services

These services, which are provided by GPs under the new contract, will be locally commissioned. Patients should expect to find these national enhanced services in every locality, but they would not be provided by every practice. Examples of this service would include more specialised minor surgery, services to violent patients, or out-of-hours services. Practices wishing to provide them would opt into enhanced clinical services. *See* **GP contract**.

National Health Performance Fund

A discretionary fund, worth £500 million a year by 2003–04, set up to provide an incentive to NHS bodies and to reward them. NHS authorities and trusts will be able to access up to £5 million each from the fund to spend on new equipment, facilities and staff bonuses, depending on the organisation's annual performance and progress relative to agreed plans and targets.

www.doh.gov.uk/nhsperformance/

National Institute for Clinical Excellence (NICE)

Set up in 1999, the National Institute for Clinical Excellence was set up as a special arm of the NHS in England, with a multi-million-pound budget to develop authoritative and reliable guidance on clinical management in controversial areas of medicine, alongside its more high-profile role of assessing the value of new drugs. The equivalent body in Scotland is the Scottish Health Technology Board.

One of the aims of NICE is to eliminate the postcode lottery of care, and the other is to ensure that the public are empowered by gaining access to the same high-quality information as their doctors, so that they are then able to make informed choices about their care. Paternalism within healthcare systems limits this choice, as some doctors aim to 'protect' patients from unsettling information. Some doctors also fear that NICE puts too much emphasis on cost cutting, and that it encourages uniformity of consultations, thus preventing clinical freedom.

NICE appraises what are considered to be the best interventions and treatments, and produces guidelines to ensure a faster, more uniform uptake of treatments which work best for patients. It forms one strand of clinical governance. It offers authoritative guidance on the highest standards of care, and aims to improve the nature and completeness of data held on primary care by:

• appraising technology

• developing clinical care programmes

• promoting monitoring of clinical performance through:

  – audit

  – referral protocols

- procedural manuals
- nursing benchmarks
- disease management protocols
- integrated care pathways
- clinical guidelines that are multi-disciplinary, formally evidenced, clinically effect-ive, cost-effective and applicable to the majority.

The National Institute for Clinical Excellence has a remit to produce and disseminate evidence-based clinical guidelines, and the Commission for Health Improvement will contribute to this. By March 2001, NICE had appraised 22 technologies, 19 of which were eventually approved for NHS use. Of these, clinical benefit was cited in all cases, but cost per quality-adjusted life-year was only cited in 50% of cases, and restrictions on the use of these treatments kept the cost of this adjustment to below £30 000 in the majority of cases. The net cost of NICE decisions was less than 0.5% of annual NHS spending.[1] *See* **Evidence-based medicine**.

www.nice.org.uk
Referral guidelines are available from primary care trusts or www.nice.org.uk/pdf/referraladvice.pdf

1 *See* www.nice.org.uk for general information about clinical guidelines.

National Institute for Mental Health in England (NIMHE)
An institute that was set up to provide research and expertise to help the NHS to implement the National Service Framework on mental health. From spring 2003, the institute will co-ordinate and disseminate research and good practice, facilitate training and improve mental health services.

www.doh.gov.uk/mentalhealthczar/

National Medicines Management Services Collaborative
A pilot scheme, run by the National Prescribing Centre, that aims to tackle medicines waste.

www.npc.co.uk

National minimum wage
The lowest wage an employer can legally pay its staff in the UK (different rates are set for Northern Ireland). Currently set at £4.22 an hour for those over the age of

22 years, and at £3.60 an hour for 18- to 22-year-olds, the national minimum wage is revised annually.

www.inlandrevenue.gov.uk/nmw/

National Patient Access Team (NPAT)

The body that was set up in June 1998 to help the NHS to achieve the Government's waiting-list targets. It identifies and disseminates good practice in the field of waiting-list management, and assists staff in introducing efficient elective care processes, such as booked admissions. The National Patient Access Team is charged with achieving the patient access improvements outlined in the NHS Plan 1999, including those set, for example, by the National Booked Admission Programme. *See* **National Booked Admissions Programme**.

www.npat.org.uk/

National Patient Safety Agency (NPSA)

A Government-sponsored watchdog set up in early 2002 as part of *The NHS Plan* to improve medical accountability and patient confidence in the service. The NPSA manages a reporting system which analyses medical errors and adverse incidents, collecting information from NHS organisations, patients and carers. Where risks are identified, the NPSA will produce solutions to prevent mistakes recurring, and it will specify national goals and establish mechanisms to track progress. It ensures that lessons are learned and fed back into practice, service organisation and delivery.

The NPSA stores reports of patient errors (examples of near misses or significant event analyses sent in by primary or secondary healthcare organisations on a quarterly basis). According to the NPSA, around 10% of patients experience adverse events, and 50% of these are preventable. It has drawn up a memorandum of understanding with related professional bodies, but all material handled by the NPSA is confidential, and there are no plans to identify doctors who are reported to this watchdog. *See* **Significant event analysis**.

www.npsa.org.uk/

National Prescribing Centre

A national Government-funded body that is responsible for modernising prescribing policies and disseminating advice and guidelines on prescription medicines, new drugs and nurse prescribing.

www.npc.co.uk
For NHS web users see www.npc.ppa.nhs.uk

National Primary Care Collaborative

Set up by the National Primary Care Development Team in June 2000, this involves practices from every primary care trust in England, and is considered to be the largest health quality improvement programme in the world. *See* **National Primary Care Development Team; Quality**.

www.npdt.org/

National Primary Care Development Team (NPCDT)

A team that was established in February 2000 primarily to assist primary care organisations (practices and primary care trusts) in developing their ability to deliver rapid, sustainable and systematic improvements in the care that they provide to patients and their communities.

   The team, headed up by Dr John Oldham, is perhaps best known for its work on advanced access and the National Primary Care Collaborative. This agency addresses all modernisation requirements of the NHS. It aims to encourage streamlining of services, sharing of skills and developing of best practice, and it supports the development of, for example, specialist GPs, patient directives and National Service Frameworks.

   Contact details are as follows:

National Primary Care Development Team
Gateway House
Piccadilly South
Manchester
M60 7LP.
Tel: 0161 236 1566.
Fax: 0161 236 4857.

See **NHS Modernisation Agency**.

www.npdt.org/
www.modern.nhs.uk/

National Primary Care Research and Development Centre (NPCRDC)

A body established in 1995, which is responsible for looking at the following:

- variations in health and healthcare

- primary care organisations

- the quality of primary care.

Its work focuses on quality in primary care, governance, budgets, workforce and partnerships within primary care.

www.npcrdc.man.ac.uk

National Service Framework (NSF)

Introduced in 1998, any of the frameworks that establish a set of national minimum standards of clinical quality and access to services in a series of major care areas and disease groups. The aim is to drive up performance and decrease geographical variations in care standards. The five service frameworks produced during the period 1999–2002 cover between them around 80% of the illnesses in the UK population, which represent half of the total NHS spend, and account for the highest mortality rates. These areas and disease groups are mental health, coronary heart disease, the National Cancer Plan, older people's services and diabetes.

NSFs establish models of treatment and care based on evidence of best practice. They look for uniformity of treatment to a minimum standard, and consistency across major care areas. In providing a treatment framework for a particular disorder or group of diseases, they aim to address the following:

- healthcare improvements

- inequalities of access

- differences in outlook

- differences in outcome

- differences in quality of care

- postcode rationing.

The six components of the NSF performance assessment framework are health improvement, fair access, efficiency, effective delivery of appropriate care, user/carer experience, and health outcomes. NSFs aim to address the programme of care from primary through to tertiary and secondary care, including both prevention and rehabilitation. They advise on setting standards/benchmarks, and also give referral and clinical risk management advice. They are devised after close collaboration with relevant professional bodies and the NHS Research and Development Centre. Clinically, the aim of an NSF would be to address the best ways to assess, diagnose, record, treat and monitor a particular disease group. *See* **Clinical governance;** **Information for Health strategy**.

www.doh.gov.uk/nsf

National Shared Service Authority

A special health authority, managed by but working independently from the Department of Health, that is responsible for developing and delivering the NHS electronic staff record (ESR), a national integrated human resources and payroll system that is planned to be delivered across the entire NHS by 2012.

National Workforce Development Board (NWDB)

This replaced the Medical Practices Committee (MPC) in April 2002, and has taken on the role of monitoring and planning the GP workforce, taking into account the distribution and role of GPs and other primary care workers in the area being examined. GP workforce planning is notoriously complex (the MPC defined 63 elements that could influence workload[1]). There are also local Workforce Development Confederations, which are involved in developing workforce plans at local level. *See* **Skill mix review**.

1 Jarvis S (2001) Death of a distributor. *Primary Care Management*. **November**: 31–2.

Need

In the care sector, this is defined as a person's requirement for a service, which has been accepted by the organisation which provides that service.

Needlestick injury

The term for an accidental injury with a used needle, scalpel or stitch cutter, leading to potential contamination with body fluids. The following clinical procedures are then considered and followed:

- establishing the potential risks of the donor

- vaccination with hepatitis B/immunoglobulin

- use of antiviral prophylactic drugs

- referral to occupational health services

- taking blood samples from the donor and recipient for analysis and long-term storage with their informed consent.

See **Infection control**; **Medical Devices Agency**.

Networking

Making connections and building visibility with work colleagues both within and outside the organisation for which one works. Networkers deliberately form relationships with others – who are usually more senior or influential – by identifying contacts in a current network and targeting people whom they think can help them to achieve their aims. They behave opportunistically, show others that they share their objectives and are interested in their goals (reciprocity), and demonstrate great resilience. It requires courage to make new connections, and they often risk rejection. Networking can involve any of the following:[1]

- attending meetings outside the organisation

- speaking at conferences or making presentations

- generating new contacts

- self-marketing

- collaborating with others in one's field on a piece of work.

Networking provides employees with additional personal and professional support. It is generally thought to enhance the professional standing of the party who is making the contact.

1 Pabari M and McMahon G (2002) Networking. *Counsel Psychother J.* **13**: 38–9.

New Deal for Communities
A Government initiative to tackle deprivation by providing intensive financial and other support to run-down areas of the UK. Its aims are to tackle poor job prospects, crime, educational under-achievement, poor health, poor physical environment and sub-standard housing.

New GP contract
Negotiations on the new GP contract began between the General Medical Council and NHS Confederation members acting on behalf of the Government in 2001. The contract was accepted in principle by the profession in mid-2002, and GPs will be voting on whether or not to implement the contract fully once it is priced and finalised in 2003. The 2002 budget was set by the Government to fund the radical changes to the NHS that it was prescribing.

The national General Medical Services contract is similar in principle to the Personal Medical Services contract. It aims to target patient needs more effectively by expanding the range of primary care offered, developing new arrangements for service delivery, improving service access for patients and introducing better clinical quality. It also aims to streamline contractual arrangements, reduce the bureaucracy involved in administering the *Red Book*, and expand practice capacity without extending the partnership. Set fees will be paid for providing certain core and specialist services, and training grants, target and item-of-service payments will be replaced by an annual payment that reflects the practice population and workload.

Written to reflect Government priorities, the aim of the contract is for general practice to be:

- run on a fixed budget

- rewarded for a quality-driven service and faster and better patient access

- developing skill mix within practices

- developing specialist GP services.

The underlying principle of the new contract is to give GPs the choice of whether to provide only core essential services (directly treating those who are ill, or who believe themselves to be ill), or whether to opt into providing a larger range of additional and enhanced clinical services. Additional services may be defined as health promotion (e.g. cervical cytology or vaccinations and immunisations). Enhanced clinical services would be adopted where practices opt to provide, for example, a specialist GP service or minor surgery.

Start-up and infrastructure costs associated with quality and outcomes will be funded. Quality markers will be tiered in three levels, with confirmation of achievement ranging from accepting level one standards (organisational quality markers) to the types of audits expected of practices that achieve National Service Framework standards at the premium level three.

In asking GPs to adopt the new contract standards, the expectation is that they will accept national clinical standards, accountability and a clinical governance structure, with the overall aim of rewarding quality, not quantity.

www.gmc-org.uk

New Opportunities Fund

The body responsible for distributing National Lottery money to health, education and environment projects in the UK.

www.nof.org.uk

NHS Act 1999

Introduced as part of the Labour Government NHS modernisation plan, this was designed as a plan for investment and reform. Some of its core principles are that the NHS would:

- continue to provide a publicly funded, universal service for all, based on clinical need

- provide comprehensive, clinically appropriate, evidence-based and cost-effective services

- be patient centred – shaped around patient need and preference

- continue to improve quality and reduce errors

- support and value its staff

- work to provide seamless care by developing partnerships with patients, their carers and their families, between health and social care, and between the voluntary sector, public and private organisations

- work with other public sector departments to reduce health inequalities

- provide open access to information about services, treatment and performance.

The Act is supported by a document, *The NHS Plan*,[1] that sets out how these object-ives are to be achieved, using ambitious targets. It introduced for the first time the idea of extending Personal Medical Services, the clinical accountability framework, and targets for improving access. It also set out a plan for changing the NHS skill mix, by developing the nurse and therapy roles so that they could take more respons-ibility for patient care and decision making. *See* **NHS Plan**.

www.modern.nhs.uk

1 Department of Health (1999) *The NHS Plan: a plan for investment, a plan for reform*. The Stationery Office, London.

NHS Alliance

An organisation which sets out to represent primary care, primary care organisations and the staff, professionals and managers working within them. The NHS Alliance aims to be an independent organisation that champions primary care trusts (and their equivalent organisations in Scotland, Wales and Northern Ireland). It advocates local empowerment and equal working relationships, equity, inclusiveness, co-operation, democracy and multi-professional working.

The NHS Alliance plays a major role in supporting and developing primary care trusts, and provides opportunities for its members to network at regular meetings and seminars. It grew out of the locality commissioning movement that set up in opposition to fundholding in the mid-1990s.

www.nhsalliance.org

NHS Appointments Commission

A body that was established in 2001 to make all chair and non-executive appoint-ments to NHS trusts, primary care trusts and health authorities. It was recently delegated the powers to appoint members to the Council for the Regulation of Health Care Professionals.

www.nhsconfed.org/nexus/welcomepack/appointments.htm

NHS Centre for Reviews

A centre that was established in 1994 to provide the NHS with information on the effectiveness of treatment and the delivery and organisation of healthcare. Its role has since been taken over by the more widely publicised National Institute for Clinical Excellence (NICE). *See* **National Institute for Clinical Excellence**.

www.york.ac.uk/inst/crd/welcome.htm

NHS Direct

A telephone helpline and website that gives access to a 24-hour nurse advice and health information service, providing confidential information on the following:

- what to do if you or members of your family are feeling ill
- specific health conditions
- local healthcare services, such as doctors, dentists or late-night-opening pharmacies
- self-help and support organisations.

Devised as one way of improving patient access, it aims to act as the first point of contact for all patient queries, especially out of hours. By 2004, NHS Direct will also be referring people directly to their local pharmacy for help (trials in Scotland are already in progress).

www.nhsdirect.NHS.uk
www.nhsdirectwales.nhs.uk/

NHS Directory

Billed as the gateway to complementary and alternative medicine for the NHS, this directory provides contact details for CAM disciplines that wish to forge closer links with GPs. It is free to all NHS professionals who wish to contact practitioners in the UK. *See* **CAMs**.

www.nhsdirectory.org

NHS History

A website that charts the history and development of the NHS from the 1920s to the 1990s.

www.hsj.co.uk/timeline/index.htm

NHS Leadership Centre

A body that was set up to develop the capabilities of leaders at all levels within the service in order to achieve improvement. Working under the umbrella of the NHS Modernisation Agency, it aims to identify and promote good leadership behaviour and to develop management skills in the NHS. It will work with both clinicians and managers. *See* **NHS University**; **Workforce development confederations**.

www.modern.nhs.uk
www.nhs.uk/modernnhs

NHS Lift

A Government scheme that was established to take up public–private equity–stake companies to overhaul GP premises. Originally set up to cover six areas, in early 2002 it was extended to a further 12 areas, despite criticism from the Commons Health Select Committee for failing to evaluate the existing schemes.

www.doh.gov.uk/pfi/nhslift.htm

NHS Litigation Agency

A special health authority which handles up to 5000 claims annually and indemnifies NHS bodies in the event of clinical negligence and non-clinical risks.

www.nhsla.com

NHS Modernisation Agency

An agency that was set up to address the modernisation requirements of the NHS. It aims to bring together healthcare improvement and leadership development in one place, to meet patient needs, and to help local clinicians and managers to meet that need. This agency encourages streamlining of services, sharing of skills, developing best practice, and national protocols and care pathway plans. The National Primary Care Development arm, whose team is headed up by Dr John Oldham, is best known for its work on advanced access.

The NHS Modernisation Agency works on issues such as clinical governance, changing workforce patterns, Beacon projects, management education and training schemes.

Update reports produced by the modernisation board can be found at www.doh. gov.uk. *See* **National Primary Care Development Team**.

www.modern.nhs.uk/

NHS National Information Authority (NHSNIA) (previously Information Management Group)

Previously known as the Information Management Group, but now renamed, this organisation is responsible for the provision of national products, standards and services to support the sharing and best possible use of information throughout the health service, via local implementation of the *Information for Health* strategy. It is in charge of NHSnet and *Information for Health*. *See* **National Electronic Library for Health**.

The NHSNIA website is www.nhsia.nhs.uk. NHS intranet users can access the site at www.avoca.co.uk

NHSnet

The secure national electronic intranet network for the NHS, enabling all parts of the service to communicate over the Internet. It is run by the NHS, to support the NHS. The aim was to have the network on every desk by December 1999, but due to technological difficulties (the original network used outdated and cumbersome X400 technology) this target was moved back to a time when the latest SMTP/broadband technology could be used. Its services include an NHS message handling service, high-speed Internet access and a national email system and electronic address book. It is hoped that every NHS employee and contractor will have their own named email address that will remain unchanged regardless of where that person works nationally. *See* **NHS National Information Authority**.

www.nhsia.nhs.uk/nhsnet/

NHS Plan

The controversial and radical plan for modernisation, investment and reform that was set out by the Government in July 2000.[1]

This 144-page document sets out new ideas for funding and investment in healthcare, and changes in relationships between clinical staff, the NHS and the private sector and social care. The five key challenges it proposed were across partnership, performance, professions and the wider NHS workforce, patient care and prevention. The aim was to make the NHS more user friendly, to improve the quality of service and minimise errors, to support and value staff, and to build a seamless service for patients. The plan discusses the ways in which this would be achieved, through additional funding and investment in staff, developing national service standards, improving clinical performance and empowering patients. A key factor was the aim of removing old-fashioned demarcations between staff, and barriers between services.

www.nhs.uk/nhsplan

1 Department of Health (1999) *The NHS Plan: a plan for investment, a plan for reform.* The Stationery Office, London.

NHSplus

A network of occupational health services based in NHS hospitals, which provides an occupational health service to NHS staff and sells services to the private sector. Services include pre-employment screening, health checks, immunisation, drug and alcohol screening, and ergonomic advice (advice on manual handling of loads, lifting and VDU operation).

www.nhsplus.nhs.uk/

NHS Purchasing and Supply Agency (PSA)

An agency that was formed in April 2000 alongside its sister organisation, the NHS Logistics Authority, to replace the NHS Supplies Authority. Its role is to act as a centre of expertise and knowledge in all purchasing and supply matters for the NHS. It contracts nationally for products and services critical to the NHS, and it buys in bulk where savings can be found.

www.pasa.doh.gov.uk/

NHS University (NHSU)

This organisation will set up a programme of learning accessible to everyone employed in health, in partnership with social services, the voluntary sector, private bodies and patient organisations, in England. The main focus is to drive forward the modernisation of the NHS, helping to deliver a patient-centred and devolved service with the emphasis on teamwork. NHSU is a national body that aims to influence policy and play a leading role in developing frameworks of national standards. It will provide support and encouragement to adults in the NHS, and will encourage interest in healthcare careers for school and university leavers.

The Government hopes eventually to accredit the NHSU with full university status.

www.doh.gov/uk/nhsuniversity

Non-verbal communication

Non-verbal signals such as gestures, touch, silence, tone of voice and delivery, which represent around 85% of communication context, and help to describe the content of the words. Facial expressions, timing and speed, body language and word choice serve to underline or undermine the verbal message. These signals tell us whether the situation is public or private, formal or informal, and serious or relaxed.

Non-verbal communication can contradict a verbal message or alter its meaning. Dress code, the apparent wealth and status reflected in the surroundings, and the use of time and space all clarify the meaning of verbal communication or increase its impact. Non-verbal signs of dominance and status are demonstrated by those who acquire or hold the largest space. A more equal, less oppressive stance is created by those who listen more than they speak, who use less discriminatory or oppressive language, and who create a less formal environment. *See* **Communication**; **Listening skills**.

Norm

A common or standard value or pattern for a given group or type. In statistics, it refers to the representative value for a group of scores.[1] *See* **Mean**; **Median**; **Mode**.

1 Samuel O, Grant J and Irvine D (1994) *Quality and Audit in General Practice: meanings and definitions.* Royal College of General Practitioners, London.

Normal distribution

The statistical term for a graphical display showing a curve which is bell-shaped and symmetrical around its *mean* (mid-point). If a significantly large number of observations or measurements is made, the distribution naturally approximates to this normal distribution. Mathematically, the distribution of means of samples taken from any population will tend towards the normal distribution as the number of samples taken increases. For example, human heights and IQ are distributed in this way.[1]

1 Robson C (1975) *Experimental Design and Statistics in Psychology*. Penguin, Harmondsworth.

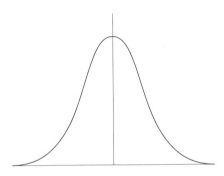

The normal distribution curve.

Normalisation policy

A policy that enables someone with a physical or mental disability to live as full a life as possible and to have access to all public services.

Not-for-profit organisation

A term that originally hailed from the USA, and which refers to a voluntary sector or charity sector organisation.

www.nonprofits.org/

Nurse prescribing

From May 2001, the Government extended independent nurse prescribing to allow more nurses to prescribe medication for a wider range of medical conditions, such as minor injuries and palliative care. Training is available to develop nurses in this way to further extend their role in general practice and the community.

www.doh.gov.uk/nurseprescribing/

Nursing home

A residential home that has qualified nursing staff available to provide nursing care for elderly people. Their work is monitored by local authority registration and inspection units. *See* **Residential home**.

www.rnha.co.uk
www.ncha.gb.com/

Objective

The *goal* is the end point (the final achievement aimed for), the *aims* are the priorities set (what the plan is) and the *objectives* specify how you will achieve those aims (how you will map the outcome).

Ideally, objectives are:

- brief

- realistic and achievable

- verifiable

- time bound (it is known when they are to be achieved)

- quantifiable (the quality can be indicated)

- quantifiable (measurable, the cost of achieving them can be prescribed)

- challenging

- easy to prioritise.

An example of criteria for good objectives is given below.

Goal:	to identify and meet the health needs of our elderly population.
Aim:	for all clinicians to update patient details at consultation.
Objectives:	1 team meeting to agree clinical coding and level of morbidity, mortality and consultation data by X
	2 to run an age/sex/diagnosis review in X
	3 X to conduct a literature review to compare our data with regional and national data held by public health.

Setting objectives involves the following steps:

- identifying priorities, costing them and staging them
- noting how success will be measured once the objective has been achieved
- noting who is responsible for achieving the objective by when: using basic 'who, why, what, where, when' headings.

Note any critical success factors, and build in a system for monitoring whether or not the objectives have been achieved. *See* **Goal setting**.

Organisational analysis and development

An applied behavioural science approach to planned change and development of an organisation.[1] It is concerned with attempts to improve the overall effectiveness and efficiency of the organisation. It looks at how organisational structure and the motivational climate (those within the organisation, their attitudes and their level of morale) can hinder achievement of its goals.[2] Organisational analysis examines how the organisation works and how its aims are defined and communicated. It aims to bring the organisation up to a level where it works optimally, thereby benefiting the employers, staff and other stakeholders (the patients, primary care organisations, trusts and allied Government bodies within the NHS).

The study of organisations is closely associated with the following:

- organisational culture
- organisational climate
- employee commitment
- organisational conflict
- change management
- management development.[3]

In order to bring about change, organisational analysis and development makes use of a number of approaches, including survey research, feedback and teambuilding. *See* **Organisations**.

1 Mumford E (1986) Helping organisations through action research: the socio-technical approach. *Qual Work Life*. **3**: 329–44.

2 Harvey DF and Brown DR (1988) *An Experiential Approach to Organisational Development* (3e). Prentice-Hall, New Jersey.

3 Mullins LJ (1999) *Management and Organisational Behaviour* (5e). Financial Times/Pitman Publishing, London.

Organisational context

The shape and size of an organisation, its position in relation to its stakeholders, and the interactions that it has with its external environment.

Organisations come in all shapes and sizes (consider the differences between a bank, a hospital, a leisure centre, a general practice and an airport). However, there are common factors. There are always two broad categories of resources:

- non-human – physical assets, materials, equipment, facilities

- human – people's abilities and skills, and their influence.

In all organisations we see the efforts and interactions of people working to achieve objectives through a structure which is directed and controlled by management. Formally, organisations operate through organisational charts, policies and procedures. Informally, they operate through personal friendships, grapevines, emotions, power games, informal relationships and leadership. The basic components of an organisation are the *operating component* (consisting of the people who actually do the work or provide the service, such as the clinical and reception team) and the *administrative component* (consisting of the managers and their team of supervisors). *See* **Organisations**.

Organisational culture

As a collection of traditions, values, policies, beliefs and attitudes that constitute a pervasive context[1] (a basic underlying assumption) for everything that is thought of and done in an organisation. All organisations are influenced by external cultural factors (e.g. language, values, religion, education, the law, economics and politics) and by internal value-driven systems (dominated perhaps by religion, conservatism or ecology).[2] In each case, authority is legitimised differently. In traditional organisations, authority is permitted by custom and by a longstanding belief in the natural right to rule. In charismatic organisations, authority is justified by a belief in the personal qualities of the leader. In bureaucratic organisations, authority is based on formal rules and impersonal principles.[3]

Some key influences on NHS culture[4]

- History – when and why the NHS was formed.

- How GPs are seen in relation to their consultant colleagues.

- The primary function of hospitals and general practice.

- The importance of reputation and the range of services provided.

- The primary goals and objectives of the NHS.

- Size and location.

continued overleaf

- Communication difficulties that present.

- Opportunities for development.

- Management influences.

- Response to change.

- Routines and rituals and the stories that are told.

- The symbols that are used.

The Government's view is that the prevailing culture within the NHS is hierarchical and patriarchal and that, in terms of work, self-interest dominates. Clinicians and managers regard power inequalities within the NHS as natural, necessary and beneficial. They attach little value to having a supportive superior, and they support a medical ascendancy model of management,[5] in which a doctor's professional autonomy and attitudes are seldom questioned by those outside the medical profession, and few doctors feel that financial or managerial decisions affect their professional practice in any meaningful way. *See* **Institutional racism; Leadership**.

1 McLean A and Marshall J (1993) *Intervening in Cultures*. Working paper. University of Bath, Bath.

2 Welford R and Prescott K (1994) *European Business: an issue-based approach* (2e). Pitman Publishing, London.

3 Weber M (1964) *The Theory of Social and Economic Organisation*. Collier Macmillan, London.

4 Mullins LJ (1999) *Management and Organisational Behaviour* (5e). Financial Times/Pitman Publishing, London.

5 May A (1998) Streets ahead on quality. *Health Service J.* **10 December**.

For more information about NHS culture and ways to work with it, see the following:

- Phillips A (2002) *The Business Planning Toolkit*. Radcliffe Medical Press, Oxford.

Organisational environment

The 'surface' influences on general practice, consisting of external influences (e.g. the Government, economic activity, scientific advances, social and cultural influences) and internal influences (e.g. patients, technology, formal goals, facilities, rules and regulations). The behavioural aspects (e.g. attitudes, personality conflicts and political behaviour) are more covert. It is the manager's role to understand and integrate the influences of their organisational environment – to co-ordinate, encourage and improve systems and individuals and to ensure that people's work needs are satisfied.[1] *See* **Organisations**.

1 Hellriegel D, Slocum JW and Woodman RW (1998) *Organizational Behaviour* (8e). Thomson Learning, London.

Organisational structure

The structure devised by management to create order, to help to establish relationships between people, and to direct the efforts of the organisation towards the goals that they have established.

The ideal organisational structure is usually hierarchical, and may look something like this:

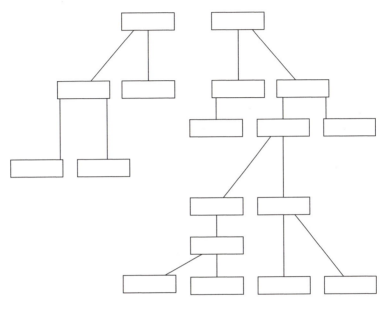

Organisational structure.

Structural problems occur when a sensible hierarchy is not followed. Inconsistent and arbitrary decisions, poor delegation and a lack of policies and procedures will lead to low morale. Poor time management and poor communication then lead to failure to make decisions or re-evaluate past decisions. Conflicting goals, cross-purposes and lack of clarity about objectives and priorities lead to conflict and poor co-ordination.[1]

1 Child J (1988) *Organisation: a guide to problems and practice* (2e). Paul Chapman, London, p. 4.

Organisation

A structure for containing the workplace and the workforce. It functions in context, so a full understanding of what an organisation is requires a broad understanding of the following:

- the organisational context (the interactions with the external environment)
- the organisational structure
- management processes

- people – and why they behave as they do, their motivations, aims and goals, and their position within a group.

Traditionally, organisations can be distinguished in terms of two generic groups, namely private enterprise and the public sector. General practice and private medicine straddle the two uncomfortably as there will always be an inherent tension between the care-taking quality and the need to make money.

Our Healthier Nation

An umbrella term for the work involving a variety of partner agencies in the pursuit of better health for the nation, namely the Department of Health, the Health Development Agency, the Local Government Associations and the National Council for Voluntary Organisations.

The White Paper entitled *Saving Lives: Our Healthier Nation* was a comprehensive Government-wide public health strategy for England, published in July 1999 with twin goals:

- to improve health

- to reduce the health gap (health inequalities).

The strategy is still current, and aims to prevent up to 300 000 untimely and unnecessary deaths by the year 2010. *Our Healthier Nation* brings together information on national priorities, Health Action Zones, NHS Beacons and current associated research. *See* **Health Action Zone**.

www.ohn.gov.uk
www.archive.official-documents.co.uk/

Outcome

The result or visible effect of an event.[1] Donabedian's definition applies more specifically to health: 'A change in the patient's current and future health status that can be attributed to antecedent health care'.[2] Donabedian adds social, psychological and functional domains to his construct of health, broadening it to include patient satisfaction, knowledge and behaviour. This illustrates how health outcome is often difficult to ascertain, as health change may be the result either of healthcare changes or of other changes such as environmental and lifestyle influences.

In clinical audit, the definition of an *outcome measure* has been refined as: 'a set of criteria which can be used to describe a health state which has been influenced by healthcare in terms of change over time'.[3]

This needs to reflect some measurable relationship to a process performed on a patient, but recognises that either a positive or a negative outcome can occur as a result of a whole range of environmental and lifestyle influences, not all of which are under clinical control.

The term *health outcome* is used to describe the result of one or more health interventions. If health change does occur as a result of clinical interventions, the validity and reliability of the change can be enhanced if the change can be duplicated, and standards can be defined.

The complexity of outcome measurements is further illustrated by Lohr, who stated that 'outcomes can be short term, long term or anything in between, and the classifications can be quite arbitrary'.[4]

A *proxy outcome* measure is one that is not definitive, but which has a valid and established (evidence-based) link with an outcome measure, so that it can provide similar information.[3] In medicine, most proxy measures are used to establish a (non-scientific) link with an outcome measure (e.g. a parent stating how much sleep a child has lost due to illness).

1 Brown L (ed.) (1993) *New Shorter Oxford English Dictionary.* Clarendon Press, Oxford.

2 Donabedian A (1980) The definition of quality: a conceptual exploration. In: *Explorations in Quality Assessment and Monitoring.* Health Administration Press, Ann Arbor, MI.

3 Samuel O, Grant J and Irvine D (eds) (1994) *Quality and Audit in General Practice. Meanings and definitions.* Royal College of General Practitioners, London.

4 Lohr KN (1988) Outcome measurement: concepts and questions. *Inquiry.* **25**: 37–50.

Out-of-area treatment (Oats)

A single episode of care relating to emergency or specialist treatments carried out in an NHS setting that is outside the patient's home health authority and that is not covered by existing service agreements. It often occurs when holidaymakers require urgent treatment. Each recorded 'Oat' results in the financial allocation to the home primary care trust being adjusted downwards, and that of the primary care trust in which the treatment is carried out being adjusted upwards.

Out of hours (OOH)

The term used for GPs providing medical cover outside normal surgery times (e.g. early morning, evening, night and weekend work). GPs will be able to opt out of OOH if they accept the terms of the new contract, and primary care trusts will be responsible for providing OOH cover. These 24-hour responsibilities are now more frequently being taken over by local GP co-operatives, Healthcall or NHS Direct.

Outpatient

A patient who attends hospital for treatment, consultation and advice, but who does not require a stay in hospital.

Outsourcing

Awarding a contract to a private, public or voluntary sector organisation to supply a service previously run by a public sector body such as a council or hospital.

Over-the-counter medicines

Medicines and medical appliances that are bought directly from the pharmacist, and are available to the public without a prescription. The Government is continually looking to extend the range of these medicines as part of their drive to improve patient access. *See* **Prescription-only medicines**.

Ownership

This is obtained once people who are undertaking a project feel that the task is both appropriate and of personal relevance.

P

PACT (Prescribing Analysis and CosTs) data

Practice reports that are sent out regularly by the Prescription Pricing Authority in Newcastle, giving an analysis of all scripts issued by GPs in England and Wales. The scripts are analysed in terms of different clinical indications and cost, and may be requested by individual GP or by type of drug.

www.npc.co.uk
For NHS web users, visit www.npc.ppa.nhs.uk

Palliative care

The physical, psychological, social and spiritual care of patients whose disease is no longer curable (e.g. those with HIV/AIDS, cancer, and some degenerative neurological disorders). Palliative care was developed by and is still largely provided by voluntary hospices, but some hospitals have specialist palliative care teams, which aim to provide the best possible quality of life for these patients.

www.hospice-spc-council.org.uk

Paperless practice

A GP practice that no longer uses paper filing systems for patient records, but which stores patient information on computers. Such practices need to ensure that patient records are available to others who are involved with the care of the same patient, and they have to store paper-based information from other parties (e.g. laboratory results). Electronic medical records (EPRs) have different characteristics to their paper-based equivalent. For example, they can be accessed simultaneously by different people, audits are easier and alert warnings are improved. However, they do also have disadvantages.

Paper records allow for considerable freedom of expression, as computer codes never reflect the breadth of normal written communication. Security is less problematic and easier to maintain. Practices that are seeking to go paperless apply to their primary care trust for approval. They need to consider a slow migration, how to construct and use interim records, and take into account factors such as accessibility, capacity and confidentiality. Simultaneous access to both paper and electronic systems will be needed for at least two years. *See* **Caldicott; Electronic medical record**.

www.nhsia/nhs.uk/

Paramedic

Ambulance paramedics in the UK are highly experienced ambulance technicians who undertake clinical training in anatomy and physiology, advanced trauma management, life-saving procedures, and the treatment of serious medical emergencies. Paramedics use a range of invasive skills and administer a wide range of drugs.

www.asa.uk.net

Parkinson's law

The maxim that 'work expands so as to fill the time available for its completion.'[1] General recognition of this principle is found in the proverb 'It's the busiest person who has time to spare.' Among other features of organisational practice that Parkinson discusses are the nature of committees and the Law of Triviality, which means that in a committee the time spent on any agenda item will be in inverse proportion to the sum involved.

1 Parkinson CN (1986) *Parkinson's Law*. Penguin, Harmondsworth.

Participative management

A leadership/management style in which people participate in and help to formulate a decision, so that they support decisions instead of fighting them, and they work hard to make it work, because it becomes their idea. The organisation thus benefits from a rich array of good information and ideas. This is now thought to be by far the best way of leading, as group discussion improves decision making, and may actually help to avert disaster. Individuals are encouraged to develop, and they contribute more to the organisation as a result. They also develop a sense of personal achievement and value. People work better and more enthusiastically when they are given a high level of freedom with regard to their contribution.

On the negative side, this style of management requires an enormous amount of time, which is often not available in the NHS. It can be inefficient if it is used inappropriately (if people are not bright or committed enough to take on board the responsibility that it releases). If it is not handled well, it can result in a complete loss of managerial control. *See* **Leadership**.

Partnership

Working with and alongside others. The Government aim, outlined in the 1999 NHS Plan, is for the NHS to work *strategically* in partnership with social care, education, transport and the voluntary sector to reduce health inequalities, and for GPs to work *operationally* in partnership with other healthcare colleagues in the wider primary care and secondary care team (e.g. social workers, therapists and consultants), in order to achieve a seamless standard of care for patients.

Partnership agreement

A partnership deed which details agreed general practice administrative and financial arrangements, such as holiday entitlement, sick pay allowances, voting arrangements and permitted periods of notice. It is sensible for all non-salaried GPs (both Personal Medical Services and General Medical Services partnerships) to have a partnership deed, which usually also covers the following:

1 financial aspects:

   • partnership assets – including property investments, equipment, sale of good-will

   • tax – needs to refer to the current tax regime and include reference to reserve accounts and the nominated partner

   • income and expenditure – allocation of allowances, profit shares, including ownership expenses, golden hellos and goodbyes, primary care trust work, out of hours, locums, Medical Defence Union cover, absence from the practice allowances

2 leave – references to maternity, paternity, adoption, sabbatical or compassionate leave

3 retirement issues – flexibility, suspension, notice periods, resignation from medical list

4 Personal Medical Services contract – restrictions and breaches and withdrawal notices

5 any restrictive covenants.

The British Medical Association and the General Medical Council both give detailed guidance on partnership agreements, and supporting advice can be obtained from Local Medical Councils. GPs should also obtain independent legal and accountancy advice. It is important that the agreement or deed is current and valid.

Patient Advocacy and Liaison Service (PALS)

A service designed to help the public to air concerns about their treatment, care and support. It was set up after the dissolution of local Community Health Councils. PALS has direct access to trusts' chief executives, as well as strong negotiating powers. Their aim is for staff to be available to patients, carers and their families to help to resolve complaints and concerns quickly. *The NHS Plan* announced the commitment to establish PALS in every trust by 2002. The first wave of PALS 'Pathfinder' sites became operational in April 2001.

The aims of PALS will vary in different localities, but include the need:

- for patients to have their concerns dealt with in a conciliatory manner

- to liaise with local primary care trusts with regard to PALs activity, gaps in services and any training needs

- to inform local people about the NHS, and to refer them on to specialist advocacy services if necessary.

PALS is central to the new system of patient and public involvement. It does not replace the existing specialist advocacy services, such as mental health and learning disability advocacy, but will be complementary to these services. *See* **Commission for Patient and Public Involvement in Health**; **Patient participation**.

www.doh.gov.uk/patientadviceandliasonservice/index.htm

Patient empowerment

A self-management approach for patients with chronic diseases, which research has shown gives rise to improvements in health outcomes with a consequent reduction in demand on the health service. For example, the *Heart Manual*, which was developed by the British Heart Foundation Rehabilitation Research Unit at the University of York, reaches about 5000 patients in the UK each year. It has been proved to be clinically effective in demonstrating improved psychological adjustment, fewer visits to GPs and a significant reduction in rates of readmission to hospital in the first six months following a heart attack. Empowering patients with chronic illnesses to undertake increased monitoring of their condition has been shown to lead to reduced severity of symptoms, a significant decrease in pain, improved life control and activity and increased life satisfaction. *See* **Doctor–patient partnership**; **Expert Patient Project**.

Patient Group Directives

Documents written to enable certain non-medical professional groups, such as nurses and pharmacists, to prescribe named medicines to particular and identified patient groups. They are used in cases where the presence in the population of a particular illnesses or condition significantly increases the workload of GPs (e.g. an influenza epidemic, increased demand for anti-smoking medication or the morning-after pill). The aim is to improve patient access, assist GPs with workload reduction, and enable allied professionals to take on some of the clinical responsibilities for patients.

Such directives stipulate the following:

- under what circumstances and criteria action will occur

- which staff group it will be applied to

- whether there is a need to apply additional local guidelines

- training requirements

- communication arrangements (e.g. when and how the responsible GP will be informed, and who will be copied in)

- consultation arrangements.

www.npc.co.uk
For NHS web users, visit www.npc.ppa.nhs.uk

Patient participation

An umbrella term for the various methods of involving 'service users' (patients) in discussions about healthcare provision, the aim being that they can constructively contribute to local difficult or unpalatable rationing decisions. Primary care contributes to this process by developing projects such as the following:

- patient voice projects (discussion/focus groups)

- patient participation groups

- informal feedback systems (e.g. suggestions boxes)

- health panels

- citizens' juries

- open meetings

- rapid appraisal (gathering information from key local informants)

- disease support groups

- interviews

- opinion polls

- neighbourhood forums

- public consultation exercises (involving patients in a particular service development)

- practice-based annual surveys

- appraisal systems (e.g. customer panels)

- postal questionnaires.

Patient participation works on the premise that patients know their experience of illness better than anyone else. If patients feel empowered, they will develop more choice and are more likely to take control of their own illnesses. They also learn and so become better informed and less passively dependent on the NHS. By participating in the discussion, patients become better educated and develop a broader understanding of public health issues and the patterns of health and disease. *See* **Patient Advocacy and Liaison Service; Patient survey; Patients' forum; Survey**.

For some more ideas and a broader understanding of such methods, see the following:

- Lilley R (2000) *The PCG Toolkit*. Radcliffe Medical Press, Oxford.

Patient prospectus
An A4-size fold-out leaflet produced by primary care trusts and sent to every household annually. These prospectuses are designed to provide information on the availability and quality of local health services. They also contain feedback from patients, and set out the top priorities for trusts in response to those views.

www.doh.gov.uk/patientprospectus

Patient survey
A survey that is either locally or nationally constructed, and which measures the following:

- access
- availability
- interpersonal care
- continuity of care
- trust
- referral
- co-ordination of care outside a practice.

The best patient surveys ensure that all questions are relevant, unambiguous, simple, flow in a logical order in a language that the studied population understands, and give simple choices of response. They do not make assumptions, ask leading or biased questions, use complex, inappropriate or offensive language, or assume that all answers will be honest. The sample size is important, as is the relevance of the sample population. It is useful to invest in specialist help when constructing a patient survey. *See* **Patient participation; Survey**.

www.npdt.org/

Patient transport service (PTS)

A service that transports patients with non-urgent conditions to and from a range of treatment settings, including outpatients, disablement service centres, routine discharges and admissions, geriatric and psychogeriatric day care, and non-urgent inter-hospital transfers. It is staffed by ambulance care assistants, who are trained in first aid, driving skills, and lifting and handling techniques.

www.asa.uk.net

Patient's unmet needs (PUNs)

Looking at the patient's unmet needs (PUNs) is one way in which clinicians can identify their own learning needs. If patient needs are not met, this may be due to a deficiency in the clinician's knowledge or skill – thus identifying the doctor's unmet needs (DUNs). PUNs can be identified by transcribing and analysing difficult and unsatisfactory consultations, and identifying where and at what point the communication between doctor and patient broke down. *See* **Learning needs**.

Patients' Forum

Every healthcare trust has a patient forum. Their aim is to monitor and review services and to influence and inform decision making. Forum members elect one of their number as a Non-Executive Director of the Trust Board.

Pay-and-reward system (performance-related pay)

The system by which staff are paid. Pay-and-reward systems may be traditional (salaries with automatic incremental pay rises), or more flexible (with a single spine scale and rewards for job development, responsibilities and initiative, rather than for age and seniority).

Any intrinsic (value-based) non-pay awards are best demonstrated by allowing individuals to use their creativity and control, allowing them to build their own jobs (job enrichment), and recognising each individual's orientation to work. Extrinsic rewards, which are measured more formally, can be demonstrated in additional holiday for long-term service, training, etc. Such flexible pay enhancements develop initiatives outside the constraints of the common pay scales. They are based on identified service needs and reflect the local position.

Pay-and-reward systems should offer terms that recruit, retain and motivate appropriately skilled staff, and which offer reasonable internal pay relativities. They should be seen as long-term pay strategies which take into account the informed view of staff as well as managers.

Pay review

This is a review of all the pay elements of a job and includes:

• a statistical analysis of the workforce

- gathering information on all elements of pay

- determining which jobs involve equal work, i.e. are same work or work of equal value

- a comparison of all elements of pay for the men and women doing equal work

- determining whether any differences identified are based on sex and whether they can be objectively justified.

In small organisations such as general practice it may not be practicable to implement all the detailed provisions of an equal pay review. The Equal Opportunities Commission (EOC) is in the process of producing tailored advice on equal pay reviews for the small business sector which is due to be launched in mid-2003. *See* **Equal Pay Act 1990**.

www.eoc.org.uk/

Pay review body (PRB)
Any of the independent panels that take evidence annually from the Department of Health and staff unions before making a recommendation on remuneration to the Secretary of State for Health, who (usually) accepts and authorises the recommended pay rise. There are two panels – one covering doctors and dentists and the other covering nursing staff, midwives, health visitors and professions allied to medicine. Pay review bodies are currently being phased out.

www.doh.gov.uk/reviewbodies/

Payroll giving
A method of giving to charity through an employee's pay packet. Donations come straight from the employee's gross pay before tax, effectively making the donation cheaper for the person donating. Until April 2003, the Government promised to add 10% to all payroll donations.

www.inlandrevenue.gov.uk/payrollgiving/

Primary Care Data Quality (PCDQ) programme
This project, supported by the NHS National Information Authority, was commissioned in recognition of the problems that GP practices have with data management. Its MIQUEST software allows extracted data to be standardised, anonymised and pooled from a variety of proprietary GP systems.

The PCDQ programme provides a mechanism for capturing the quality data required to support clinical governance and the National Service Frameworks. Using a set of queries written by this system, and following a data collection plan, GP practices are able to build their own disease registers and monitor their patients' treatment. The programme has been devised to highlight the importance of good-quality data input and management. See **MIQUEST**; **PRIMIS**.

www.nelh-pc.nhs.uk
For those on the NHSnet, visit http://nww.nelh-pc.nhs.uk

Peer appraisal
See **Appraisal**.

Peer review
The consideration or appraisal of performance by colleagues within the same profession, or by another group with comparable skills and experience. Changes in behaviour have been found to be greatest among those who were in most disagreement at the outset of the peer-review process.[1]

1 Grol R (1990) Peer review in primary care. *Qual Assurance Healthcare*. **2**: 119–26.

Performance assessment framework
There are six components of the National Service Framework (NSF) performance assessment framework, namely health improvement, fair access, efficiency, effective delivery of appropriate care, user/carer experience and health outcomes.

National Service Frameworks establish models of treatment and care based on evidence of best practice. They look for uniformity of treatment to a minimum standard, and for consistency across major care areas. They provide a treatment framework for a particular disorder or group of diseases, and aim to address the following:

- healthcare improvements

- inequalities of access

- differences in outlook

- differences in outcome

- differences in quality of care

- postcode rationing.

See **National Service Framework**.

Performance indicator
A predictor of overall performance. In general practice, the term is used interchangeably with 'medical audit standard'. The Government, health authorities and primary care organisations have developed performance indicators:

- as a measuring aid

- to inform the clinical governance agenda

- to support them in dealing with patient complaints as part of their risk management procedure.

There are performance indicators in place as administrative audits (failure to apply for Postgraduate Educational Allowance, comparisons of item-of-service payments, complaints, patient removal requests) and also clinical indicators (e.g. in prescribing, or standards of medical record summaries). *See* **Audit**; **Standards**.

Performance management

The underlying principle of this style of management is to support and reward well-performing individuals and effective systems by using priority setting, targets, timescales and outcome measurements.

There is an opposing argument that performance and outcomes are notoriously difficult to measure, as the number of variables makes objective measurement impossible, and the review becomes too subjective. *See* **Performance review**.

Performance-related pay

A method of salary enhancement that is related to an individual's performance in the job. It is now rarely used as it is generally thought to be demotivating and unfair. Any intrinsic (value-based, non-pay) rewards are best demonstrated by enabling individuals to use their creativity and control, allowing them to build their own jobs (job enrichment), and recognising each individual's orientation with regard to work. *See* **Pay-and-reward system**.

Performance review

Continuous performance monitoring undertaken as part of the management cycle to ensure that effective practice is maintained. In audit, it refers to activity concerned with data collection and analysis, and applying the information to introduce change. In management, it refers to the appraisal of an employee's work. In both instances the audit cycle is followed, where performance is measured and compared with a pre-ordained standard, the aim being to bring the performance closer to the standard.[1]

1 Horder J, Mourin K, Pendleton D *et al*. (1986) Terminology of performance review. In: D Pendleton, T Schofield and M Marinkar (eds) *In Pursuit of Quality: approaches to performance review in general practice.* Royal College of General Practitioners, London.

Personal development plan (PDP)

A personal, confidential folder that describes a learning plan set out over a short period of time. For clinicians, it should contain descriptions and demonstrations of the following:

- current practice

- chosen fields of work or specialties, and time approportioned to this
- continuing educational and professional development
- good clinical care, good relationships with patients and colleagues
- audit results
- appraisal
- any complaints or plaudits
- any significant events (including critical incidents)
- criminal convictions or disciplinary hearings
- any breaks in registration
- any conditions set, erasure or suspensions.

PDPs aim to address not just academic but also operational competence. They will eventually replace the Postgraduate Educational Allowance mechanism. It is expected that GPs will make any learning and recording integral to their working day. Practices will be expected to provide a multidisciplinary training and development plan as part of the core practice professional development plan (PPDP).

A PDP should reflect the culture of a GP's working environment as well as the skills and knowledge relating to their post. It should:

- identify noted weaknesses in knowledge, skills and attitudes
- identify what has been learned from mistakes, and how
- note changes in role or responsibilities which create new learning opportunities
- prioritise learning needs and set outcomes
- set goals and describe how these will be achieved over a set period of time
- justify the selection of these goals
- describe the plan to evaluate outcomes.

See **Competence assessment scheme; Learning plan; Practice professional development plan; Revalidation.**

Personality

Personality differences can be a source of great strength and creativity, or of conflict. People and organisations each have their own personality. Personalities differ from each other in terms of the following:

- attitudes
- values

- beliefs

- culture.

People also demonstrate a whole range of abilities and talents (musical, interpersonal and communication skills, self-knowledge skills, spatial ability, sports achievements, artistic and creative abilities), all of which combine to make up what we call personality. Personality is influenced by early developmental experiences (social, family and cultural) as well as by adult experiences. *See* **Belbin RM; Group; Myers–Briggs Type indicator.**

Personnel management
The short-term, operational level of people management, involving the direction and control of people through policies and procedures (induction, disciplinary procedures, interview, etc.).

It is a simplistic model of people management which seeks to direct and control, and unless human resource management principles are applied, it tends to view people as dispensable assets.

Personnel management is concerned with first-line staff management; a more complex system is employed by human resource managers. Personnel managers are responsible for the following:

- human resource planning and employment

- payroll administration, including related rewards (e.g. holiday and maternity pay)

- organisational design

- management of work patterns

- observing current and future employment legislation and legal requirements

- training and development

- staff relations, services, welfare and safety.

This will involve the organisational development of the following:

- job descriptions

- contracts of employment

- disciplinary procedures

- grievance procedures

- annual appraisals

- training and development policies

- additional services (e.g. pensions, occupational health or counselling schemes for staff).

See **Human resource management**.

PEST analysis (political, economic, sociocultural and technological analysis)
A popular technique for analysing the general environment, which looks at the potential (future) impact of political and other variables on an organisation (e.g. legislation, demographic changes, shifts in values and culture, State investment and technological developments).

Peter principle
In the study of occupational incompetence and hierarchies, this refers to the situation where competent employees tend to be promoted until a position of incompetence is reached. The analysis of hundreds of cases of incompetence led to the formulation of the principle that 'in a hierarchy every employee tends to rise to their level of incompetence.'[1]

1 Peter LJ and Hull R (1970) *The Peter Principle*. Pan Books, London.

Planning cycle
A cycle that involves the following steps:

- identifying the problem
- collecting the data to quantify the problem
- analysing the problem
- organising and co-ordinating a plan of action
- implementing the plan
- reviewing
- monitoring.

Planning involves objectivity, realism, flexibility, logical thinking and wide communication. It needs everyone's involvement through delegation and team work. The process of planning enables the individual or organisation to evaluate and clarify some of the wider issues facing it, and it helps to formulate goals and identify the resources and action necessary to achieve those goals. Planners work methodically using a variety of methods, such as audit, mapping or charts (which map the goals graphically on the vertical axis, and show the timescale on the horizontal axis), to set out the plan of action.

PMR

A commonly used abbreviation for a personal medical record.

Personal Medical Services (PMS)

Introduced via the NHS (Primary Care) Act 1997, Personal Medical Services allow primary care providers such as GPs, nurses and community trusts to test different ways of delivering services. For GPs, PMS contracts replace the standard national GP contract, and doctors are paid according to performance against targets based on meeting local health needs. PMS also allow GPs (who have traditionally been self-employed) to work on a salaried basis as employees of the local NHS authority.

The PMS contract was developed following Government surveys in the late 1990s which showed that the traditional model of independent contractor status, with its financial and managerial responsibilities, together with the 24-hour responsibility for patient care, was a major contributor to stress and a significant barrier to GP recruitment. The PMS contract is designed to be more flexible than the GMS contract. It is being sold as suitable for anyone wishing to:

- target more precisely the needs of a particular group of patients

- expand the range of primary care offered

- develop new arrangements/organisations for the delivery of services

- provide more flexible employment options for GPs

- give other primary care professionals greater career scope and opportunities

- expand practice capacity without extending the partnership

- streamline their contractual arrangements

- develop better human resource management systems

- develop enhanced financial management and accountability frameworks

- improve service access for their patients

- reduce the bureaucracy involved in administering the *Red Book*

- address local recruitment and retention problems

- improve the equity of GMS resource allocation.

The Government envisaged GPs benefiting from flexible working patterns, a steady cash flow, a reduction in bureaucracy, and being able to negotiate their own salary and terms of service.

A PMS contract can be formed from the following:

- a single practice

- a group of practices

- a whole primary care group.

PMS contracts may be either:

- *PMS*: provision of those services which patients could normally be expected to receive from any GP (e.g. General Medical Services)
- *PMS-PLUS*: provision of a wider range of services over and above that normally provided as General Medical Services, such as non-core services or elements of hospital and community health services.

The principles of PMS can be summarised as follows.

- they reward quality, not quantity
- they adopt accepted national clinical standards
- they account for local Health Improvement Programmes
- they accept a clinical governance structure
- they aim to empower local services to change
- they should be developed in partnership with all stakeholders
- they should ensure seamless and integrated care.

PMS contracts set minimum standards around accessibility, staffing, clinical governance and accountability. Practices with a large list size may be reluctant to increase partnership size, but PMS flexibility allows practices to receive growth monies not taken up for extra partners to develop salaried doctor and nurse practitioner posts, thus increasing career opportunities and satisfaction. PMS contracts also allow for the development of outreach work with other agencies. Community nurses can be employed directly, giving a return of flexibility for local innovation.

PMS-PLUS schemes will bring further benefits to patients as services transfer from secondary care, and improve the equity of GMS resource usage (e.g. by improving services to deprived areas).[1] *See* **Primary care**.

www.doh.gov.uk/pricare/pca
www.bma.org.uk
www.nhsalliance.org

1 NHS Executive (2000) *Personal Medical Services Pilots Under the NHS (Primary Care) Act 1997: a comprehensive guide* (3e). NHS Executive, Leeds.

Population

In healthcare, this term is often used to describe an entire group of people, objects or events (e.g. all of the asthmatic patients in a practice, or all of the nurse referrals undertaken in a year).

Postcode lottery

The term used to describe the inequalities in care that can be found in different parts of the UK, due to different resource priorities. As with local Government allocation, the Government allocates resources using different measures of deprivation, weighted capitation, etc. These resources are distributed at a local level according to a mix of local and national priorities, which may differ from one county to the next.

Postgraduate Educational Allowance (PGEA)

An annual allowance that is paid to GPs who undertake to attend a certain number of training events each year, to include a range of both clinical and management topics. PGEA approval is sought and obtained from the local GP regional training office prior to such an event being organised. The PGEA scheme will eventually be replaced by another funding source under the terms of the new contract and revalidation. *See* **Fees and allowances; Revalidation**.

Post Registration Education and Practice (PREP)

A continuing education programme for nurses that is an essential element of maintaining registration on the UKCC central register. It became mandatory under law in 1995. The standards are not dissimilar to those of the current *continuing medical education* and the new revalidation proposals. The core aim is to drive up nursing standards, and the programme includes details of registration renewals, breaks in service, standards for professional development and a *personal professional profile* (*PPP*), similar to a personal development plan. There is a UKCC recommendation that all nurses in practice should be supported or mentored by colleagues, and that time should be set aside to allow reflection on practice.[1] *See* **Revalidation**.

1 Richardson A (1998) Personal professional profiles. *Nurs Standard.* **12**: 35–40.

Practice activity analysis

The recording and analysis of common data held in general practices, so that doctors and managers can compare individual or group performance and activity with pooled data from other practices. Such analyses are usually undertaken within or between practices.

Practice allowance

An allowance that forms part of the payments made to non-Personal Medical Services GPs for General Medical Services. The allowances are graded according to the number of patients on the list (basic practice allowance), a designated area allowance, seniority payments, and an initial practice allowance for newly qualified doctors. There is also a GP assistant or associate allowance. Other allowances are given for having locums, agreeing to attend postgraduate educational sessions (Postgraduate Educational Allowance) and providing an out-of hours service. *See* **Fees and allowances**.

Practice manager

A manager who is employed by the GPs within a practice, and whose role is to manage the business and the GPs themselves. As general practice is run as a small business, and the main bulk of the income is from contracted NHS work, this may involve all of the following:

- *financial management*: cashflow forecasting, managing debt, partnership tax, simple book-keeping (practice accounts up to trial balance level), budgetary controls, costs and pricing, long-term planning

- *information and technology*: IT and presentation skills, knowledge of spreadsheets and data analysis packages, using IT for audit and research

- *estates and premises management*

- *product management*: stock control, production control, measuring systems

- *selling and marketing*: customer relations, prospecting, promoting the business.

The practice manager's role has changed considerably over the years, and the NHS now demands very highly developed management skills from its managers. The most frequently encountered problem in general practice is that employing doctors in the past often underestimated the level of management skill required. It is still not unusual to find managers appointed from within the business who were previously receptionists with very good organisational and interpersonal skills, but no experience of business planning or organisational analysis and strategy.

A practice manager needs to have excellent interpersonal skills, a high level of self-awareness, and an ability to research and analyse. Increasingly, practice managers are found to be more actively involved in strategic and clinical management (planning, monitoring and advising the partnership on clinical governance, systems management, alternative clinical management paths and business development).

The key tasks of the practice manager are as follows:

- understanding, supporting and maintaining the practice ethos

- representing the practice to all professional and public bodies

- facilitating consensus between partners, enabling decisions and ensuring that they are acted upon

- supporting the interests of all groups within the practice

- communicating effectively by means of writing, reading and presentation

- being responsible for day-to-day decisions

- meetings – preparing, chairing and achieving results

- consultation – using internal and external resources

- negotiation – formal and internal bargaining

- developing people – selection, planning succession, training and developing staff, appraisal, counselling, promotion and managing conflict

- managing teams – understanding psychology, motivation and organisational culture

- managing change

- people management – dealing with stress, planning and using time, investing in and supporting staff

- taking control – managing the bosses, managing problems, decision making

- co-ordinating, implementing and monitoring within the practice.

Practice professional development plan (PPDP)

A business plan that practices are required to produce which includes the individual practice personal development plans (PDPs), and the business, clinical and development aims and objectives for the next few years. Practice professional development plans enable personal development plans and learning needs to be linked to outcomes.

The document that is produced, the exact content of which is defined by the local primary care organisation, feeds into the local workforce planning document (the Health Improvement Programme). PPDPs are normally produced annually, and may also contain the relevant appraisals and revalidation documents for all staff. *See* **Business plan**; **Personal development plan**.

Premises improvements

GP premises can be improved using a variety of funding schemes, including improvement grants, cost rent schemes, personal finance initiatives (PFIs) using independent developers, or Local Improvement Finance Trusts. *See* **Local Improvement Finance Trusts**.

Prescribing formulary

A formulary that sets out the recommended drug type and dose for commonly presenting clinical problems. It may be devised at either practice or locality level, following discussion with its intended users and local pharmaceutical colleagues and prescribing advisers. The discussion will focus on dosage, cost, volume, efficacy, palatability, adverse reactions and side-effects, as well as patient compliance, concordance and convenience. The following issues will also be considered:

- drug licensing

- controlled drugs and drug dependence

- setting sensible targets to achieve change

- areas where patient education can achieve change

- the evidence base

- secondary care initiatives

- circumstances where variations can be explained by repeat prescribing cycles.

A formulary is devised following discussion of current 'best practice', which may include recommendations about doctor compliance, using better tolerated, cheaper or more effective drug dosages or volumes, as well as successful best management systems (e.g. when to review opportunistically, who to alert if exceptionally high spends are expected). Also included in the discussion would be a system of review to accommodate emerging new drugs.

www.npc.co.uk
For NHS web users, visit www.npc.ppa.nhs.uk

Prescribing incentive schemes

Schemes that are run by primary care organisations in order to assist General Medical Service-contracted GPs who are unhappy about spending time and money on what they consider to be initiatives that benefit neither the patient nor themselves. Prescribing incentive schemes aim to give these GPs the financial (and clinical) incentive to effect change in their prescribing habits, the idea being that any money saved through cost-effective and efficient prescribing outweighs that allocated to achieve the target.

Incentives vary across the country, but may include any of the following:

- targeting high-spending practices by using visiting pharmacy advisers, specialist GPs, local community pharmacists or facilitators who can assist with analysis of prescribing patterns

- managed care solutions, where pharmacists link with practices to change select drug groups

- encouraging GPs to use an IT solution – a system which analyses individual and collective prescribing patterns and encourages a formulary approach

- naming and shaming – the use of practice-identifiable league-tables that give information on local and individual prescribing rates and costs

- production of a local formulary

- making Brown Bag reviews one of the qualifying arms of the scheme

- providing regular education events

- increasing the distribution of patient education leaflets to practices

- finding out which drug companies are willing to sponsor product change.

See **Prescribing indicators and targets**.

www.npc.co.uk
For NHS web users, visit www.npc.ppa.nhs.uk

Prescribing indicators and targets

The NHS supports GP practices that wish to reduce prescribing costs, and to further this aim, primary care organisations have set up prescribing indicators using national recommendations. The indicators usually fall into specific, commonly used drug groups (e.g. antibiotics, hypnotics, antifungals, anti-inflammatories), or generic versus brand use. The targets will take into account specific local issues that affect prescribing costs adversely, as well as the effects of new staff or systems destabilising the use of the formulary. For example, the following factors are considered:

- the instigatation of nurse prescribing

- whether the practice population is stable or transient

- high-cost patient groups

- high levels of hospital-initiated prescribing

- an unusual environment that creates additional or associated clinical costs.

See **Prescribing incentive schemes**.

www.npc.co.uk
For NHS web users, visit www.npc.ppa.nhs.uk

Prescribing protocols

Locally agreed protocols that include information about the clinical or management systems needed to reduce prescribing risk. Within this, educational standards are set for clinicians and staff, and agreements are made concerning who prescribes what, where and why, with the aim of achieving consistency. With the aim of reducing clinical and administrative risk, administrative standards may also be set, defining the following:

- patient access

- systems for preventing fraud

- systems for ensuring secure storage

- standards set for the time period between receipt and production of scripts

- time limits for prescription collection, if scripts are available by email or telephone, or if patients can obtain them without being seen

- the use of educational leaflets and posters on reducing drug use

- agreements for signatures, counter-signatures, additions or corrections
- type and frequency of updating of records.

See **Prescribing formulary**.

www.npc.co.uk
For NHS web users, visit www.npc.ppa.nhs.uk

Prescribing strategy

Local health organisations have such strategies, which include the use of prescribing indicators, formularies, protocols, prescribing targets and patient directives. Prescribing strategies are produced after discussion and agreement with local stakeholders. The main issue for GPs is usually target setting – the main hinge for this is the prescribing incentive scheme.

www.npc.co.uk
For NHS web users, visit www.npc.ppa.nhs.uk

Prescription-only medicines (POMs)

Medication that is available by prescription only. *See* **Over-the-counter medicines**.

Prescription Pricing Authority (PPA)

An organisation that sends out monthly, quarterly or annual reports which analyse doctors' prescribing habits. Doctors can request a particular level of analysis, level one being the first, simple level, and level three being the most complex. By means of such analyses, doctors can monitor their own and their partners' prescribing habits and costs, and see whether their particular prescribing pattern matches that of the locality, or whether it deviates from the national norm. The PPA is particularly concerned with highlighting the use of high-cost or high-use drug groups. PACT data shows the doses prescribed as well as the number, type and cost of drugs. Analysis of their PPA reports by a partnership forms part of the wider prescribing formulary discussion.

www.npc.ppa.nhs.uk

Presentation skills

The mainly one-way communication skills that are required for presenting. Presenters need to have a prior understanding of their audience, what they are expecting from the presentation, and their prior knowledge of the subject. They will ascertain the purpose of the presentation (e.g. whether they are aiming to inform or persuade). A good presentation will:

- have a preface outlining its topic, purpose, duration and shape

- introduce the speaker, seeking common ground with the audience
- give a brief outline of the present situation, why there is a need for change, etc.
- look at the main alternatives that the audience will want to consider
- summarise the facts/arguments
- propose a recommended course of action
- admit the limitations of any proposals, and then make persuasive points about them
- invite questions.

See **Facilitation**.

For more information on presentation, including advice on techniques and how to deal with difficult audiences, see the following:

- Phillips A (2002) *Communication and the Manager's Job.* Radcliffe Medical Press, Oxford.

Primary care

Services provided by family doctors, dentists, nurses, midwives, health visitors, pharmacists, optometrists and ophthalmic medical practitioners, as well as other community staff such as community physiotherapists, speech and language therapists, and occupational therapists. See **Primary care trust**.

www.doh.gov.uk/pricare/index.htm

Primary Care Division of the National Health Executive (NHE)

The body that works on all the main elements of the Government's modernisation programme for primary and community care.

www.doh.gov.uk/pricare/index.htm

Primary care group (PCG)

Forerunner of the primary care trust, any of the voluntary GP-led groups that have a range of duties, from advising the local health authority on commissioning care for their local population to commissioning care themselves. All primary care groups are expected to become primary care trusts by April 2004. See **Primary care**; **Primary care trust**.

Primary care organisation (PCO)

The generic term for primary care groups and primary care trusts. Some primary care groups will be in place until April 2004, when they will become trusts responsible for all of the operational functions of the health authorities that they replace. See **Strategic health authority**.

Primary care trust (PCT)

Evolved from primary care groups, PCTs are free-standing statutory bodies that provide primary and community services to their local population. They co-ordinate and manage the work of family doctors and community nursing and therapy services. PCTs will have responsibility for 75% of the entire commissioning budget for healthcare from April 2003, to enable them to commission secondary (hospital) care on behalf of their local population. *See* **Primary care group**.

www.doh.gov.uk/pricare/pcts

Prime service provider (PSP)

Following the publication in 2002 of the Government's IT strategy outlined in the document *Delivering Twenty-First Century IT: support for the NHS*, prime service providers are the companies that will be selected to provide the new NHS computer systems. *See* **Computing in healthcare; Electronic medical record; Electronic staff record**.

PRIMIS (Primary Care Information Services)

A scheme that aims to help practices to improve patient care by making more effective use of their clinical support systems. PRIMIS is supported by the NHS National Information Authority, and schemes are currently being set up nationwide, with the aid of local facilitators, as part of the NHS modernisation programme.

PRIMIS aims to assist practices and their primary care organisations in making constructive use of their data for audit, governance, and planning and commissioning purposes. PRIMIS facilitators assist with training, data analysis and interpretation, the idea being that consistent and complete recording of clinical data supports:

- improved patient care
- easier prevention and health promotion
- better follow-up
- more effective multidisciplinary care
- better chronic disease management
- improved practice organisation
- easier data extraction and manipulation.

In order to implement PRIMIS, the facilitator supports and trains practices in the following:

- information management skills
- Read codes

- system functionality

- confidentiality and data protection queries

- the use of MIQUEST data extraction tools.

See **NHS Modernisation Programme**; **NHS National Information Authority**.

www.primis.nhs.uk
www.primis.nottingham.ac.uk

Priority despatch

A system of telephone triage used by ambulance services to ensure that the most urgent emergency calls, such as heart attacks, receive priority treatment. The system enables the call taker in the ambulance service control room to classify the telephone request into one of three categories – A (life-threatening), B (serious but not life-threatening) or C (minor emergencies).

Traditionally, all 999 calls are answered immediately by sending an ambulance with paramedic crew. If they were used to full capability, these despatch criteria would allow the service to delay sending an ambulance to category C calls, or to refer the caller to another agency, such as NHS Direct. *See* **Paramedic**.

www.doh.gov.uk/emergencycare/index.htm

Private finance initiative (PFI)

A public/private initiative whereby primary care premises are developed using independent (private) developers. It is a method of providing new public buildings and projects, such as schools, hospitals, roads and homes, by using private sector money up front that is later repaid with interest by the State. Under rules for the initiative introduced in 1992, a private sector consortium designs, builds, finances and operates the new building or project for a period of at least 25 years. The consortium will be regularly paid from public money depending on its performance throughout that period. *See* **Premises improvements**.

www.centre.public.org.uk/briefings/

Proactive management

The use of planning ahead (being proactive) as a management device to aid clarity and vision in the following:

- time management

- personal organisation

- organisational development.

In contrast, reactive management is crisis ridden. The reactive person responds to influences or a crisis, but does not plan ahead to manage the risk of such an event occurring.

Procurement
The process of buying in goods or services from an external provider. It covers everything from determining the need for new goods to buying, delivering and storing them.

Prodigy (Prescribing Rationally with Decision Support in General Practice)
A computer-guided decision-making tool for GPs. It is a decision support system designed to run alongside a practice clinical computer system, now under the auspices of the National Institute for Clinical Excellence (NICE), that is intended to provide GPs with peer-reviewed, evidenced-based prescribing guidelines for around 200 commonly occurring conditions. It integrates with the patient electronic record, and can thus check for contraindications and drug interactions. It includes patient–doctor shared-decision screens, patient advice leaflets and reference sources for information on the following:

- non-drug treatments

- epidemiology

- definition of the condition

- complications

- references in the literature.

Information is provided for guidance only, and drug choices are made primarily on the basis of efficacy, safety and their side-effect profile.

www.npc.co.uk
For NHS web users, visit www.npc.ppa.nhs.uk

Professions supplementary to medicine (PSM)
See **Allied health professional; Health Professions**.

Provider
A body that provides health or social care under contract arrangements with a purchasing body.

Person specification
See **Job specification**.

Postcode lottery
The term that is applied when each NHS commissioning organisation defines which treatments are available to whom under which circumstances. In order to address this, the Government has funded National Service Frameworks, the National Institute for Clinical Excellence, the Commission for Health Improvement, NHSnet and the National Electronic Library for Health, with the aim of standardising the type and level of care available to the public. When each individual organisation defines its own treatments, the situation leads to a 'postcode lottery' of prescribing and care.

Between them, the above organisations provide a framework that evaluates the levels and types of clinical care available, and they make recommendations on the best outcome-based treatments that are currently available. Supporting management teams within the commissioning organisation involve clinicians in applying the principles set by the Government, assisting them in defining their own commissioning needs and solutions in relation to those set by the Government. *See* **Commissioning**.

Professional Executive Committee (PEC)
The formal means by which GPs and nurses have a say in their primary care trust.

Professionalism: a code of practice for doctors
Working to a common set of standards of good practice that have been set by a professional body. Doctors are being asked to adopt and respect new professional values which encourage professional development, such as the following:

- working well with others, and embracing teamworking

- adopting a certain level of qualification and service quality

- self-regulation

- aspiring to have a standard of behaviour that is based on a complex body of knowledge

- viewing the doctor–patient relationship as more of a partnership

- accepting public accountability

- being business-like – being highly organised and performing well

- constantly reviewing and reflecting on work

- having a clear set of values and beliefs.

An integral part of being a professional is working to a set of standards – the first of which, for doctors, was the Hippocratic oath. The word 'professes' can be interpreted as a public commitment to a set of values, such as this oath.[1] The nature of this professionalism is changing as doctors are being encouraged to become publicly accountable and less paternalistic. In October 2001, the General Medical Council produced guidelines (*Good Medical Practice*) that highlight the importance of putting patients first. Sir Donald Irvine, when he was president of the General Medical Council spoke of the cultural flaws in the profession that hamper this ambition, citing 'excessive paternalism, lack of respect for patients and their right to make decisions about their care, secrecy and complacency about poor practice'.[2]

An important characteristic of a professional is the sharing of ideas and knowledge and a constant desire to keep abreast of new developments. Doctors are being encouraged to build on the concept of professionalism through continuing professional development, more rigorous self-regulation, continued implementation of recertification or revalidation, and accepting accountability for their work.

1 Solotti R (2001) What is it that makes GPs professionals? *Doctor*. **11 October**: 42.

2 Laurance J (2001) The new professionalism. *Doctor*. **11 October**: 65.

Professionalism: a code of practice for managers

The Institute of Health Service Management (IHSM), which represents the majority of practice managers, has published a code of management practice that defines professional management behaviour. Their aim is to promote professional standard setting and good practice, and to encourage professional development. The recently published code builds on the first one, published in November 1992, which stipulates (in addition to giving a guide to management function) that members should uphold the good standing and reputation of the profession of management by:

- having due regard for and compliance with relevant law

- not misusing or abusing their power or position

- providing information on request in order to investigate any alleged breach of practice.

The IHSM definition of a professional is someone who justifiably claims to provide an expert service that is of value to society, by maintaining high standards of education, training and practical judgement and honouring the special trust placed in them by clients, employers, colleagues and the general public. Professionalism in this context also involves the acceptance and habitual exercise of ethical values such as truthfulness, integrity, conscience, openness, transparency, honesty, loyalty and fairness. Other recommendations are that IHSM members should:

- pursue integrity and competence in all managerial activity

- take active steps with regard to continuing professional development

- take responsibility for safeguarding the security of confidential information
- openly declare any personal interest which might be seen to influence managerial decisions
- agree and uphold proper lawful policies and practices within their organisation
- avoid entering into arrangements which unlawfully or improperly affect competitive practice
- never offer or accept any gift, favour or hospitality intended as, or having the effect of, bribery and corruption.

See **Continuing professional development; Management code of conduct.**

www.ihm.org.uk

Project brief
A written summary that takes the reader step by step through the process of a project as follows:

- the proposal
- details of the project
- ways of evaluating the performance.

See **Risk assessment/management.**

Prospective audit
The process of gathering data as an event or process happens, usually over a pre-scribed and defined period of time and using a predetermined number of cases and purpose-designed data-collection forms (recording sheets) or computerised data entry. This has advantages over retrospective audits in that the completeness of the data can be controlled. The disadvantage of prospective audit is that participants may be tempted to alter the data in order to meet a personal agenda, thereby bringing in a research bias. *See* **Audit; Sample.**

Protocol
A formal policy or set of guidelines to be followed for a given procedure; an accepted or established procedure that has been developed from broad principles for local (either individual or group) application. Although it is often synonymous with the words 'procedure' or 'guideline', the term 'protocol' is more often used when the procedure is evidence based. *See* **Guideline.**

Public health

Public health concerns itself with examining and monitoring environmental health. Public health experts recognise that health is broadly affected by social and economic factors (e.g. poverty, unemployment, social exclusion), environmental factors (e.g. air and water quality, housing, food and safety) lifestyle choices (e.g. diet, physical activity, use of alcohol and drugs, sexual behaviour) and access to good-quality services (e.g. education, social care, health, local transport and leisure), as well as by fixed factors (e.g. age, sex, genetic make-up).

Those involved in public health consider that responsibility for the population's health exists at many levels – at the individual, practice and community level as well as nationally and globally.

Environmental health officials maintain links with other public and private sector workers who are key to the process of maintaining public health (e.g. social care, the voluntary sector, housing, transport, education, local shops and businesses).

www.pho.org.uk
www.nelph.net/

Public Health Information Scotland (PHIS)

An initiative that aims to increase understanding of the factors that determine health and ill health, helps to formulate public health policy, and increases the effectiveness of the public health endeavour.

www.show.scot.nhs.uk

Public–private partnership

The situation that occurs when an organisation, such as a council or government department, strikes a deal that allows the private sector to deliver a public service. The term can cover anything from the building of a Private Finance Initiative hospital to a contract for a business to collect domestic rubbish. There is some debate as to whether or not the act is one of privatisation, as public bodies are involved in setting standards for the work. *See* **Local Improvement Finance Trusts**; **Private Finance Initiative**.

www.society.guardian.co.uk
www.4ps.co.uk

Purchaser

Any budget-holding body that buys health or social care services from a provider on behalf of its resident population or service users.

Quality

A measure of the degree of technical excellence, but in the context of medicine and healthcare it may also be defined as value for money (effectiveness, efficiency and economy), fitness for purpose (relevant, acceptable) or customer satisfaction (equitable, accessible).[1] Quality means different things to patients, providers and purchasers. For example, human qualities (e.g. kindness) and pain relief may be more important to some than achieving a perfect clinical outcome.

The provision of a *quality service* requires commitment and example from management, an approach which focuses on the customer, and a participative environment and teamwork. *Quality organisations* are those which pursue continuous improvement, with the organisation existing to meet the needs of the patient, not itself.

Some of the steps taken by the present Government to improve the quality of NHS care have the introduction of the following:

- National Service Frameworks

- the National Institute for Clinical Excellence

- the Commission for Health Improvement

- NHSnet

- the National Electronic Library for Health.

Between them, they provide a framework that evaluates the levels and types of clinical care, and makes recommendations on the best outcome-based treatments that are currently available. *See* **Clinical governance; Total quality management**.

1 Maxwell R (1984) Quality assessment in health. *BMJ.* **288**: 1470–2.

Quality-adjusted life-year (QALY)

A measure used by health economists to assess the potential health benefits and cost-effectiveness of a particular healthcare intervention (e.g. an operation, or a course of drugs) by taking into account its effect on a patient in terms of subsequent quality and length of life.

QALYs are used by health planners to prioritise treatment (e.g. in the deliberations of the National Institute for Clinical Excellence in determining which procedures should be made available on the NHS). *See* **National Institute for Clinical Excellence**.

Quality assessment

The measurement and comparison of the technical and interpersonal aspects of care against predetermined standards. In healthcare, the National Primary Care Research and Development Centre in Manchester works to assess quality of care in general practice.

www.npcrdc.man.ac.uk

Quality assurance

In healthcare, this was defined by the World Health Organization as follows: 'To assure quality is to ensure that patients receive such care as is most likely to produce the optimal achievable outcome … consistent with biological circumstances … concomitant pathology ... compliance with recommended treatment … minimal expense … lowest achievable risk to patient … and maximal satisfaction with process and results'.[1] Ovretveit has an all-encompassing definition, namely 'all activities undertaken to predict and prevent poor quality'.[2]

Quality assurance goes one step further than quality assessment, as it aims to continually monitor and improve standards of care by systematically checking the levels of quality by means of a performance review or audit cycle process. *See* **Quality assessment; Quality control; Total quality management**.

1 World Health Organization (1989) The principles of quality assurance. *Qual Assurance Healthcare.* **1**: 79–95.

2 Ovretveit J (1992) *Health Service Quality: an introduction to quality methods for health services.* Blackwell Scientific Publications, Oxford.

Quality circle

A small, organised group of people who do similar work and who meet together weekly in order to identify, analyse and solve work-related problems. Quality circles have specific methods, and they only flourish when the culture of the work environment has evolved to encourage participation and the admission of mistakes. *See* **Group; Team; Total quality management**.

Quality control

An alternative term for *quality assurance*. It is the process by which quality performance is measured and improved. *See* **Quality assurance; Total quality management**.

Quality improvement
A term that is used interchangeably with medical audit.

Quality Protects
A Government programme, launched in 1998, that aims to transform children's services by 2004. Local authorities must show that they are meeting 11 key objectives which cover children in need, looked after children and children in need of protection. Each council must produce an annual management action plan outlining their strategy for transforming their services in order to receive a share of the children's service grant (worth £885 million over five years) that supports the initiative. Councils must work in partnership with the NHS and the voluntary sector.

www.doh.gov.uk/qualityprotects/

Quality team development (QTD)
A technique devised by the Royal College of General Practitioners. Linking with the Commission for Health Improvement and Health Improvement Programmes requirements, quality team development supports the new culture in addressing performance. It puts patients first, and looks for clinicians and managers to work together. The scheme asks general practice to examine, for example, the ease of obtaining appointments, the quality of premises, the level of confidentiality within the practice and the use of patient surveys. A quality team will have assessed the need for and developed broad health promotion contracts, such as linking with other community agencies (e.g. youth services for sexual health work) or with the council on green issues (e.g. transport, clean air, recycling policies), or they may identify a special client group to which they are to provide a service, and make special access plans to include them.

For example, quality team development might be used to improve primary care access to learning-disabled patients by:

- reviewing screening requirements and including annual screening for mental/ visual/thyroid problems
- updating and improving the protocol for determining consent for treatment
- Listing local support groups and specialist services available.

See **Access**.

Quango
A quasi-autonomous, accountable non-Government organisation, sometimes referred to as a non-departmental public body; an organisation that is set up to address specific current issues that would normally be addressed by the (less independent) Civil Service.

Open to public scrutiny, quangos are part of national Government, but they operate at arm's length from Government departments. There are around 1000 such organisations in the UK, which between them spend more than £24 billion. Examples within the NHS include the Audit Commission and the Health and Safety Executive.

www.cabinet-office.gov.uk/central/1997/consult/quchap1/

Quarry House

The seat of the NHS Executive, which arbitrates on applications for Personal Medical Services, trust status, etc.

www.hse.gov.uk

R

Race Relations Act 1976

Part of a whole raft of anti-discrimination legislation, this prevents employers from discriminating against employees on grounds of race. A recent amendment (in 2002) to the act requires GPs to collect data (on ethnic group, country of birth, language spoken and read, religion and interpretation needs) for the ethnic minorities in their practice. The requested target is for practices to have 'ethnically' coded at least 75% of these patients by March 2005.

The 2002 amendment takes steps to deal with racism in the public sector by forcing all public bodies, such as councils, hospitals and schools, to take steps to promote good race relations. *See* **Discrimination**.

www.hmso.gov.uk/

Random case analysis

The statistical term for an on-the-spot audit – that is, a detailed review of the care of a particular patient, such as a review of the care pathway, chosen at random from a list of cases. This review may be a peer group activity or part of the tutorial technique of a clinical teacher. It is often the starting point for identifying a subject to be audited.[1]

1 Samuel O, Grant J and Irvine D (eds) (1994) *Quality and Audit in General Practice: meanings and definitions.* Royal College of General Practitioners, London.

Rapid response

An intermediate care service model designed to prevent avoidable acute admissions by providing rapid assessment and diagnosis for patients referred from GPs, Accident and Emergency, NHS Direct or social care. It provides rapid access to short-term nursing and therapy support on a 24-hour basis. *See* **Intermediate care**.

Re-accreditation

See **Accreditation of healthcare**.

Reactive management

Responding to an effect, influence or crisis without planning ahead to manage the risk of it occurring. It is the opposite of being proactive and planning ahead. *See* **Proactive management**.

Read codes

A numeric coding system, developed by Dr James Read, that is used to develop common terminology and protocols for the electronic communication of patient records and other clinical information. Read codes are also known as clinical terms. The Government plans eventually to replace Read codes with a simple American coding system.

www.nhsia.nhs.uk/

Red Book

The General Medical Service GP 'Bible', which contains information on the fees and allowances available to GPs to resource their practice. It is to be replaced by a less bureaucratic system of payments under the new GP contract proposals. *See* **GP contract**.

www.doh.gov.uk/pricare/

Reference

A statement, theory, result or procedure that is utilised when conducting research or writing, and is credited to its source. The reader is thus enabled either to ascertain what is the author's own opinion, or to find their way to the work that has already been done in the area of research referenced. References are conventionally written in alphabetical or numerical order, in the sequence of author's name, year of publication, title of article, title of journal, volume number and page range (first and last pages) of the article.

Reference costs

A national schedule that itemises the cost of individual treatments across the NHS in areas of major hospital activity (e.g. hip operations), allowing trusts to increase efficiency by comparing costs with similar providers. *See* **Commissioning**.

www.doh.gov.uk/

Referral

A written or spoken request for help for someone in need of an assessment, usually made by a service provider for a service user, although in some services patients can self-refer.

Region

England has nine official Government administrative regions, namely north-east, north-west, Yorkshire and Humberside, East and West Midlands, east of England, south-west, south-east and London.

www.regions.dtlr.gov.uk

Regional co-ordination unit (RCU)

Established in 2000 as the national headquarters for nine regional offices, the RCU was formed to ensure that a range of Government programmes are delivered coherently at a local and regional level. The RCU brings together the English regional services for the following:

- the Home Office
- the Department for Culture, Media and Sport
- the Department for Environment, Food and Rural Affairs
- the Department for Education and Skills
- the Department of Trade and Industry
- the Department for Transport
- the Department for Work and Pensions
- the Department of Health
- the Office of the Deputy Prime Minister.

Together the RCU and local government offices aim to cut through bureaucracy and add value to delivery, bringing together key stakeholders and local partners, using knowledge gained at local level to influence policy design in Whitehall.

www.rcu.gov.uk

Registrar

A qualified doctor who has undergone junior training and is now working towards specialising as either a consultant or a GP. *See* **Vocational Training Scheme**.

Regulation

The establishment by various regulatory bodies of independent standards of training, conduct and professional competence. The aim is to protect the public, guide workers and employees, and ensure personal accountability for maintaining safe and effective practice. Regulation includes effective measures to deal with individuals whose continuing practice presents an unacceptable risk to the public, or who are otherwise unfit to be registered members of the profession. *See* **Council for the Regulation of Healthcare Professionals; Health Professions Council; Self-regulation**.

Reliability

The statistical term for the extent to which a measurement that is made repeatedly in identical circumstances will yield concordant results.[1] The term relates to the consistency of performance of an instrument or method of measurement.[2] The reliability of an individual measure is increased by basing the measure not on a single observation but on a whole series of observations (e.g. using the mean).[3]

1 Brown L (ed.) (1993) *New Shorter Oxford English Dictionary*. Clarendon Press, Oxford.

2 Samuel O, Grant J and Irvine D (eds) (1994) *Quality and Audit in General Practice: meanings and definitions*. Royal College of General Practitioners, London.

3 Robson C (1975) *Experimental Design and Statistics in Psychology*. Penguin, Harmondsworth.

Repeat script

A prescription that is reissued in the same or a similar format by a doctor or nurse. In the average large group practice, up to two-thirds of all GP prescriptions may be repeats, which represents around 80% of total prescribing costs.[1]

1 Phillips A (2002) *The Business Planning Toolkit*. Radcliffe Medical Press, Oxford.

Replication

See **Reproducibility**.

Reproducibility

The statistical term for the likelihood of obtaining the same results when repeating the same measurement (or action) under different circumstances.[1] This reproducibility depends on the variability of findings over time (which is in turn influenced by variables) and on the robustness and consistency of the measuring method. In experiments, the term *replication* may be used instead of reproducibility.

1 Samuel O, Grant J and Irvine D (eds) (1994) *Quality and Audit in General Practice: meanings and definitions*. Royal College of General Practitioners, London.

Research

A rigorous and systematic investigation with the aim of establishing facts or principles or collecting valid information on a subject.[1] It is similar in approach to audit, but the latter uses established knowledge and facts to improve care, whereas research aims to explore new ideas. Furthermore, although audit also uses some research tools (e.g. data collection, analysis), it is not tied to research methodology. Scientific research methods are about proving facts in a way that can be replicated by other people using the same method. Research requires a hypothesis and a control or a statistically significant sample. *See* **Audit**.

1 Samuel O, Grant J and Irvine D (eds) (1994) *Quality and Audit in General Practice: meanings and definitions.* Royal College of General Practitioners, London.

Residential family centre

A centre in which a family lives for a set period. The children remain under their parents' care while living in the centre.

Residential home

A home that provides personal (but not nursing) care and other services and whose work is monitored by local authority registration and inspection units. *See* **Nursing home**.

www.ncha.gb.com/

Residential rehabilitation

A short-term programme of therapy in a residential setting, usually following an acute hospital stay or referral by a GP, rapid response team or social care services. This model of care is suitable for medically stable patients who require a short period of rehabilitation to enable them to regain sufficient confidence and physical functioning to return home safely. It takes place in a unit such as a nursing home, residential care home, community hospital or rehabilitation centre. *See* **Intermediate care**.

Respite care

Care that is provided by a day centre, day hospital, residential centre, hospice or family. It is usually provided by the State to support the carer and give them a break from full-time caring.

Restraint

A controversial means of control, intended to prevent a person from harming him- or herself or other people, commonly used in mental healthcare. It may be physical (e.g. laying hands on the patient), mechanical (e.g. strapping the patient into a chair) or medical (e.g. sedating or tranquillising the patient).

Restricted funds

Funds that are subject to specific requirements outlined by the giver (e.g. the Government giving a sum of money to a primary care trust to spend on prescribing a particular drug for a particular group of patients). *See* **Ringfencing**.

Retrospective audits

An audit which reviews records in order to gather facts about past activities. This may involve examining existing records whose data may be incomplete, and only making judgements on what is actually recorded.

Any bias can be overcome by planning to collect data prospectively, using specially designed data-collection forms or enhanced records. *See* **Audit**; **Sample**.

Revalidation

Part of the Government's plan to organise additional rapid and robust mechanisms for dealing with poor and under-performing doctors. In the first phase, they concentrated on secondary care, in the second, they concentrated on primary care. The General Medical Council's GP compulsory revalidation programme means that:

- clinical audit will be compulsory

- all contracted doctors will be required to participate in annual appraisal

- non-principals and locums will need to be named on a local register

- all doctors working in primary care will be subject to clinical governance arrangements

- there is agreement to take part in mandatory schemes for reporting significant healthcare events

- GPs must keep personal portfolios that demonstrate their professional and educational development (personal development plans).

GPs will be assessed in a rolling programme. The assessment will be conducted by a local revalidation group consisting of local informed stakeholders such as a locally elected GP, a medical director, a GP educationalist and a lay person. If the group is concerned about failing performance, they will have the authority to refer the individual with a recommendation that he or she should be revalidated.

This system aims to acknowledge and reward clinical progress and achievement, while identifying and supporting those whose performance has deteriorated. It aims to detect and support those doctors who have failed to keep up to date, who are discourteous to patients, who work poorly with colleagues, or who make poor or dangerous clinical decisions.

The General Medical Council members have also agreed that these revalidation folders could include the following:

- details of criminal convictions

- disciplinary hearings

- any breaks in registration that occurred during the revalidation period

- any conditions placed on the registration by the General Medical Council; any erasure or suspensions.

See **Clinical governance**; **Performance assessment framework**.

www.gmc-org.uk

RIDDOR (Reporting of Injuries, Diseases and Dangerous Occurrences Regulations, 1995)

Serious injuries in the workplace must be reported under these regulations, where 'serious' is defined by the regulations as fractures (but not to digits), injuries from falling objects, physical assault, loss of sight, electric shock or any injury lasting for more than 3 days. *See* **Health and safety**; **Medical Devices Agency**.

Ringfencing

The practice by the Government of earmarking parts of the funding that it gives to organisations for national priorities, thus effectively instructing those organisations how to spend some of their money. At present, money is ringfenced for spending in areas such as mental healthcare. *See* **Restricted funds**.

Risk assessment/management

Sometimes called *controls assurance*, a systematic approach to evaluating risk, and to reducing loss of life, financial loss, loss of staff availability, loss of safety or loss of reputation.

When applied to a clinical environment, this means looking for hazards, evaluating the risks, and building in mechanisms to avoid mistakes involving people and property. Thus it involves managing the risk of error arising from clinical or organisational mistakes. The main areas include the following:

- *people and risk*: staff need to be protected from the effects of stress, violence, ill health or damage from poor handling procedures

- *healthcare risks*: risk management during clinical procedures is primarily directed at patient outcome, but risks to clinical staff should also be considered

- *the working environment*: this includes equipment, utilities, lighting, flooring, VDU workstations, food hygiene, space, noise and hazardous substances.

When applying risk management principles to a project, goals and objectives are prioritised with specific indicators, namely *must do*, *could do*, *high impact* and *low impact*. One of the most reliable ways of measuring risk is through continual audit.

Risk assessment is good (and required) management practice aimed at improving morale, reducing repair bills and insurance premiums, and saving time. Primary care organisations will support such initiatives and assist practices in improving security, both in their cost rent and improvement grant schemes and in GP support schemes. Arrangements are made for GPs who so wish to take on seeing known violent patients for their colleagues locally. *See* **Clinical governance; Health and safety; Medical Devices Agency**.

www.croner.co.uk
www.medical-devices.gov.uk/

For further information on clinical governance and risk management, see the following:

- Phillips A (2002) *The Business Planning Toolkit*. Radcliffe Medical Press, Oxford.

- Lilley R (1999) *The PCG Tool Kit* (2e). Radcliffe Medical Press, Oxford.

- Lilley R with Lambden P (2000) *Making Sense of Risk Management*. Radcliffe Medical Press, Oxford.

Robust

Within the NHS, the technical term used to describe a scientific, clear and decisive action or measurement. Targets, goal setting and league-tables form robust measurements; evidence-based medicine is also robust. *See* **Performance management**.

Royal College of General Practitioners (RCGP)

An organisation that represents GPs in England, Scotland and Northern Ireland. The RCGP provides its members with information on current relevant research, learning and education opportunities, events, awards, etc. It has a library and publishes its own journal, the *British Journal of General Practice*, which is also available to members online.

www.rcgp.org.uk

Salaried GPs

The White Paper entitled *The New NHS: modern, dependable* signalled this Government's desire to offer GPs a salaried option. More GPs, especially younger ones, are taking up a salaried option, a choice which brings women in particular more freedom to pursue a life outside work. The salaried option also suits those who wish to avoid the trials and responsibilities of partnership. Where disputes and conflicts occur, it is less important for salaried GPs to evaluate their position and work together as doctors in partnership have to in order to achieve their common core aims and objectives.

Local Negotiating Committees have been set up in some areas of the country in response to the growing number of GPs contracted for salaried services to primary care trusts. These are viewed as a particularly effective way of representing salaried GPs' interests. *See* **GP contract**.

Sample

The process whereby samples of data are taken and analysed during the audit cycle or research. Relevant material has to be selected so that inferences about that group of people, events or objects can be made. For example, if the organisation undertaking the audit has a specific age/sex/ethnic bias to its population, their sample must represent this. If material is selected with a predisposition towards one particular view, this will clearly distort the results.

The method of choosing a sample for any study is of crucial importance, and its size must be sufficient for the purposes of the study. When sampling, material may be selected randomly, sequentially, systematically or as a 'one-off'. Because it is important for samples to be representative, and in order to reduce bias, samples are often taken at random, which reduces the opportunity to select particular examples from memory. The best random samples are generated using random numbers taken from a computer. The size of the sample is immaterial – what is important is that the audit or research team is convinced of the representativeness and relevance of the data presented to them. Samples are expected to be complete, representative, relevant and valid, with confidentiality maintained.

The different types of sampling include the following:

1 *sequential sample*: where cases are taken in their original order

2 *stratified random sample*: where distinct subgroups are identified and random samples are then drawn from each of them

3 *systematic sample*: where one starts at an arbitrary point in a list and chooses cases at regular intervals after that point

4 *random case analysis*: often used as a teaching tool in medical audit, where the case of a particular patient is chosen at random.[1]

See **Audit**; **Sample**.

1 Samuel O, Grant J and Irvine D (eds) (1994) *Quality and Audit in General Practice: meanings and definitions*. Royal College of General Practitioners, London.

Scottish Council for Voluntary Organisations (SCVO)

A membership organisation for Scotland-based charities and voluntary and campaign groups. It provides charity management services and advice, as well as representation to the Scottish Executive and other interested bodies.

www.scvo.org.uk/membership

Scottish Health Care

The Scottish Executive Health Department runs independently from the Health Department in England. This website provides online health information for NHS Scotland. It runs a health management information service for NHS professionals and advises on the latest clinical strategies.

www.show.scot.nhs.uk

Scottish Health Technology Board (SIGN)

The Scottish version of the National Institute for Clinical Excellence, its role is to develop authoritative and reliable guidance on clinical management in controversial areas of medicine, alongside its more high-profile role of assessing the value of new drugs. *See* **National Institute for Clinical Excellence**.

www.htbs.co.uk/

Seamless care

This operates at many levels. Clinically, seamless care results when teams from both acute and community sectors in health, social care and education come together to support the patient in intermediate care schemes. Seamless care results when multi-disciplinary teams work together in collaborative care planning, or from joint commissioning, joint project or joint funded work at a strategic level. The ultimate aim is to develop partnerships with patients, their carers and their families, between health and social care, and between the voluntary sector, public and private organisations.

Secondary care

Specialist care, typically provided in a hospital setting or following referral from a primary or community health professional. *See* **Primary care**.

www.doh.gov.uk/

Selection interviewing

The process by which a group of interviewers chooses a candidate for a job. Such interviews should be standardised and have a system for evaluation of results in order to avoid the risk of bias. The purpose of selection interviews is to persuade the candidate to do the talking in a controlled way on topics under your direction, to help them to clarify the various options that are open to them, and to ascertain how they may satisfy the job requirements. Selection interviews should be non-directive, diagnostic and reflective, rather than interrogative. They should be non-threatening, and ideally the questions asked should encourage joint problem solving.

The purpose of a selection procedure is to choose a person with the qualifications, skills, experience and personal attributes that would allow him or her to perform a predetermined role. The selection of new members of staff is a crucial decision, as the consequences of a good or bad appointment will remain within the organisation for the duration of the employment of that member of staff.

Selection procedures need to be seen to be fair, consistent and effective – the selection process is an important public relations vehicle. Procedures must be both effective and legal. This involves the following:

- staff profiling and workforce planning
- complying with legal requirements and recommended codes of practice
- job analysis
- job descriptions.

For more information on interviewing skills, see the following:

- Phillips A (2002) *Communication and the Manager's Job.* Radcliffe Medical Press, Oxford.

Self-assessment

A means by which people can set out their own estimation of their needs for support, usually on a standardised form.

Self-help group

A group of people with similar problems who meet together regularly for mutual support and to campaign for improved services.

www.patient.co.uk/selfhelp/

Self-managed learning

A method of learning through reflection. Personal development plans are designed for self-managed learning, where individuals take personal responsibility for their own learning, and evaluate their own learning needs through reflection and observation. By documenting a problem situation, the learner can reflect on what they have learned, how they problem solved, and how they managed the changes required to avoid a recurrence of the problem.

Learning sets are another way in which self-managed learning can occur. Although it is empowering, some people find self-learning difficult, because they feel that others should be responsible for their development, or else they believe that they have nothing to learn about anything. See **Continuing professional development**.

Self-regulation

A number of healthcare professionals, including doctors, dentists, nurses, midwives, health visitors, opticians, pharmacists, osteopaths, chiropractors and allied health-care professionals, such as occupational therapists, physiotherapists and speech and language therapists, currently operate under self-regulation. The various regulatory bodies establish independent standards of training, conduct and professional competence for the protection of the public, to guide workers and employees, and to ensure personal accountability for maintaining safe and effective practice ('fitness to practise'). They include effective measures to deal with individuals (through either exclusion or training recommendations) whose continuing practice presents an unacceptable risk to the public, or who are otherwise unfit to be registered members of their profession. See **Council for the Regulation of Healthcare Professionals**; **Regulation**.

Sensory impairment

Partial or complete loss of the ability to hear or see.

www.sense.org.uk/

Service and Financial Framework (SAFF)

An annual planning round in which new services are developed. It is to be replaced by a three-year Local Delivery Plan.

Health authorities submit annual service and financial frameworks to the NHS Executive, committing them to meeting ministerial targets within the available resources. These frameworks set out agreed activity levels and funding, and are underpinned by a series of service level agreements between commissioning bodies (including health authorities, primary care groups and primary care trusts) and hospital trusts.

www.doh.gov.uk/

Service level agreement

An agreement between organisations and/or agencies setting out how services must be provided, what their standards will be and how monitoring will take place. They were developed as a commissioning tool, and the Government has introduced new service level agreements as part of their NHS financial reforms[1] which cover payments by result, nationally agreed prices for procedures and episodes of care, and commissioning based on case-mix-specific volumes. New service level agreements will define what resources are available, the mix of services provided and the changes of service delivery and quality of service that the provider is agreeing to make. They will ensure payments by result. *See* **Commissioning**; **Healthcare resource group tarrif**.

www.doh.gov.uk/nhsfinancialreforms/

1 *Reforming NHS Financial Flows. Introducing payment by results: 2002 consultation document.* www.nhs.uk.

Service user

An individual who uses, requests, applies for or benefits from health or local authority services. They may also be referred to as a client (by social services and the voluntary sector) or as a patient or consumer (within the NHS).

Seven-Point Plan

An interview plan[1] which looks at physical make-up, achievements, general intelligence, special aptitudes, interests, disposition and circumstances. It has now been superseded by the equal opportunities interview process.

1 Rodger A (1970) *The Seven-Point Plan* (3e). Originally devised for the National Institute of Industrial Psychology, and now available from the National Foundation for Educational Research. *See also* Mullins LJ (1999) *Management and Organisational Behaviour*. Pitman Publishing, London, pp. 750–1.

Sex Discrimination Act 1975

Part of a raft of employment laws to prevent sexual harassment of or discrimination in the workplace against women (especially pregnant or married women), equal access and contractual rights for all employees. It was recently amended by the Indirect Discrimination and Burden of Proof Regulations 2001. The burden of proof now lies with the employer, who must show that they did not legally discriminate against the applicant who makes the claim against their employer.

www.acas.co.uk

Shared medical record

A common database of information that is accessible by all healthcare sectors (community, acute and intermediate care). The shared medical record holds common medical information such as main diagnoses, height, weight, immunisation status, screening results, any allergies, prescriptions and at-risk details (e.g. smoking status or social risk factors). Other medical information includes assessment dates, individual care plans, significant results and discharge letters, as well as core administrative data such as referrals. The information is held by and accessible to all of the patient's main carers, thus promoting seamless care. If properly used, it avoids the patient having to duplicate information by giving it to many people on many different occasions.

Shifting the Balance of Power

The programme of change brought about in order to empower frontline staff and patients in the NHS. It is part of the implementation of *The NHS Plan*, and has already led to the establishment of new structures. Its main objective is to foster a new culture in the NHS at all levels which puts the patient first.

The main feature of change has been giving locally based primary care trusts the role of running the NHS and improving health in their areas. This has meant abolishing the previous health authorities and creating new ones (strategic health authorities) that serve larger areas and have a more strategic role. The Department of Health is also refocusing in order to reflect these changes. This includes the abolition of its regional offices.

www.doh.gov.uk/shiftingthebalance/

Short-term contracts

A short-term contract is a time-limited employment contract document, where the employee is contracted to work for a short period – usually between one month and 3 years, but sometimes more. Workers on short-term contracts have full employment rights under current employment legislation, including rights to sick pay, annual leave, pensions, etc.

Short-term contracts and flexible working patterns are becoming more common and desirable throughout the working world, as people no longer feel such a strong need to conform to work values. The social function of work is becoming less important. *See* **GP contract; Salaried GPs**.

Sickness absence

Time away from work due to ill health. Self-certification gives employees some responsibility with regard to deciding the severity of a short-term illness, but the employer has the right to make certain enquiries concerning the length of the illness. It is permissible in law to dismiss an employee should their attendance be unsatisfactory, even if this is due to illness, provided that disciplinary procedures are followed. The length of absence should be balanced against the employer's needs, and advice should be sought from an occupational physician and a human resource manager.

Significance

A statistical term for the level of probability of an occurrence. If an action has caused a change to be induced in an experiment, and the chance of it happening due to chance or random errors is very low, the change is said to be statistically significant.

Significant event

An episode in the care of a patient in which a specific action by a healthcare worker has a particularly beneficial or detrimental outcome.

In medical audit, significant events are used to focus attention on aspects of healthcare which might benefit from review. Significant event audit is a detailed review of the significant events that occur during the care of either a single patient or a group of patients.[1] See **Confidential enquiry**; **Critical incident technique**; **Significant event analysis**.

1 Samuel O, Grant J and Irvine D (eds) (1994) *Quality and Audit in General Practice: meanings and definitions*. Royal College of General Practitioners, London.

Significant event analysis (SEA)

Analysis of important clinical or administrative events (significant healthcare events) that in retrospect proved risky to the patient, doctor or organisation. These are events from which important lessons could have been learned. Significant events may range from a missed diagnosis, missed visit or unexpected death to the theft of a script pad, a staff upset or a patient complaint. Significant event analyses work on the premise that if it is not acknowledged that mistakes can be made, no learning or personal development can occur. Significant events can be examples of when things go right as well as of when they go wrong, and team discussion and analysis enable learning and change to occur.

Significant event analyses ask the following questions.

- What are the facts?

- What went well?

- What went badly?

- How could I improve?

- What action should be taken?

- How should the event be recorded?

Healthcare organisations are required to report significant events, and a single database for analysing and sharing lessons learned from incidents and near misses is being developed. A *confidential enquiry* is a term often used to describe a significant event audit[1] where data are collected with the aim of identifying the circumstances that lead to adverse or unusual events. This is often used in general practice as a review of individual cases. *See* **Significant event**.

1 Bradley CP (1992) Turning anecdotes into data: the critical incident technique. *Fam Pract.* **9**: 98–103.

Single regeneration budget (SRB)

Now discontinued as a national scheme, the single regeneration budget was created in 1994 to narrow the gap between deprived and wealthy areas by funding local regeneration initiatives. Local partnerships of community, voluntary and business groups received money for schemes that aimed to improve employment prospects, address social exclusion and crime, and support economic growth.

www.regeneration.dtlr.gov.uk/

Skill mix review

Following a staff profiling exercise, this procedure maps out the key skills and the hours required to do the job against the available skills and time of the staff. Skill mix review involves noting the following:

- the names of staff

- the whole-time equivalent (wte) hours worked by them

- their job title, grade and pay per hour

- a brief synopsis of their skills

- any training needs.

The following steps are then undertaken:

- mapping out the required tasks

- noting any discrepancies

- matching those staff members who are best suited and graded for the job required

- identifying who the job would best be done by, and when.

This techniques requires ruthless honesty and objectivity, and a realistic appraisal of the job needs, followed by further discussion with all of the interested parties. If jobs are to be changed, the usual changes involve any of the following:

- making job changes when staff leave and need to be replaced
- reformulating the job to the hours and tasks that best suit the staff
- upgrading roles and pay to a smaller number of more highly skilled staff
- downgrading roles and pay to a larger number of less skilled staff.

Nurse triage is one example of a common change that is implemented following a larger skill mix review after a national workforce planning exercise.

Skill mix reviews work in organisations that are trying to save money or to overcome persistent recruitment and retention difficulties.

Smart-card

Lifetime patient records that are held on a credit-card-sized card, which is retained by the patient, allowing personal medical information to be accessed by NHS institutions electronically.

Social exclusion

The situation where either individuals or a geographical area suffer from poverty caused by a combination of adverse factors such as unemployment, high crime rates, low incomes and poor housing.

The Government's approach to regeneration is based on tackling the problems posed by social exclusion as a whole, rather than simply focusing on its individual elements. The Social Exclusion Unit (SEU) was set up in December 1997 to help to reduce social exclusion. It works with Government departments to research, implement and promote policies that tackle social exclusion and poverty.

www.cabinet-office.gov.uk/seu/index

Social model

A model or philosophy of health that works on the premise that illness has sociological and psychological causes, and can therefore be cured either by structural changes within society or by psychological intervention (e.g. tackling poverty and social exclusion and/or providing help through the talking therapies to those who need it). *See* **Medical model**.

Social regeneration

The process of tackling the social problems that lead to deprivation, such as crime and drugs. The process is different to physical regeneration, which tackles run-down buildings and communal areas, and economic regeneration, which is aimed at creating jobs and wealth.

www.regeneration-uk.com

Social services departments

Established under the Local Authority Social Services Act 1970 in England and Wales, these local authority departments are responsible for the provision of personal social services. They combined the former children's, health and welfare departments. The services that they provide include social work, home care and community care. *See* **Social work**.

www.adss.org.uk

Social work

The provision of personal help to resolve a range of social and economic difficulties. The term was first adopted by social theorists in the early 1900s, and began to be used more widely in the 1970s following the establishment of social services departments and the British Association of Social Workers. Social workers work across the range of age groups, from infants and children to the very elderly. Their work is increasingly linked with health, education and the criminal justice system. *See* **Social services departments**.

www.basw.co.uk/

Span of control

In line management, the number of subordinates who report directly to a manager or supervisor. It does not refer to the total number of subordinate operating staff. For this reason the terms 'span of responsibility' or 'span of supervision' are sometimes deemed more appropriate. At lower levels in the organisation, where responsibility is more concerned with operational performance, the span can be larger. If the span is too wide, it becomes difficult to supervise adequately and there is a slowness to adapt to change. If it is too narrow, there may be a problem of consistency in decision making and co-ordination. Staff morale may suffer if there is too close a level of supervision, and administrative costs may increase. The ideal span depends on the nature of the organisation, the complexity of work and the personal qualities of the manager.

Special health authorities

Health authorities with unique national supra-regional functions which cannot be effectively undertaken by other types of NHS bodies, such as the NHS National Information Authority or the National Institute for Clinical Excellence.

www.doh.gov.uk/

Specialist GPs

The Government plan is to devolve specialist care down to local levels, which is cheaper, improves access for patients and reduces waiting times. It is facilitating the introduction of specialist GPs who are able and willing to take on some of the more complicated work that is usually undertaken in hospitals (e.g. colposcopies, ECGs and vasectomies). GPs with special interests in areas such as diabetes care, elderly and palliative care, dermatology, mental and sexual health, ENT, cardiology, orthopaedics and rheumatology are also expected to be in demand.

The Royal College of General Practitioners has specified that GPs may work for their own practice population, or provide a wider service to surrounding practices within their primary care trust. Draft specialist accreditation frameworks for GP specialists ask that primary care trusts check GPs for the following:

- evidence of training and/or acquisition of competencies

- arrangements for induction, support and continuing professional development

- appropriate facilities and service delivery

- monitoring and clinical audit arrangements.

Primary care trusts must be satisfied that any appointment fulfils local community and clinical governance needs. GPs with special interests are expected to assist in the commissioning and development of services as part of a generalist or specialist team.[1] See **Intermediate care**.

www.nhsalliance.org
www.bma.org.uk
www.rcgp.org.uk

1 Solotti R (2001) RCGP drafts framework for specialist GP service. *Doctor*. **27 September**: 26.

Specialist library

Under the umbrella of the National Electronic Library for Health network, specialist libraries are to be set up within three years. Specialist library teams will be established that are broadly based, to include a network of information specialists, patient organisations and professional bodies from the healthcare community. See **National Electronic Library for Health**.

www.nhsia.nhs.uk/nelh/

Specialist registrar

A junior doctor who has finished their basic specialist training as a house officer, and who has embarked upon higher specialist training in the area of medicine in which they wish to specialise in the future. Specialist registrars can become consultants after at least six or seven years. GP registrars are junior doctors who are training to become GPs. *See* **House officer**.

www.bma.org.uk/

Springboard Development Programme

Originally developed by two UK consultants, and used extensively throughout the NHS, this programme is designed to develop female employees by providing an opportunity for women to acknowledge and value their skills and qualities, develop their confidence and set themselves goals for the future.

The programme consists of a structured workbook with a series of exercises, case studies and activities centred on ten topics, including goals and objectives, the world about you, knowing yourself, finding support, the assertive you, more energy – less anxiety, managing your image, blowing your own trumpet and making it happen.

The programme is very popular and successful, and has been adopted by public sector organisations throughout the UK.

www.brazentraining.co.nz

Staff charter

A charter that is produced in consultation with staff and which describes some of the fundamental rights frequently sought by employees. Such a charter could be developed as part of an Improving Working Lives standard initiative, as it shows that staff are both informed and consulted about matters which are likely to affect their employment. Thus staff should have the following rights:

- to be treated fairly, with courtesy and understanding, to ensure equity for all and respect for individual differences
- to be fully and properly trained to do the job that they are employed to do
- to be rewarded fairly for the contribution that they make to the organisation, taking into account effort, skill and achievement
- to comment or complain to their employers without fear or prejudice
- to be able to feed their ideas and views back to a management structure that will listen to and act upon them
- to be informed and consulted about matters that are likely to affect their employment.

Staff profile

A prerequisite for completing a skill mix review, this profile documents the following:

- the names of staff

- their whole-time equivalent (wte) hours worked

- their job title, grade and pay per hour

- a brief synopsis of their skills

- any training needs.

Stakeholder

Any person who has an interest in an organisation, its activities and its achievements, including customers, partners, employees, shareholders, owners, Government and regulators. Stakeholders influence the direction and culture of an organisation, and they have an interest in and/or are affected by the goals or activities of the organisation. Stakeholders within the NHS may belong to Government groups (local councils, primary care trusts), pressure groups (the press, patient voices, professional associations), employees (managers, trust staff) or business partners (patients, provider units, allied professionals, drug companies).

Any consultation or analysis of an organisation is usually 'stakeholder focused'. *See* **Stakeholder analysis**.

Stakeholder analysis

An investigation of the concerns and interests of stakeholders, with the aim of finding out whether there are any conflicts of interest, so that the organisation can work to minimise them.

There are ethical concerns that NHS stakeholders are interested in workers' rights, patient safety, whistleblowing, research, doctors' remuneration, discrimination, privacy and security of data. An example is shown below.

GP stakeholders and their concerns

- Employees (who have joint needs with their employers)

- Providers of finance, both public and private (who expect a fair service for bearing the risk of investment)

- Consumers – customers and patients (who want value for money, good care, efficiency, full service access)

- Community and environment (which are concerned with the siting of buildings, pollution, transport, waste, research)

- Government (which both assists and limits through money and directives)

Healthcare strategy is still partly governed by profit (in general practice in particular), and partly by broader public policy issues such as politics, monopoly supply, bureaucracy and finite resources. The power and influence exercised within the NHS should also be tempered by responsible and ethical management. NHS organisations by default accept and assume responsibility for the public good.[1] *See* **Forcefield analysis**; **Stakeholder**.

1   Mullins LJ (1999) *Management and Organisational Behaviour* (5e). Financial Times/Pitman Publishing, London.

Stakeholder pension

A low-cost, flexible pension aimed at low or middle earners, often in charities and campaign organisations. It was launched in April 2001. All organisations that employ five or more people must offer a pension facility, either internally or externally.

http://www.stakeholder.opra.gov.uk/

Standards

In audit, an accepted or approved example of something against which others are judged or measured. During audit, standards are set using a specific, measurable criterion as a benchmark. In this context, standards must be precise and measurable, and must specify 'an adequate, acceptable or optional level of quality'.[1] Standards do not have to be a measure of excellence or quality, but of acceptability. If the present standard of care provided for patients is satisfactory, this may be acceptable to the audit team, and the standard may not need to be changed. However, standards are usually raised or altered (reset) in order to achieve better results. The best audits define both minimum and optimum standards. Ownership of standards is a vital stage in accepting the validity of an audit.

In medicine, the term 'standard procedures' is often used interchangeably with 'criterion' , 'guideline' and 'protocol'. Here it describes a professionally considered range of acceptable variation from the norm. A *minimum standard* would be considered to be a standard of performance below which performance is unacceptable. An *optimum standard* would be the best standard obtainable with the available resources and conditions. During *standard setting*, standards of care are negotiated and developed within partnership of a group of local clinicians, or from the work of a national standard-setting body such as the National Institute for Clinical Excellence, or set by an external body (e.g. practice performance targets for cytology screening or immunisation rates). If developed nationally, the standards are often adjusted to the local situation. Again ownership is vital, as they are more likely to be accepted if they are defined by those who will use them.[2]

Statistically, a *standard deviation* describes a widely used measure of variability,[3] namely how far a subject is placed from the mean or average scores. The larger the standard deviation, the further the subject score is placed from the average. *See* **Audit**; **Criterion**.

1   Donabedian A (1982) Explorations in quality assessment and monitoring. In: *The Criteria and Standards of Quality. Volume 2*. Health Administration Press, Ann Arbor, MI.

2   Samuel O, Grant J and Irvine D (eds) (1994) *Quality and Audit in General Practice*. Royal College of General Practitioners, London.

3   Robson C (1975) *Experimental Design and Statistics in Psychology*. Penguin, Harmondsworth.

Star ratings
The annual grading system (from zero to three stars) by which NHS acute trusts are measured against a range of performance indicators (e.g. waiting times, ward cleanliness). The system is designed to give an illustration of their clinical and managerial effectiveness. Three-star trusts are allowed more managerial freedom. Zero-star trusts are placed on 'probation' and given between 3 and 12 months to improve or face the threat of being taken over by alternative management.

Statutory authority
An organisation that is required by law to provide public services and which receives central or local government funding (e.g. trusts, health authorities, local authorities). *See* **Statutory services**.

Statutory maternity leave
All pregnant women, regardless of the amount of hours worked or length of service, are entitled to a period of maternity leave of at least 14 weeks. Of this, 6 weeks is paid at 90% of full salary. *See* **Statutory maternity pay**.

www.acas.co.uk

Statutory maternity pay (SMP)
The pay that is given to pregnant women, the amount and period (currently just under £50 per week for 18 weeks) of which is defined by law. During this time the pregnant woman retains all of her contractual rights, and she cannot be dismissed because of any pregnancy-related illnesses.

Statutory services
Services provided by the local authority as a matter of course (e.g. benefits, social services, hospital treatment on the NHS, schools). *See* **Statutory authority**.

www.dss.dov.uk/lifeevent/benefits

Strategic health authority (SHA)
Set up in April 2002, with the abolition of health authorities and the creation of primary care trusts under NHS *Shifting the Balance* proposals, their working boundaries mirror those of the regional health authorities that they replace.

Strategic health authorities are responsible for performance managing primary care trusts and NHS trusts, a job that was previously done by eight regional and around 95 district offices. Now 28 strategic health authorities will report to four Directorates of Health and Social Care and will be expected to provide feedback to ministers.

Their old role of commissioning health services for their local communities has been passed to primary care trusts. From April 2002, strategic health authorities have provided strategic management support for primary care trusts and hospitals in improving NHS performance. *See* **Health authority**.

www.doh.gov.uk/shiftingthebalance/index.htm

Strategy

A three- to ten-year look ahead at an organisation. There are three different levels of strategy that organisations use for planning ahead:

* operational level (meetings, etc.)

* tactical level (a look at next month, a review of the quarterly returns)

* strategic level (a 3- to 10-year plan).

When forward planning, health organisations consider the forces that currently impact on their performance, and they assess the future effect of these (the economic and demographic trends, the sociological forces, and the legal and governmental developments). Strategic planners consider the overall impact on healthcare of an exponential increase in, for example, the elderly population, or poverty, or the development of new drugs that could completely cure cancer. A good strategic planner will have the ability to look ahead and see the whole picture, not just the detail.

Strategic management concentrates on overall strategies and long-term plans – that is, what the organisation goals should be between 3 and 10 years from now.

Stress management

A term used in workplaces to describe the action human resource departments take to manage stress in their workforce. Various strategies are used by employers, from providing a good occupational health service to ensuring a healthy organisational culture. Stress is most common when there is a mismatch between the worker and the work that they do. It is more likely to occur where there is a poor work culture (poor communication, irregular meetings, absence of training and development) and lack of positive feedback to the employee. Stress thrives in situations of conflict, low pay, constant insecurity, repetitive tasks and continuous change.

Structural funds

Money from the European Union aimed at regenerating the most deprived parts of the European Union. These funds can be used for a wide range of projects, including new businesses, infrastructure, training and job creation. Governments have to match the European Union's investment in order to take full advantage of the money.

www.dti.gov.uk/europe/

Structure
In management, the term for the factors that constitute the context of the organisation, such as the buildings, administrative arrangements, etc.

Substance abuse/misuse
The use of a mood-altering substance in such a way that it is either socially unacceptable or impairs social, medical and/or occupational functioning. Substance misuse is the term often used in the same context as substance abuse, which strictly means use of substances in a manner for which they were not intended.

www.drugscope.org.uk

Superannuation
The amount of money that is deducted regularly from the employee's payslip in a contributory pension scheme, or for the pension that is actually paid out to such employees. Not all NHS work is considered to be pensionable, and some independent contractors, such as GPs, argue that all work which contributes to the overall function of the NHS (e.g. education, training, project and committee work), not just clinical work, should be superannuable.

Supported discharge
A service that provides a short-term period of nursing and/or therapeutic support in a patient's home, typically with an individually tailored package of home care. *See* **Intermediate care**.

Supported housing
Accommodation for vulnerable people with care needs, such as sheltered housing for older people, hostels for the homeless, and accommodation for people with learning difficulties and mental health problems.

Sure Start
An initiative that aims to improve children's life opportunities by working with parents and parents-to-be in deprived areas and providing better access to family support, advice on nurturing, health services and early learning. It forms a cornerstone of the Government's drive to eradicate child poverty. There are already more than 150 local Sure Start programmes across England and Wales, with the number set to rise to at least 500 by 2004. Ministers are investing £580 million in the scheme for the three years from April 2001. *See* **Social exclusion**; **Social regeneration**.

www.surestart.gov.uk/home

Survey

Statistically, the systematic collection and analysis of data from a particular population at any one time. Surveys may be either *descriptive* (seeking to describe issues of concern) or *analytical* (where patterns, differences and correlations are sought from the material).[1] *See* **Patient participation**; **Patient survey**.

1 Samuel O, Grant J and Irvine D (eds) (1994) *Quality and Audit in General Practice*. Royal College of General Practitioners, London.

Sustainable development

An approach to world development that aims to allow economic growth without damaging the environment or natural resources. The Government has produced a strategy for ensuring sustainable development in the UK, and this is expected to be adhered to across the whole of the public sector as well as industry. For primary care, ethical sustainable development has to be considered within the domain of health and safety. It includes the following:

- waste production and disposal
- recycling
- use of ecologically sound materials
- water conservation
- green contracting
- use of local resources
- green transport (discouraging car use, encouraging walking, use of public transport and cycling).

See **Business ethics**; **Health and safety**.

www.sustainable-development.gov.uk
www.defra.gov.uk/environment/greening/index.htm
www.nhsestates.gov.uk/
www.sustainable-energy.org.uk

SWOT analysis

A form of business analysis, developed by Ansoff,[1] that focuses on the strengths and weaknesses, opportunities and threats of an organisation. It is commonly used when studying an organisation, as it provides a basis for problem solving and decision making.

Strengths refer to positive or distinctive attributes that provide a significant market advantage. Weaknesses are any negative aspects or deficiencies in the organisation, its image or reputation which need to be corrected. Opportunities are considered to be favourable conditions which usually arise from changes in the external environment, technological advances, improved economic conditions, etc. Threats are the opposite of opportunities, and refer to unfavourable situations or developments that are likely to endanger the operations or effectiveness of the organisation (competitors, changing social conditions, legislation, etc.).

1 Ansoff HI (1987) *Corporate Strategy*. Penguin, Harmondsworth. *See also* Ansoff HI (ed.) (1969) *Business Strategy*. Penguin, Harmondsworth.

T

Target payments

Payments made to General Medical Service GPs who manage to reach the targets set for them nationally to meet a given percentage standard of patient recall for childhood immunisations and cervical cytology (smear tests). Two rates are set (higher and lower) for each patient group. Personal Medical Service GPs are able to negotiate more realistic local targets for their practices, taking into account the local population of defaulters or non-attenders (those who will not or do not attend for their treatment). *See* **Fees and allowances**.

Team

A group of people who are working together to achieve common goals. Teamworking is used to help:

- improve communication

- learning

- develop a sense of belonging

- build co-operation

- develop mutual support

- motivate staff

- achieve more.

The management advantages of teamworking are that each person has the opportunity to contribute their unique knowledge. Individuals achieve more when working in teams than they could alone, and management can ensure that everyone agrees on the objectives and nature of the working relationship.

The way in which clinicians, managers and interrelated services are working together with specific and shared responsibilities for healthcare provision is a new approach for the NHS. The Government vision of healthcare delivery is centred on teamwork, with more integrated/seamless care, multidisciplinary teamworking and disappearing boundaries between primary, secondary and social care.

In integrated and effective teamworking, visions are shared and involvement and co-operation are obtained from everyone. Teamworking is not always easy. The team needs to find a balance between the needs of the following:

- the task – do the task objectives fit with organisational objectives?
- the team – what are the group objectives as a whole?
- the individual – who will want to contribute and challenge, and who may need authority to carry out delegated tasks?

Teams have their own growth process, like groups – they explore, experiment, and then mature, co-operate and perform. Teams progress through various stages of development, rarely in a linear or consistent fashion. As teams struggle to cope with rapidly changing internal or external events, or variations in team membership, they will progress or regress through the levels. Progress is most likely when teams consciously acknowledge or address the need to develop or tackle the reforming issues that are raised by change. Teams that do not take this into account will probably regress to earlier stages of development, despite the length of time that they have been working together, and this will inevitably affect their performance.

Teenage pregnancy unit (TPU)

A national co-ordinating body that was set up to address the growing rate of teenage pregnancy in the UK.

Telemedicine

The use of communication systems, such as video links and computers, to provide remote diagnosis and healthcare, allowing more care to be provided in the community or at home.

www.tis.bl.uk/
www.nelh.nhs.uk/

Temporary resident

A patient who is not registered with a GP practice who signs on for a temporary course of treatment (e.g. while on holiday in the area). Different fees are paid to the GP taking them on for treatment depending on the length of stay and the type of consultation. *See* **Fees and allowances**.

Termination interview (exit interview)

An interview for an individual who is leaving an organisation. The objective of this is for the manager to:

- discover the real reason for the person wanting to resign

- use what they have learned to prevent others from leaving.

T-group

A method of communication/sensitivity training,[1] which became popular in the 1960s, which provides participants with the opportunity to learn more about themselves and their impact on others, and in particular how to improve their interpersonal communication skills.

Training aims to concentrate on the process (feeling) level of communication rather than on content (informational value). Groups are usually leaderless and structureless, although trainers may guide the group, and the dynamic that is created causes individuals to act in characteristic ways. It is these responses that are examined. Feedback received by individuals from other group members forms the main mechanism for learning.

Taking part in T-groups can be a very tense and anxious experience, but it has been shown to lead to an increase in interpersonal skills, to induce change and to encourage more open and flexible behaviour, although whether this behaviour transfers outside the group is not always clear, unless additional therapy work occurs.

1 Cooper CL and Mangham IL (eds) (1971) *T-Groups: a survey of research*. John Wiley & Sons, Chichester.

Thinktank

A colloquial term which has now fallen into official use to denote a research organisation that does pieces of work on specific issues in order to promote specific aims and interests. Thinktanks inform Government and other organisational policy.

www.policylibrary.com/

Third sector

The generic collective name for charity, voluntary, non-government and campaigning organisations.

Time management

The management of limited time in the most effective and efficient way, by the following means:

- having clear objectives

- careful forward planning

- effective organisation

- defining priorities and action

- ability to delegate successfully.

Effective time managers record, conserve and cost the time, as well as managing it.[1]

1 Mullins LJ (1999) *Management and Organisational Behaviour* (5e). Financial Times/Pitman Publishing, London.

Total quality management (TQM)

A particular approach to improved organisational performance and effectiveness. The concept was inspired by Japanese management, and definitions are generally expressed in terms of the following:

- a way of life for the organisation as a whole

- a commitment to total customer satisfaction through a continuous process of improvement

- the contribution and involvement of people.[1]

The principles of total quality management can be summarised as follows:

- management through shared vision

- designing systems to liberate people

- seeking appropriate involvement and co-operation from employees

- making services customer led

- emphasis on quality

- focusing on long-term results

- becoming biased to action.[2]

In TQM, systems are made to fit people. Quick responses are aimed for, and the highest quality equates to the lowest cost. Management empowers rather than controls as people are seen to be key to quality. Human resource management and quality management converge to give total quality. TQM organisations never consider people to be dispensable, but rather they regard them as an asset.

Total quality management applied to healthcare

TQM can provide a strategic focus in the search for a culture of total quality service, which is of particular significance in the public sector. The concept of TQM in healthcare was broadened by Maxwell and McCormick,[3,4] whose premise was that TQM aimed to improve patient care by achieving high standards, reflective practice and risk management, to ensure that healthcare was:

- accessible (no physical, cultural or linguistic barriers, timely)
- appropriate (conforming to legislation, research based, meeting the needs of the population)
- effective (promoting health and recovery, research based, following good practice guidelines)
- efficient (making best use of resources, skills, money, people, buildings and equipment)
- equitable (respectful to all, providing service on the basis of need, not personal characteristics)
- relevant (responsive to the population served, adequate, balanced)
- acceptable (meeting the cultural and religious expectations of users)
- knowledge based (sound and accurate information supporting decision making)
- accountable (principally and financially, outcome based)
- integrative (involving other agencies).

Total quality management does not supplant traditional approaches, but it provides the tools with which traditional medical knowledge can be made to work better. It is concerned with achieving value for money and using resources effectively, and it aims to give workers more opportunity to contribute to the development of services. It harnesses conflict and focuses on improving processes, and it seeks to reduce inter-professional wrangling.

TQM improves not just numbers but also services. It is involved with improvement, not punishment. For example, if patients require more expensive care because they are older and more fragile, this is considered to be a defensible position for clinicians to take.

TQM changes the culture of an organisation in order to achieve tangible benefits for everyone, and it therefore fails if the leaders are uncommitted or suppress their desire for improvement. It aims not just to satisfy the needs of the patient, but to delight them. *See* **Improving Working Lives standard; Quality assurance**.

www.smartman.co.uk
www.qmuk.co.uk

1 Mullins LJ (1999) *Management and Organisational Behaviour* (5e). Financial Times/Pitman Publishing, London.

2 Carlisle J and Parker R (1990) *Beyond Negotiation: redeeming customer–supplier relationships*. John Wiley & Sons, Chichester.

3 Maxwell R (1984) Quality Assessment in health. *BMJ*. **288**: 1470–2.

4 McCormick JS (1981) Effectivenesss and efficiency. *J R Coll Gen Pract*. **31**: 299–302.

Training and Enterprise Council (TEC)

A body that is intended to develop close partnerships between local employers and educational establishments in providing vocational education and training to meet local economic needs.

www.tec.co.uk

Training policy

A policy that demonstrates the organisational attitude to training. Modern policies would ensure that everyone in the organisation was included, and budgets for continuing education would be built into the overall budget. A training policy demonstrates one route to managing the risk of staff failing to perform, adequately as staff training prompts higher standards of care, effectiveness and efficiency, reduces organisational and clinical error, increases staff motivation and reduces costs.

Once written, a training policy would be circulated widely throughout the organisation, and it would address the following:

• ongoing training as a contractual obligation

• widening training options to include wider, non-operational issues (discriminatory practice, quality issues, assertiveness training, time management, teambuilding, etc.)

• the need for an ongoing funding obligation

• the need for requests for training to be taken seriously.

Transactional analysis (TA)

One of the more popular ways of explaining the dynamics of interpersonal communication. Originally developed by Eric Berne,[1] it is now a theory which encompasses personality, perception and communication. Although Berne used it as a psychotherapy method, it has been convincingly used as a training and development tool by organisations.

Transactional analysis has three basic underlying assumptions.

• Personality consists of three ego states which are revealed in distinct ways of behaving – as child, adult and parent. We have preferred ego states.

• All of the events and feelings that we have ever experienced are stored within us and can be replayed.

- A dialogue can be analysed not only in terms of ego state but also in terms of whether the 'transaction' produces a 'complimentary' or 'crossed' reaction.

In the majority of cases at work, transactions are from adult to adult, which encourages rational, logical responses. However, if the child or parent ego states dominate, we can have over-emotional (childlike), critical (critical parent) or over-nurturing (nurturing parent) behaviour re-stimulating unwanted behaviour and leading to resentment. Transactional analysis can be regarded as a useful tool in aiding our understanding of social or difficult work situations and the games that people play both within and outside work organisations.

1 Berne E (1966) *Games People Play*. Penguin, Harmondsworth.

Triage
A process that is used in emergency departments for assessing the relative needs of patients when deciding which of them should be given priority for treatment. It is increasingly being used in GP surgeries to improve access.

www.doh.gov.uk/epcu/

Tuckman BW
Tuckman[1] is best known for his theory that groups pass through different stages in their development, classically demonstrating *forming, storming, norming, performing* and *deforming* behaviour. *See* **Group**.

Task	Activity	Features
Forming dependence	Define the nature and boundaries of task	• Group members concerned with why they are there
		• Interpersonal relationships and boundaries are tested
		• Dependency on leader develops
		• Uncertainty and anxiety are felt
		• Commitment to group is low
		• Grumbling about task
		• Behaviour meandering and ineffective
		• Suspicion of task and each other
		• Testing and confronting behaviour
		• Hesitating or avoiding task
Storming	Questioning the value of exercise	• Conflict occurs
		• Members resist task and group influences
		• Arguments about what the purpose of the group is

(continued overleaf)

Task	Activity	Features
		• Members may undermine each other and the leader
		• Authority is questioned
		• People jockey for position within the group
		• Challenging behaviour
		• Experimenting with hostility, aggression, frustration, rivalry, resentment, opposition
		• Defensive behaviour
Norming	Opening up and inviting	• New roles adopted by group members
		• Resistance to group overcome
		• Expression of intimate, personal opinions around the goal are expressed
		• Feelings of belonging to the group and identification with the group as a unit emerge
		• Commitment goes up
		• Defining tasks
		• Evaluating
		• Mutually supportive
		• Showing unity and consensus
		• Liking each other
Performing/ interdependence	Effectively pursuing the task	• Group energy directed towards completion of task
		• Creative problem solving
		• Roles become flexible and functional
		• Frequent and mutual contributions
		• Interpersonal issues now disregarded, or sorted, or used as a tool to achieve group goals
		• Feel safe and confident
		• Achieving
Ending/mourning	Facing the loss of the group experience	• Denial of ending
		• Termination phase
		• Group dissolves because task is completed
		• Group resists disintegration through social contact
		• Fantasising about the 'good old days' may begin, idealising the past history of the group – this may occur when interpersonal issues prevent the group from accomplishing its task
		• Bargaining, anger or depression may occur
		• Group may perform rituals

1 Tuckman BW (1965) Developmental sequences in small groups. *Psychol Bull.* **63**: 384–99.

Two-tier workforce
The situation that is created when a private company takes over the running of a public service (e.g. as has happened in the case of laundry workers and cleaners in hospitals). Workers who were previously employed in the public sector have their terms and conditions protected by law, but usually those newly joining currently have no such defence.

www.unison.org.uk/

U

Unison

One of the largest public sector unions, that represents many millions of healthcare workers, from administrative, clerical, ambulance, nursing and midwifery, pathology and senior management workers through to scientific, technical, dental and allied health professional staff. Some sectors, such as doctors, speech and language therapists and psychologists, have their own representation elsewhere.

www.unison.org.uk/

User involvement

Involving patients in service developments or their own treatment. The NHS requires that healthcare organisations seek to identify and meet the health needs of the population that they serve. Not all doctors are committed to this. User involvement saves the NHS money in the long term, as it helps patients to take responsibility for their own health through patient education. People who take an active interest in developing healthcare develop a broader understanding of health and disease, and they begin to understand that health is affected by the following factors:

- social and economic factors – poverty, unemployment, social exclusion
- environmental factors – air and water quality, housing, food and safety
- lifestyle choices – diet, physical activity, use of alcohol and drugs, sexual behaviour
- access to good-quality services – education, social care, health, local transport, leisure facilities
- fixed factors – age, sex, genes.

Through being involved in discussions about healthcare provision, the hope is that service users will begin to develop responsibility for their health, and will become less dependent on healthcare providers to meet their needs. Their involvement is particularly useful and welcome when making difficult or unpalatable rationing decisions.

Most healthcare providers need to develop further ways of working in partnership with patients. They could achieve this by the following means:

- patient participation groups
- informal feedback systems (e.g. suggestions boxes)
- health panels
- open meetings
- discussion/focus groups
- rapid appraisal (gathering information from key local informants)
- disease support groups
- interviews
- opinion polls
- neighbourhood forums
- practice-based annual surveys
- appraisal systems (e.g. customer panels)
- postal questionnaires.

See **Patient participation**.

For some more ideas and a broader understanding of patient participation, see the following:

- Lilley R (1999) *The PCG Toolkit* (2e). Radcliffe Medical Press, Oxford.

V

Validity

The extent to which research, experiments or audit measure what they purport to measure.

Variable

In an experiment, the experimenter investigates the relationship between two things or *quantities* by deliberately producing a change in one of them and observing the change in the other. These quantities in which changes take place are known as variables.

The variable which the experimenter deliberately manipulates is called the *independent variable*. The variable in which we are looking for consequent changes is called the *dependent variable*. It is important that the experimenter is aware of and controls as many of the variables as possible during the course of their observation.

The difficulty with much clinical research is that there are inevitably too many variables involved when studying change over time in human subjects. The experimenter may change one variable (e.g. the amount of medicine administered), and make inferences about the relationship between cause and effect. Although attempts are made to match subjects by for example, age and sex, each subject differs physiologically, psychologically and with regard to social class, what they have just eaten or what they ate yesterday, their unique genetic make-up, previous illness or predisposition to illness, etc. It is virtually impossible to control all of these variables, or to control any interaction that may occur between the variables.

Thus the type and extent of the variables are considered in experimental design, and the statistical significance is calculated once any change occurs. *See* **Experiment**.

VDU assessment

A health and safety assessment that employers are obliged to undertake using the 1992 Management of Health and Safety at Work regulations. This includes assessing computer equipment used by employees, to ensure that its use does not cause illness or injury such as repetitive strain injury (RSI) or eye strain.

The 'EC Six-Pack' gives a set of assessments which include investigating the health and safety of display screen equipment. This advises staff on ways to avoid health problems associated with VDUs (e.g. eyestrain, neck and back pain, hand, wrist and elbow pain, tension headaches, dizziness, nausea, tension and irritability). It also recommends that managers advise or pay staff who spend a significant amount of time working 'on screen' to:

- have regular eye examinations
- arrange their work area so as to provide good lighting and minimise glare
- arrange and adjust their office furniture so as to minimise strain on their eyes, neck and back
- take frequent breaks from using the equipment.

See **Health and safety**.

www.hawnhs.hda-online.org.uk/

Violence at work

The most common forms of violence at work are against people and property. They include attacks and assaults, thefts of equipment or personal possessions, and vandalism.

Various methods have been recommended for reducing violence at work and for improving security, beginning with a risk assessment. This involves identifying the risks, and then creating a plan outlining what to do in order to minimise further such events and ensure the health and safety of everyone and everything in the organisation.

Primary care organisations and local crime prevention officers provide advice on ways to improve external and internal security by introducing sophisticated locking and alarm systems and ensuring that staff have adequate business and security awareness and are trained in customer awareness. Primary care organisations will also give financial support to GP practices that wish to improve their security, and they support retainer schemes for GPs who are willing to take on seeing violent patients for their colleagues locally. *See* **Zero tolerance**.

Vocational Training Scheme (VTS)

The training that GP registrars have to undertake before they enter general practice. *See* **Registrar**.

Voluntary Training Scheme

The training that doctors undertake during their registration period in preparation for becoming a GP. *See* **Registrar**.

Volunteer

A person who gives a portion of their time, or a period of time in a year, without payment to an organisation as a worker or helper. National Government organisations and charities sometimes reimburse volunteers' travel and related expenses.

www.volunteering.org.uk/

Vulnerable children

Disadvantaged children who would benefit from extra help from public agencies to allow them to make the most of their opportunities in life.

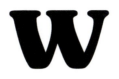

Waiting-list

The number of patients who are waiting for treatment on the NHS. *See* **Waiting-time**.

www.doh.gov.uk/waitingtimes/booklist

Waiting-time

The length of time for which patients wait for treatment on the NHS. It normally refers to the period between a GP referral and an outpatient attendance, or the time that elapses between being put on the waiting-list and the date of admission to hospital. *See* **Waiting-list**.

www.doh.gov.uk/nhsplan/

Walk-in centres

Nurse-led drop-in centres managed by the NHS that provide minor treatments, self-help advice and information on the NHS, social services and other local healthcare organisations. Set up in response to the 1999 NHS Plan, they were designed to improve patient access and reduce the GP workload. Staffed by nurses and GPs, they deal mainly with minor illnesses and are particularly popular with commuters and shoppers, as they are often based within easy access of public transport terminals and shops. Continuity of care will remain a problem until patient records are all electronically held. Preliminary research shows that the majority (68%) of patients who use walk-in centres are non-registered patients living in a different area, possibly those who cannot access their own GP easily due to work or other commitments. The vast majority (98%) of patients need either advice or treatment that can be prescribed by a nurse.

www.doh.gov.uk/nhswalkincentres/

Weighted capitation

The resource allocation formula that distributes NHS funds and aims to target resources at the most needy areas. Using basic indicators of need, the formula sets a target allocation for each region. Ministers decide annually how quickly authorities should be moved towards this target.

www.doh.gov.uk/

Whistleblowing

The disclosure by an employee or professional of genuine concerns about crimes, illegality, negligence, miscarriages of justice, or danger to health and safety or the environment, and the cover-up of any of these, whether committed by the employer or by a fellow employee.

If anyone has serious concerns about clinical malpractice, health and safety breaches or misuse of public funds, the procedure for raising these concerns is termed whistle-blowing. The Public Interest Disclosure Act 1998 aims to promote accountability and openness within organisations. Whistleblowers have legal protection under this act. It provides a framework that enables anyone who has suspicions that serious mal-practice is occurring to report their concerns in a considered and responsible way. As it is particularly difficult for anyone within a small organisation to raise such concerns, any policy that is written should reflect the dynamics of the employer–employee relationship, so that anyone should feel able to address legitimate concerns without fear of censure or of appearing disloyal. All employees, including agency staff, staff under contract for services and general practitioners, should be covered by such a policy. The latter will cover when to use a whistleblowing procedure, which pro-cedure to use for which issue, what to do, how to protect staff from victimisation and how the organisation will deal with any concerns that are raised.

For further information, contact any of the following:

- Health and Safety Executive. Tel: 020 7717 6000.
- National Audit Office. Tel: 020 7798 7000.
- Serious Fraud Office. Tel: 020 7239 7272.
- NHS fraud reporting number: 08702 400100.

See **Fraud**.

www.hmso.gov.uk/

White Paper

A statement of policy issued by the Government. White Papers are usually preceded by a consultative Green Paper, and often form the foundation of new legislation.

www.explore.parliament.uk/search/

Workforce Development Confederations

Local bodies that work under the national umbrella organisation, the National Work-force Development Board, which have taken on the role of monitoring and planning the local primary healthcare workforce. They develop workforce plans at local level by looking at local skill mix in detail, and they promote and assist individuals who wish to start or return (after a gap) to work within the NHS. *See* **National Workforce Development Board**.

www.wdconfeds.org/
www.nhs.careers.nhs.uk/

Workforce planning

The NHS Plan (Human Resource Strategy 'Working Together') makes it a require-ment for employing health organisations to consider how they are going to meet changing clinical demands. Workforce planning requires the organisation to think through the key issues that need to be considered in planning ahead to meet the needs of a given population. This involves analysing existing staff resources by keeping a staff inventory, considering the impact of losses and changes/developments among the staff, forecasting the future needs of and demands on the practice, and reconciling the supply of and demand for staff.

The workforce issues that require broader consideration include local economic and labour market analyses and looking at current trends across the local health economy (e.g. the creation of primary care trusts). The focus on staff addresses any recruitment difficulties, skills shortages, high turnover rates and staff retention prob-lems, as well as professional aspirations and jealousies and any new professional regulations.

Workforce planning:

- is linked to the local Health Improvement Programme

- is directly related to service developments

- supports plans to develop local services

- covers all staff groups

- is focused on changes in service levels and delivery patterns.

The main benefits for forward planning in this way lie in being able to apply tighter, more credible criteria to funding applications, and to be better prepared if staff shortages arise. Planners would consider the following:

- the treatments that occur in the sector under scrutiny

- the skills required

- the evidence base

- the predicted delivery models

- any foreseen impacts of new technology/treatments

- the way in which these new models affect staffing numbers/roles/working arrangements

- the staff groups involved in the patient pathways

- which of these staff groups may now, or in the future, be employed

- whether anyone else could provide the same service

- if so, the training and supervision that they would require.

A workforce plan would review the current staff and service provision and then present a chart specifying current workforce numbers and costs, grades, skills, training needs and age profiles. *See* **Skill mix review; Staff profile; Workforce Development Confederations**.

Working rights

Formal recognition and respect for people's needs and expectations at work by an organisation. These rights may be written as a code of good practice, and would include the following:

- full observance of all legal matters relating to employment

- just treatment

- fair reward for work done

- job security

- opportunities for training and development

- opportunities for career development

- a pleasant and safe working environment.

See **Staff charter**.

World Health Organization

An international non-governmental organisation, created in June 1946, which aims to promote health and healthcare worldwide. It co-ordinates international health initiatives and work on the prevention and control of disease, advises governments on strengthening health services, and also promotes the following:

- biomedical and health services research

- improved hygiene, housing, nutrition, sanitation and working conditions.

www.who.int/

Write-up
Applying the methodology used when writing up experiments to the presentation of reports. The following sections are included:

- *title*

- *introduction* – a general statement of the problem or subject under discussion, continuing with a review of any other work in the area and any associated explanations or theories. It concludes with the hypothesis (what may be anticipated as an outcome)

- *method* – in this section the reader is told exactly what was done, what information was collected and who was involved (e.g. the experimental design, subjects, apparatus or material and procedure)

- *results* – the presentation and description of results, displayed simply and clearly, preferably using titled and cross-referenced tables and graphs

- *discussion* – the results of any analysis, a description of their bearing on the original hypotheses, the relevance of the results in theoretical and practical terms, and suggestions for further work that is needed. A description of the limitations of the usefulness of the results should be included

- *references*.

Z

Zero tolerance

A Government-sponsored campaign that promotes the message to NHS employees and their patients that violence towards NHS staff will not be tolerated. The Zero Tolerance campaign was set up to address the growing problem of patient violence in Accident and Emergency and primary care services, especially GP surgeries.

Every primary care trust is working towards having in place systems and structures to ensure that all of their contracted employees, GPs and their staff are protected from violent patients. *See* **Violence at work**.

How to Think and Intervene Like an REBT Therapist

Windy Dryden

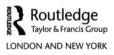
Routledge
Taylor & Francis Group

LONDON AND NEW YORK

First published 2009 by Routledge
27 Church Road, Hove, East Sussex BN3 2FA

Simultaneously published in the USA and Canada
by Routledge
270 Madison Avenue, New York, NY 10016

Routledge is an imprint of the Taylor & Francis Group, an Informa business

Typeset in Times by Garfield Morgan, Swansea, West Glamorgan
Printed and bound in Great Britain by TJ International Ltd, Padstow,
Cornwall
Cover design by Andy Ward

This publication has been produced with paper manufactured to strict
environmental standards and with pulp derived from sustainable forests.

British Library Cataloguing in Publication Data
A catalogue record for this book is available from the British Library

Library of Congress Cataloging-in-Publication Data
Dryden, Windy.
    How to think and intervene like an REBT therapist / Windy Dryden.
        p. cm.
    Includes bibliographical references and index.
    ISBN 978-0-415-48793-1 (hardback) – ISBN 978-0-415-48795-5 (pbk.)
1. Rational emotive behavior therapy. 2. Therapist and patient. 3.
Counselor and client. I. Title.
    RC489.R3D7868 2009
    616.89'14–dc22
                                                            2008048059

ISBN: 978-0-415-48793-1 (hbk)
ISBN: 978-0-415-48795-5 (pbk)

Trainee B, on the other hand, is so mindful of making an inter-personal connection with Lisa that he takes pains to show her that he understands her very accurately from her frame of reference. In doing so, the trainee uses the client's 'A'–'C' language without qualifying it in the way that the trained REBT therapist did. This had the unintended effect of reinforcing the 'A'–'C' causal model in Lisa's mind that the trained therapist avoided.

In summary, the trained REBT therapist uses two important concepts, one interpersonal and the other more technical, in a flexible way and in doing so he shows that he is mindful of the therapeutic context. On the other hand, both trainees use only one of the two relevant concepts and run into difficulties because they are not making use of the other concept when it is relevant to do so.

Forming an educational connection with a client and informed consent

At some point early in the process of REBT the client needs to be informed about the nature of this approach to counselling, so that she can give her informed consent to proceed. This does not mean that the therapist will deliver a lecture on REBT (although some REBT therapists might do this, e.g. Woods, 1991). What it means is that the client will be given some indication about what REBT is likely to entail for her and what she can reasonably expect from her REBT therapist.

While REBT is an approach to therapy that values openness and being explicit, just how much information a client is provided about REBT involves the therapist making a delicate judgement that will be influenced by a number of factors including:

- *The nature of the client's problem(s).* If the therapist is plan-ning to use a client problem to explain the REBT approach, it is easier to say how he may tackle some problems rather than others. The more explicit the client's problem, the more likely it is that the therapist can explain how he will tackle it using REBT.
- *The distress level of the client.* It is not a good idea for the therapist to inform a client about REBT when that client is very distressed. When the client is experiencing such distress,

this will interfere with her cognitive processing of the information the therapist is giving her.

- *The intelligence level of the client.* Here it is important that the therapist does not:

  a confuse a client with information that is too complicated for her to process or

  b patronise a client by giving her simplified information when she is able to process more complicated material.

Educating clients about REBT: a written example

What follows is information that I send to people who contact me by email enquiring about my approach to therapy. As I do not know at that stage what problem or problems a person will be seeking help for, the information that I provide is necessarily general.

There are a number of approaches to counselling and it is important that you understand something of the one that I practise which is known as Rational Emotive Behaviour Therapy (REBT). REBT is based on an old idea attributed to Epictetus, a Roman philosopher, who said that 'Men are disturbed not by things, but by their views of things'. In REBT, we have modified this and say that 'People are disturbed not by things, but by the rigid and extreme beliefs that they hold about things.' Once people have disturbed themselves they then try to get rid of their disturbed feelings in ways that ultimately serve to maintain their problems.

As an REBT therapist I will help you to identify, examine and change the rigid and extreme beliefs that we argue underpin your emotional problems and to develop alternative flexible and non-extreme beliefs. I will also help you to examine the ways in which you have tried to help yourself that haven't worked and encourage you to develop and practise more effective longer-lasting strategies.

At the beginning of counselling, I will teach you a framework which will help you to break down your problems one at a time into their constituent parts. I will also teach you a variety of methods for examining and changing your rigid and extreme beliefs and a variety of ways of helping to consolidate and strengthen your alternative flexible and non-extreme beliefs.

As therapy proceeds, I will help you to take increasing responsibility for using these methods and my ultimate aim is to help you to become your own therapist. As this happens, we will meet less frequently until you feel you can cope on your own.

and I suggested that we needed to think about having a vegetarian option and he just lost it. He told me that he was organising the food and that I should keep my nose out of it. He made me so angry when he said that.

[Trainee B's thinking: I know that Lisa has made an 'A'–'C' statement which I need to correct, but now is not the time to do it. I have to show her that I understand her from her frame of reference first.]

Trainee B: So, Lisa . . . Your fiancé made you feel angry when he told you to mind your own business about having a vegetarian option on the wedding menu.

Lisa: That's right he really pissed me off.

Let me now compare the thinking and intervention of the trained therapist with those of the two trainees.

The trained therapist makes a compromise between the interpersonal connection issue of showing the client that he understands her and the technical issue of helping the client to see the difference between the causal, 'A'–'C' model of anger and the correlational model of anger where 'A' is not seen as causing 'C'. The therapist knows that he needs to deal with this issue at some point, but judges that other considerations are more important at this early stage of counselling, i.e. making an interpersonal connection with the client through empathy, but – and this is the important point – without reinforcing the client's 'A'–'C' causal model of anger.

By contrast, both trainees lack the experience to take this middle ground position. They both take REBT theory too seriously. Trainee A knows that the client has made an 'A'–'C' statement and knows that he is 'supposed' to use this to teach REBT's 'ABC' model of emotions. However, he seems to think that he has to do this there and then without regard to other considerations. Indeed, these considerations are not present in trainee A's thinking or intervention. Ignoring the importance of making an interpersonal connection with Lisa results in her feeling, rightly or wrongly, that the trainee is against her.

than reinforcing her causal model (e.g. 'He made you angry . . .'). If the therapist considered it important to mention her causal model as a way of conveying understanding, it is important that he stresses that this is her view of events not how things were in reality. He can do this by saying something like:

- 'As you saw it, he made you angry . . .'
- 'From your perspective, he made you angry.'

Note, however, in none of the responses made or attributed to the trained therapist, did he challenge Lisa's causal model of emotions. He will do this later when he considers he has made a sufficiently good interpersonal connection with Lisa.

Now I will consider how two trainees might think about and respond to the same client statement.

Lisa and trainee A

Lisa: Well, the other day we were talking about the catering arrangements for our wedding menu and I suggested that we needed to think about having a vegetarian option and he just lost it. He told me that he was organising the food and that I should keep my nose out of it. He made me so angry when he said that.

[Trainee A's thinking: Oh! Lisa has made an 'A'–'C' statement, I'd better challenge that.]

Trainee A: Actually in this type of therapy we say that he doesn't make you angry. Rather, you make yourself angry about his behaviour.

Lisa: So it's my fault and not his. That's what my fiancé says. Now I have two people against me!

Lisa and trainee B

Lisa: Well, the other day we were talking about the catering arrangements for our wedding menu

- How can I structure the session and get the client to use this structure?
- When is the best time for me to use the 'ABCs' of REBT to assess a specific example of the client's problem?

An example

Here is an example of how a trained REBT therapist and trainee might differ in their thinking and interventions in one of the above areas.

Lisa and a trained therapist

Lisa is discussing her relationship with her fiancé in her first session of REBT. In this segment she is working with a trained REBT therapist.

> *Lisa:*   Well, the other day we were talking about the catering arrangements for our wedding menu and I suggested that we needed to think about having a vegetarian option and he just lost it. He told me that he was organising the food and that I should keep my nose out of it. He made me so angry when he said that.
>
> *[REBTer's thinking: I want to show Lisa that I understand her from her frame of reference, but here is also an opportunity to teach her about the 'B'–'C' connection and correct her 'A'–'C' thinking. I really haven't shown that I understand her so that is my priority and as I do so I will avoid reinforcing 'A'–'C' thinking, but I don't want to go into a big spiel about the 'B'– 'C' connection yet.]*
>
> *REBTer:*   So, Lisa ... You felt angry when your fiancé told you to mind your own business about having a vegetarian option on the wedding menu.

Note that the REBT therapist uses the phrase 'You felt angry about . . .' In doing so he puts forward a correlational relationship between Lisa's fiancé's behaviour and her feelings of anger rather real risk that the client experiences concept burn-out, which means that because she hears a rational concept many times, either she becomes bored with this concept and/or it loses its meaning for her. To combat this, the experienced REBT therapist endeavours to enliven the process and keep the client engaged in REBT by using the same concept in novel ways. As this is an advanced therapist skill it lies beyond the scope of this book, but it is worthy of a mention in a comprehensive overview of therapeutic engagement (see Dryden, 1986a).

Forming an interpersonal connection with a client

When a client comes to a first session with a trained REBT therapist, that therapist engages in the following kind of thinking which often takes the form of questions since the therapist knows very little about the client at that point. I will also present the kind of thinking that a trainee might engage in on the same issue.

The thinking of a trained REBT therapist

Although the trained REBT therapist has been schooled in the active-directive, structured nature of REBT, he also knows that he needs to be very mindful of more generic working alliance considerations while attempting to form an interpersonal connection with the client (Dryden, 1999a).

To reflect these dual concerns the following thoughts are typical of a trained REBT therapist at the outset of therapy.

- How can I encourage the client to talk while I keep the session as structured as possible?
- How can I show the client that I understand what she is saying without reinforcing 'A' causes 'C' statements?

The thinking of a trainee

By contrast, the trainee tends to favour technical thinking over interpersonal connection thinking, as shown below:

1   An interpersonal connection
2   An educational connection
3   An outcome connection
4   An enlivened involved connection.

Engagement I: an interpersonal connection

It is important that the therapist involves the client as a full participant in the process of change. Making an interpersonal connection with the client is important, particularly at the beginning of the process. From the client's point of view such a connection is enhanced when she considers that the therapist:

- Encourages her to express herself
- Understands her
- Accepts her.

Engagement II: an educational connection

This second connection points to the client understanding the main salient features of REBT such as the 'ABC' model of psychological disturbance and health and the roles that she and her therapist are likely to perform during the therapy (Dryden, 2006). This educational element is a prerequisite of the client giving informed consent to proceed, for the client cannot give her consent if she has not been informed.

Engagement III: outcome connection

All therapy is purposive in that both client and therapist are mindful or should be mindful of the outcome of their meetings. In putting forward his reformulation of the concept of the working alliance, Bordin (1979) argued that therapy is enhanced when the client and therapist agree on the client's goals for change. I will discuss this issue in Chapter 7.

Engagement IV: an enlivened involved connection

REBT has a number of concepts that the client is likely to become familiar with during the therapeutic process. As a result there is a

Chapter 1

Thinking and intervening related to engaging clients in REBT

Whatever the technical merits of Rational Emotive Behaviour Therapy (REBT), it should not be forgotten that techniques employed by both the therapist and the client are done so within a relationship that forms and develops between them. There is a great deal of research pointing to the importance of the quality of this relationship to the outcome for the client in all forms of psychotherapy (Wampold, 2001) and REBT therapists generally acknowledge this importance. Indeed, REBT's position on the place of the relationship in this approach to psychotherapy has not changed over the years (Dryden, 1987).

It is that a good relationship between therapist and client is desirable, but neither necessary nor sufficient for therapeutic change to take place. It is important to note that this view is from an REBT theoretical perspective and clients may have a different view. It may be that clients are more concerned about how they will get on with their counsellors and how helpful they think they will be to them than the REBT position recognises in its view on the place of the relationship in REBT.

Having said this, it is my view that unless the therapist engages the client in the process of REBT at the outset and helps sustain the client's engagement throughout this process, then he will face an uphill struggle to help the client and perhaps more importantly to encourage the client to help herself.

The concept of engagement in REBT

I have used the term 'engagement' here deliberately because it captures four important connections between therapist and client within REBT:

distinctive features of REBT (Dryden, 2008), REBT therapists do differ amongst themselves on a number of issues, a fact that was brought out in a book I edited entitled *Idiosyncratic Rational Emotive Behaviour Therapy* (Dryden, 2002).

Thus, while I have been mindful of the danger that I am really writing about how *I* think and intervene as an REBT therapist, I do acknowledge that this work is influenced by my personal views about REBT. Please bear this in mind as you read this work. Note also that for clarity I have used 'he' for the therapist and 'she' for general references to the client in this work; this usage is not meant to suggest that therapists are more likely to be male or clients female.

Windy Dryden
London and Eastbourne
September 2008

In the course of giving feedback to one such participant, I found myself saying that it was important that the person think like an REBT therapist while conducting the peer counselling session. This idea seemed to resonate with the rest of the membership of that supervision group and also more widely with participants in the practicum as a whole. In particular, participants were keen to learn how to think like an REBT therapist before intervening like an REBT therapist. This level of interest provided the impetus for the present work.

So what I plan to do in this work is to articulate the thinking that REBT therapists engage in at various junctures in the therapeutic process and show how this thinking affects their interventions. In doing so, I will compare the thinking and interventions characteristic of a skilful, trained REBT therapist with those of a trainee making errors characteristic of a person at the introductory level. Please bear in mind that by adopting this approach I am not saying that all trained REBT therapists are skilful and all trainees make the errors outlined in this book. What I am saying and attempt to show throughout this book is that trained REBT therapists make better use of the working alliance between them and their clients than do trainees and apply REBT theory more flexibly than trainees. The latter tend to neglect the alliance in their thinking and interventions and tend to stick rigorously and sometimes rigidly to therapeutic guidelines they learn from REBT texts and during the course of REBT training practica.

Although I will touch on issues of some complexity in this book, my main goal is to write for those who have recently been introduced to REBT rather than for seasoned REBT practitioners. As such, I will not include such advanced issues as helping clients to generalise change and ending the process of REBT.

When I told a colleague about this project, they said that I was really writing on the theme 'How to think and intervene like Windy Dryden'. While this was partly said in jest, it also had a serious point. Although I am very classical in my approach to teaching REBT at the primary practicum level in that I follow closely the teachings of the founder of REBT, Albert Ellis, I have my own emphases even at this level. For example, I am particularly careful to help practicum participants keenly distinguish between rational beliefs and irrational beliefs, using language that brings out the essential differences between these two sets of beliefs (see Chapter 5). While there is a consensus of views about the more classical,

Introduction

This work was conceived during a supervision session that I was conducting at the January 2008 Primary Practicum on Rational Emotive Behaviour Therapy (REBT) at the Albert Ellis Institute in New York. The primary practicum is often the first extended training experience that people have in REBT and as such it is important that they are exposed to the fundamentals of REBT theory and practice. The teaching is geared to this end, but even more important are the opportunities afforded participants to practise REBT under supervision. This is done by supervised peer counselling which is a cornerstone of the practicum.

In supervised peer counselling participants counsel one another in pairs live in front of peers in their supervision group and in front of the group's supervisor. When adopting the role of client, participants are instructed to discuss a real-life emotional or behavioural problem, an issue that they really want to address. And when they adopt the role of counsellor, participants are instructed to identify a specific example of their 'client's' problem and work with this using the 'ABCs' of REBT that they have been taught in the lecture sessions.

In these peer counselling sessions, the supervisor's task is to help the counsellor practise REBT when dealing with the client's problem. Participants in these practica have usually had prior training in general cognitive behaviour therapy (CBT) and/or in other approaches to counselling. Particularly when they have had training in general CBT, participants taking the role of counsellor tend to respond to their 'clients' using strategies and techniques derived from general CBT rather than from the classical REBT approach they have signed up to learn and that they have been taught in the practicum.

Contents

Educating clients about REBT: comparing the thinking and interventions of a trained REBT therapist with those of a trainee

It is not always possible or desirable to send a client brief written material about REBT prior to a first session. Therefore, the therapist needs to find an appropriate time to give the client sufficient information about REBT that will enable her to give her informed consent about proceeding.

Until a person has given her informed consent to proceed with REBT, she is best considered to be an applicant for a service rather than a client of that service. From this perspective, the person becomes a client when she gives her informed consent to proceed (Garvin and Seabury, 1997).

Karen has come to therapy for help with her procrastination problem. In the first session, she has talked about her problem in general terms and the impact it has had on her life and she has given a specific example of her problem. In that example, it emerges that Karen procrastinates when she thinks she won't be able to understand a topic.

[REBTer's thinking: Now would be a good time to educate the client a little about REBT and get her informed consent to proceed. But I first want to make sure that she is ready for such an explanation. If so, I want to stress that she has other alternatives should she think that REBT is not an approach for her.]

REBTer: Would it be helpful for me to outline the approach that I'll be using to help you so you can judge whether or not it's for you?

Karen: That would be good.

REBTer: In doing so, I want to stress that this approach is not the only one on offer, but it's the one that I use. If it's not for you we can talk about alternatives and a possible referral. OK?

Karen: Fine.

[REBTer's thinking: I could talk about REBT in general terms, but I want my explanation to be more closely related to the client's problem. Let's see how she responds when I do so.]

REBTer:	You mentioned in your example that you procrastinate when you think that you may not understand a topic. Is that right?
Karen:	Yes.
REBTer:	My approach would help you to look carefully at this and use what we call the 'ABC' model. 'A' is what you are responding to in the situation. So, here your 'A' would be your prediction that you won't understand what you are about to read straight away. 'C' represents your feelings or in this case your behaviour in the situation. So here 'C' is procrastination. Are you with me so far?
Karen:	Yes.
REBTer:	Now we argue in this model that 'A' does not cause 'C'. The missing ingredient is 'B' or your beliefs about 'A'. A belief can either be flexible or rigid. Now a flexible belief in the situation you have outlined might be: 'I want to understand the material straight away before I get down to work, but it's not necessary that I do so' and a rigid belief would be: 'I must understand the material straight away before I get down to work'.

[REBTer's thinking: I need to involve Karen here and I'll do so by seeing if she can see the different effects of holding these two beliefs.]

REBTer:	Which of these two beliefs will lead to procrastination and which to getting down to work?
Karen:	Well, the rigid belief would lead to procrastination.
REBTer:	Right. So a major goal in REBT would be to help you to identify rigid beliefs like this that lead to procrastination and to develop flexible alternative beliefs. There are many ways of helping you to do that but that is the major strategy. What do you think?
Karen:	That makes sense. So we don't have to go into my childhood then?

REBTer: Only if it is relevant to do so.
Karen: That's a relief.

[REBTer's thinking: I think that Karen is ready to give her informed consent to proceed, but I need to see if she has any questions first that I can answer.]

REBTer: Do you have any questions about what I've said?
Karen: No, I think it's straightforward.
REBTer: So would you like to proceed with me using this approach?
Karen: Yes.

Now let's see how a trainee might think and respond in the same situation.

Trainee: Would it be helpful for me to outline the approach that I'll be using to help you so you can judge whether or not it's for you?
Karen: Yes it would.

[Trainee's thinking: Great! I'll outline the basics of REBT and then we can get going.]

Trainee: What we do in REBT is to help you to identify, challenge and change the irrational beliefs that underlie your problems and help you to change them to rational beliefs. How does that sound?
Karen: I am not sure. I already know that I am being irrational when I procrastinate, but knowing that doesn't help me. In fact it makes me feel worse.

[Trainee's thinking: Now Karen is revealing her problem about her problem. I know in REBT we should start with that, so I will target that for change first.]

Trainee: What are you telling yourself to feel worse about your procrastination?
Karen: I'm sorry I don't understand your question.

Let's compare the thinking and intervention of the trained therapist with the thinking and intervention of the trainee.

The trained therapist uses the client's problem and the factors that the client has already revealed about it when outlining his likely approach in using REBT. He puts flesh on the bones as it were. By contrast, the trainee does not do this. Rather he outlines a general approach to REBT using the language of irrationality and rationality. Taken out of context, it is a risk to use such words and in the trainee's example it clearly backfires. Note, in contrast, that the trained therapist does not use this language. Rather he contrasts a rigid belief which he takes from what the client has said about her specific problem and contrasts this with its flexible alternative. Most importantly, he helps the client to see the different effects these different beliefs are likely to have on the client's relevant behaviour (i.e. a rigid belief leads to procrastination while a flexible belief leads to non-procrastination). Helping the client to understand the relevance of these beliefs to her problem and healthy alternative (or goal) increases the chances that she will give her informed consent to proceed. This she does in response to the trained therapist's approach.

When we consider more closely the trainee's thinking and responses in this situation, we see that while he understands the need to explain REBT to the client, his thinking and responses lack the sophistication of the trained therapist. Thus, as explained above, he does not tailor his explanation to the client's particular problem and his thinking shows that he is not aware of the need to do so.

When giving his general explanation, the trainee emphasises the role of irrational beliefs in people's problems and the need to change these to rational beliefs. While this is theoretically correct, the client is unlikely to understand what this means and Karen reveals this very point when she says in reply that she knows she is being irrational when she procrastinates, but this only makes things worse. The trainee does not seem to understand that the two are at cross purposes even though it is clear that they are using the term 'irrational' in different ways (Dryden, 1986b).

At this point, the trainee probably needs to backtrack and use different language to explain the REBT approach. Instead the trainee takes the client's statement that she feels worse when she realises that her procrastination behaviour is irrational as evidence that she has a 'meta-emotional' problem and his thinking and response show that he allows himself to get sidetracked by beginning to assess this secondary problem.

At this point, the trainee has departed from his main task, which is to inform the client about REBT and elicit the client's informed consent about proceeding, Indeed, by beginning to assess what he sees as the client's meta-emotional problem (feeling worse when she is aware that she is acting irrationally), the trainee has actually proceeded with therapy without gaining such informed consent. By contrast, the trained therapist clearly asks for and gets such consent.

Thinking and intervening related to therapeutic style

Different approaches to counselling and psychotherapy make different recommendations concerning the style to be adopted by their practitioners (Dryden, 2007). REBT practitioners are advised to adopt a therapeutic style characterised by the following:

- being active
- being structured
- creating a focus
- being specific
- directing the client to salient issues.

Having said this, it is important that the therapist is mindful of the working alliance between him and his client and to recognise that there may be times when the therapist has to be more passive and less active to preserve this alliance.

I am going to demonstrate the thinking and interventions of a trained REBT therapist concerning the need for specificity and compare these with the thinking and interventions of a trainee in the same area.

Thinking and intervening related to specificity

There is a popular game called Cluedo where players have to guess the identity of a murderer and say which implement he or she used and where he or she committed the crime. This serves as a good model for REBT therapists who often need to encourage their clients to be specific in order to help them effectively. Such specificity is important, for example, if a detailed specific 'ABC' assessment is to be made.

I will first discuss how a trained REBT therapist thinks and intervenes when a client is not specific enough in her disclosure and then consider how a trainee might think and intervene in similar circumstances.

Kay has come to therapy because she is anxious about her health. Her trained REBT therapist has asked for a specific example of her problem.

REBTer:	Can you give me a specific example of your anxiety about your health?
Kay:	Well I get anxious whenever I find a lump or lesion on my body.

[REBTer's thinking: I need to find a way of encouraging Kay to be more specific. Let me see if she is currently anxious about her health.]

REBTer:	Is there anything you are currently anxious about regarding your health?
Kay:	Yes.
REBTer:	What are you anxious about at this time?
Kay:	I am anxious about a skin lesion on my arm.

[REBTer's thinking: Now let's see if I can get a specific example of her anxiety about her skin lesion.]

REBTer:	Can you tell me of a specific episode of your skin lesion anxiety?
Kay:	I can't think of one. There are so many.

[REBTer's thinking: Let me see if asking her to look at the lesion now leads to her making herself feel anxious.]

REBTer:	Kay, would you feel anxious if you looked at the lesion now?
Kay:	Very much so.

[REBTer's thinking; It would be great if she would agree to look at it now. It would help me be accurate in my assessment of her problem. Let me explain what I am doing first.]

REBTer: Kay, having a specific example of your anxiety will help me enormously to understand the factors that comprise this anxiety. For that reason would you agree to look at the lesion now?

Kay: Well, I'd rather not. I'm too scared to.

[REBTer's thinking: Well, I've got my specific example now since Kay is potentially feeling anxious here and now and presumably is dealing with that anxiety by avoiding looking at the lesion.]

REBTer: So right now you would feel anxious if you looked at your skin lesion. So how are you dealing with your feelings right now?

Kay: By not looking at it. But now the lesion is in my mind, I am also anxious if I don't look at it. Does that make sense?

[REBTer's thinking: So by focusing on her feelings of anxiety of the moment I am getting the material I need to assess a specific example of Kay's problem.]

REBTer: Yes it does. Shall we focus on your feelings of anxiety now so we can both understand what's going on?

Kay: OK.

Now let's see how a trainee may think and intervene in the same situation.

Trainee: Can you give me a specific example of your anxiety about your health?

Kay: Well I get anxious whenever I find a lump or lesion on my body.

[Trainee's thinking: I need to ask my question again because Kay hasn't told me of an example.]

Trainee: Can you give me a specific example?

Kay: Well there are so many that they all merge together.

[Trainee's thinking: This is getting difficult. Let me ask her about the last time it happened.]

Trainee: When was the last time you felt anxious about a lump or lesion on your body?

Kay: I'm always anxious about my health.

[Trainee's thinking: I am going round in circles. So I will have to deal with this as a general issue.]

Let's consider the differences between the trained therapist and the trainee here. Both asked Kay for a specific example of her anxiety in keeping with REBT practice. In response, Kay struggled to identify one specific example claiming that there were too many to choose from. While the trainee persisted with his strategy of asking for a specific example in the 'there and then', the trained therapist was more successful in using a 'here and now' approach. In doing so, the client became anxious and began to give the therapist the specific information that he needs to carry out an assessment of a specific example of the client's target problem in line with the REBT's treatment recommendations.

It is clear from the trainee's thinking and interventions that bringing the issue of the client's health anxiety into the here and now did not occur to him. In short, he lacked the creativity shown by the more experienced, trained therapist. Consequently, the trainee considered that having exhausted his repertoire of attempts to have the client identify a specific example of her problem, he had no option but to deal with the issue in a general way.

Thinking and intervening related to structure and focus

One of the problems of much counselling and therapy that is ineffective is that it tends to be unstructured and lack a working focus. A good REBT therapist tends to be structured and focused in his work with his clients unless there is a good reason not to be. What follows is an example of how a trained REBT therapist thinks and intervenes when the issue of being structured and creating a focus becomes salient. I will contrast this with how a trainee might think and act in the same situation.

An example of structuring and focus

Hattie has come to therapy for help with a number of problems including performance anxiety, work procrastination and relationship problems. After taking a brief history, the therapist asks Hattie how he can help her.

Hattie: I don't know. I have so many problems I don't know where to start.

[REBTer's thinking: I can structure the process for Hattie by asking her to briefly outline her problems and then later I will ask her to focus on one at a time.]

REBTer: Let's make a brief list of them and then we can decide which one we will focus on. Does that make sense?

Hattie: Yes, it does. Well I get very anxious whenever I have to give a presentation at work. I've always been like that but it's got worse recently.

[REBTer's thinking: I need to intervene quickly here otherwise she will get into the problem before I have constructed a problem list. I will explain to her now what I intend to do.]

REBTer: OK, let me make a note of that problem. What I am doing is beginning to construct a problem list so that we both know what we need to cover in therapy. OK?

Hattie: OK.

REBTer: So apart from anxiety about giving presentations at work, what other problems are you seeking help for?

Hattie: I find it hard to get down to work and to do my chores. I leave things to the last minute then get stressed when I get overwhelmed with all the things that I have put off.

REBTer: So you have a problem with procrastination. Shall I add that to the problem list?

Hattie: Yes.

REBTer: Any other problems?

Hattie: Well the one that I'm most troubled by is that I have rows with my friends.

[REBTer's thinking: I am going to have to be careful. I want a bit more information, but don't want Hattie to open up too much on this issue at this stage.]

REBTer: Is there any recurring theme to these rows?
Hattie: Well, let me think . . . The rows tend to happen when I think that they are being intrusive.

[REBTer's thinking: It would be useful if I could identify the feeling that Hattie experiences when she makes the inference that people are being intrusive.]

REBTer: And when they are being intrusive, how do you feel?
Hattie: I get really mad.
REBTer: And when you get mad do you row with them?
Hattie: Yes.
REBTer: Would you row with them if you didn't get mad with them over this?
Hattie: I guess not.
REBTer: So are the rows due mainly to their intrusion or to you getting mad about their intrusion?
Hattie: Well I wouldn't get mad if they weren't intrusive.
REBTer: That's correct, but what is in your control, their intrusion or your angry reaction to their intrusion?
Hattie: My reaction.
REBTer: And since your angry reaction leads to the rows, as you said before, shall we add your anger about their intrusion to your problem list?
Hattie: Put like that, yes.
REBTer: Any other problems to add to your problem list?
Hattie: Not at the moment.
REBTer: OK, but as a problem list is fluid we can add and subtract items as we see fit. OK?
Hattie: OK.

[REBTer's thinking: Now would be a good time to summarise the items on Hattie's problem list. Then I will create a focus by asking her which problem she would like to start with.]

REBTer:	OK. So let me recap. We have three problems on your problem list. First, your anxiety about giving presentations at work. Second, your procrastination and finally, your anger about other people's intrusiveness that leads to you rowing with them. Have I understood you?
Hattie:	Yes.
REBTer:	Are there any other problems that you have that need to be added to the list?
Hattie:	No that's it for the moment.

[REBTer: Now I have a great opportunity to create a focus by asking Hattie which problem she would like to begin with. But first I have to make a case for dealing with problems one a time.]

REBTer:	Before we start, do you think that your problems are best dealt with one at a time or all at once?
Hattie:	One at a time.
REBTer:	In which case which problem should we begin with?
Hattie:	I would like to·deal with my anger when others are intrusive.

Now let's see how a trainee might think and respond to the same situation.

Once again, after taking a brief history, the trainee asks Hattie how he can help her.

| Hattie: | I don't know. I have so many problems I don't know where to start. |

[Trainee's thinking: To develop the working alliance I am going to suggest that Hattie begins where she wants to begin.]

| Trainee: | Where would you like to start? |
| Hattie: | I'm not sure. Everything is all mushed together in my mind. I just go round and round in circles trying to make sense of everything. But the more I try to do that the more dizzy I get. I'm going a bit dizzy right now just talking about it. |

> *[Trainee's thinking: I'd better help to get her focused. I'll do this by asking her which problem she would like to start with.]*
>
> Trainee: One good way of countering such confusion is to focus on one problem at a time. So which of your problems would you like to begin with?
>
> Hattie: ... Er ... I'm sorry, I just tuned out there. What did you say?
>
> Trainee: I said which of your problems would you like to begin with?
>
> Hattie: I'm not sure ...

Let me discuss the differences here between the thinking and responses of the trained therapist and the thinking and responses of the trainee.

When the client indicates that she is not sure where to start, the trained therapist views this as an opportunity to propose a structure to the client. He suggests that they develop a problem list. This strategy was developed by Aaron T. Beck and some of his cognitive therapy colleagues in the treatment of depression (Beck *et al.*, 1979). It is particularly helpful when clients are confused and/or overwhelmed by their problems or when they tend to see their problems as an undifferentiated mass. By developing a problem list the therapist helps Hattie engage in the therapeutic process by bringing a sense of order to that process. In order to do this successfully the therapist manages the development of Hattie's problem list by discouraging her from getting into any one problem until the list is completed. He does this by explaining what he is doing and eliciting Hattie's agreement to maintain the structure. This enables the therapist to interrupt Hattie without threatening the working alliance between them. Once the trained therapist has structured the process and helped Hattie to develop her problem list, he then creates a therapeutic focus by encouraging Hattie to work on one problem at a time. Notice how he does this, he does not assert that this is the best way of dealing with her problems. Rather, by asking Socratic questions, the therapist helps Hattie to see that working with one problem at a time is the best way forward.

By contrast, the trainee responds to Hattie's uncertainty about where to start by encouraging her to start where she wants. This only serves to increase Hattie's confusion rather than alleviating it as the trained therapist does.

In response the trainee asserts that the best way forward is to focus on one problem at a time and asks Hattie which of her problems she wants to work on first. Notice, however, that by this time Hattie is so confused that she cannot process what the trainee is saying and the trainee's attempts to bring order to Hattie's confusion come too late. What the trainee fails to do is to introduce structure into the process at a time when Hattie could benefit from it, i.e. at the outset when she first indicated that she was confused.

What the trained therapist did was to introduce structure and then create a working focus. By contrast, the trainee failed to introduce structure when it was needed and thus his attempts to create a working focus were too late to be helpful.

Having dealt with the important issue of engaging clients in REBT, I will, in Chapters 2–7, show you how to think and intervene like an REBT therapist in the assessment process. This involves taking specific examples of a client's problem and putting it into REBT's 'ABC' framework within a situational context. I will start by considering how a trained REBT therapist thinks about the context in which a specific example of the client's target problem occurs and how this thinking affects his interventions. I will contrast this with how a trainee might think and act in response to the same topic area.

Chapter 2

Thinking and intervening related to placing client problems in context

Every psychotherapist and counsellor makes sense of what clients say to them about their problems. When this understanding is formalised it is known as assessment when applied to specific client problems and case formulation when applied to an overall under-standing of the 'case' or how clients' problems fit together within the overall context of their lives.

In this chapter and in Chapters 3–7, I will outline the thinking that trained REBT therapists engage in when they are assessing their clients' problems and compare this thinking with that of trainees learning how to become REBT therapists.

The importance of context

If you think about it, clients experience their problems within some kind of context. This context can be located within space and time and it is very helpful to keep the game of Cluedo in mind when thinking about the context. As mentioned in Chapter 1, Cluedo is a game in which players have to guess who committed a crime, where it was committed and with what implement. When thinking about clients' problems it is useful to think in a similar way:

- Where was the client when she experienced the problem?
- When did the client experience the problem?
- Who was she with when she experienced the problem?

The context in which the person experienced the problem can be real or imagined. Here are examples of what I mean.

- At Sunday lunch, Peter felt depressed in the kitchen when his mother told him that his brother had just won a scholarship to Oxford.

  (Here it is apparent that Peter felt depressed about what his mother told him there and then in the kitchen. This is an example of disturbance taking place in a real context.)

- At Monday morning in the College coffee bar sitting on his own, Peter felt depressed when he thought about the fact that his brother had just won a scholarship to Oxford.

  (Here it is apparent that Peter felt depressed when he thought about what his mother told him in the kitchen the day before. This is an example of disturbance taking place in an imagined context.)

Descriptions of contexts are important

It is important to help the client to describe the context in which she disturbed herself. As we will see later, a person disturbs herself about a particular aspect of the real or imagined situation that provides the context for her disturbance. It is useful, therefore, to know the 'facts' of what actually happened in this context so that these can be compared later with the person's inferences about what happened. I have put 'facts' in inverted commas here, because while it is possible to say whether a person's description of what happened is descriptive rather than inferential, it is not possible to say whether or not the person's description is accurate (see the example below).

When an REBT therapist asks a client to describe the situation she was in when she disturbed herself, he listens very carefully to her response. Here is an example of what the REBT therapist thinks in this situation:

> *REBTer*: So can you describe the situation you were in when you felt depressed?
>
> *Harriet*: I was with my friends and we were all talking, but Jackie was ignoring me.
>
> *[REBTer's thinking: Is my client describing the situation or is she adding inferential meaning to what happened? The word 'ignored' suggests that this is an inference so let me ask a relevant question to clarify this.]*

REBTer: Can you describe what Jackie actually did or
              failed to do that led you to conclude that she
              was ignoring you?

Harriet: She did not look at me or address any remarks
              to me.

*[REBTer's thinking: That is Harriet's description of Jackie's
behaviour. It may be accurate or inaccurate, but it is descriptive. Therefore 'Jackie was ignoring me' is an inference.]*

When a person reveals her inferences, these are important to
consider when attempting to understand what she was most disturbed about in the situation at hand. But first we need to discuss
the nature of the client's disturbed emotions which occur at 'C' in
the 'ABC' framework and concentrate in doing so on the thinking
and interventions of both trained therapist and trainee.

Chapter 3

Thinking and intervening related to emotional 'Cs'

In REBT we use an 'ABC' framework to assess our clients' problems. As I have discussed above, it is useful to understand the context in which a client has disturbed herself and a brief description of that context frames the 'ABC' assessment that is to be done.

While you may think that the term 'ABC' points to the preferred order in which 'ABC' variables are to be assessed (where 'A' is the aspect of the situation about which the client is most disturbed, 'B' is her irrational beliefs about 'A' and 'C' is the emotional, behavioural and thinking consequences of 'B'), you would be wrong. The term 'ABC' is used in that order because it makes sense to clients and is best remembered by both clients and therapists alike.

However, when assessing an instance of a client's emotional problem, REBT therapists are most likely to use a 'CAB' order or an 'ACB' order. My own preference in therapy is to employ the 'CAB' order and I also recommend its use to trainees.

Consequently, when discussing how to think like an REBT therapist, I will start considering such thinking when it comes to working with clients' 'Cs'. Because this is an introductory text, I will concentrate on emotional 'Cs' in this work and will refer to behavioural and thinking 'Cs' as they help to illuminate emotional 'Cs'.

Thinking and intervening with respect to unhealthy negative emotions at 'C'

Clients come to therapy largely because their lives are not working in one or two specific areas or more generally across different areas. Thus, they may be experiencing problems in the work area of their life or in the relational area. REBT's viewpoint is that as long as clients are emotionally disturbed in whichever area or areas their problems are located, they will be handicapped in adequately addressing these problems. Thus, the REBT therapist's initial focus is to help clients to address their emotional problems as these are manifest in these other more practical problems before they help them effectively address their practical issues.

The client may not share this view and thus the REBT therapist first needs to present a rationale to the client that her emotional problem needs to be addressed before her more practical issue.

Discussing with clients the importance of addressing emotional problems first: a straightforward example

Michael has sought counselling because he is having trouble dating women. The dates that he does have are, by his account, unsuccessful and a woman rarely agrees to see him for a second date. On assessment, it transpires that Michael lacks social skills (for example, he has poor eye contact, rarely smiles, and finds it difficult to engage people in conversation) and he is also very anxious in the presence of women. In REBT, his lack of social skills is regarded as a practical problem and his anxiety as an emotional problem. Here is how a trained REBT therapist thinks, having carried out his assessment of Michael's problems.

[REBTer's thinking: So Michael has two problems: a practical problem and an emotional problem. It's unlikely that Michael will be able to put into practice his newly acquired social skills with women when he is anxious in their presence so I am going to put this to him when discussing the order in which we will address his problems.]

REBTer: So, Michael, here is my suggestion concerning how we should go forward. Let me know what you think. OK?

Michael: OK.

REBTer: As we have seen, you have two problems which contribute to difficulty dating women. You lack certain key social skills which I can help you learn and practise and you are anxious in the presence of women which I can also help you to

address. My view is that as long as you are
anxious in the company of women, your anxiety
will get in the way of putting your newly
acquired skills into practice. So I suggest that we
tackle your anxiety first and then help you to
acquire and apply those key social skills. What
do you think?

Michael: I see what you are saying, but if I really learn
these social skills and apply them wouldn't that
mean that I wouldn't be anxious when I am with
women? I would rather start learning those
social skills straight away.

*[REBTer's thinking: I need to ask Michael for his permission
to pursue my point, otherwise, doing so without permission may
threaten the working alliance and as we have just begun
therapy, the alliance may not be very strong at present.*

*Assuming I get Michael's permission, I need to show him
that no matter how skilled he becomes at relating to women his
anxiety will interfere with him demonstrating these skills where
it matters – in the presence of women. I need to find a way of
putting this to him so that he can understand it. However, if he
insists on starting with his practical problem for the sake of
sustaining the working alliance, I will go along with it and see
what happens.]*

REBTer: Will you allow me to put my case a little
differently?

Michael: OK.

REBTer: I can tell that learning social skills is very
important to you and I agree that they will
definitely help you to develop relationships with
women. My concern is helping you to maximise
your learning and that's why I suggest that we
start by tackling your anxiety. Let me put it like
this, trying to put into practice your developing
skills while you are anxious is like walking up a
hill with a ball and chain around your leg. You
can do it, but it isn't very efficient. Dealing with
your anxiety first is like taking the ball and chain

> off your leg so that you can walk freely. What do you think?
>
> *Michael*:   Put like that, it makes sense to start with my anxiety problem first.

Now let's see how a trainee would think and respond to Michael's wish to start addressing his practical skills problem before his emotional problem. I will assume that the trainee has already put forward the same rationale as the trained therapist concerning starting with Michael's emotional problem first (see above).

> *Michael*:   I see what you are saying, but if I really learn these social skills and apply them wouldn't that mean that I wouldn't be anxious when I am with women? I would rather start learning those social skills straight away.
>
> *[Trainee's thinking: Well I have made a case for starting with Michael's emotional problem first, but he has not accepted it. I know I am not supposed to threaten the working alliance so I am going to go along with Michael's request and start addressing his practical problem first.]*
>
> *Trainee*:   OK, Michael. Let's start helping you to develop better social skills.

Let's compare the trained therapist's thinking and response with those of the trainee regarding the client's point that he wants to start with his practical problem before his emotional problem.

As you can see, the trained therapist demonstrates in his thinking and in his interventions that he is mindful of the working alliance between him and Michael and that he is also keen to encourage Michael to address his emotional problem before his practical problem. Notice that after the therapist explains the reasons for this preferred order he does not acquiesce to Michael's wish to address his practical problem first. Rather he asks for permission to put his point in a different way and makes a more persuasive case the second time around. His thinking reveals that if Michael still wanted to address his social skills first after this second rationale, then the therapist would at that point have gone along with the client, albeit reluctantly.

By contrast, the trainee shows in his thinking that he is mindful of the desirability of starting with the client's emotional problem first and of the need to sustain a good working alliance with the client. When Michael does not accept his initial rationale to begin with his emotional problem, the trainee acquiesces to the client's wish, showing in his thinking that working alliance considerations have become more salient than making a second attempt to encourage the client to target his emotional problem before his practical problem.

Understandably, the trainee lacks the sophistication of the trained therapist in practising REBT and attending to working alliance considerations. In his thinking and behaviour the trained REBT therapist indicates that he can make a more persuasive attempt to encourage Michael to prioritise his emotional problem having asked for permission to do so. The manoeuvre based on such thinking bears fruit in that Michael gives such permission and is persuaded by the REBT therapist's second attempt to have him address his emotional problem before his practical problem in therapy.

By contrast, the trainee's thinking indicates that making a second attempt at persuasion does not cross his mind. As such, he is disadvantaged in starting with the client's practical problem.

Discussing with clients the importance of addressing emotional problems first: a more complicated example

Keith has come to counselling because he keeps being passed over for promotion at work and wants help to get promoted. This raises a number of issues for the REBT therapist. First, as Keith's goal is outside his control, it is difficult for the REBT therapist to accept this goal. Rather, the REBT therapist can only realistically accept as a goal one that is in Keith's direct control, i.e. his performance and behaviour on the job and the associated emotions that might be relevant. On questioning, Keith reveals that his appraisals have pointed to two factors that are impeding his promotion prospects:

1   the fact that he often loses his temper on the job and
2   his poor presentation skills at in-house conferences.

The client also reveals that he is depressed about his latest failure to be promoted and this is affecting his performance on the job.

So Keith has three problems, all of which are impacting negatively on his promotion prospects:

- poor presentation skills
- losing his temper at work
- feeling depressed about his latest job promotion failure.

I am going to outline what an REBT therapist is likely to think about how to proceed with Keith and compare this to how an REBT trainee might think.

[REBTer's thinking: So Keith has three problems. My hypothesis is that as long as he keeps losing his temper at work, he is unlikely to get promoted no matter how much progress he makes on his presentation skills. But as long as he is depressed about his lack of promotion, he is unlikely to be committed to working on either of these problems so I am going to provide the client with a rationale for tackling these problems in this order:

1 feeling depressed about his latest job promotion failure
2 losing his temper at work
3 poor presentation skills.]

[Trainee's thinking: I know in REBT that we are supposed to deal with emotional problems before practical problems so I will ask the client which of his emotional problems he wants to start with.]

Note the following similarity and differences between the trained REBT therapist's thinking and that of the trainee. Both know that in REBT it is recommended that clients' emotional problems are addressed before their practical problems. However, note that the REBT therapist is more sophisticated in his thinking than the trainee on this point. First, the trained therapist is applying this principle with due regard to the client's two emotional problems and the order in which they need to be tackled. By contrast, the trainee plans to ask the client which of the two emotional problems the client wants to tackle first. The trainee is implementing the correct REBT principle, but without due regard to the nuances of the client's actual situation. This shows the importance of thinking about REBT principles while taking into account the idiosyncratic nature of the client's situation.

Let me now show you how the differences in thinking of the trained REBT therapist and the trainee affect how they are likely to have responded to the client.

Keith:	So how do think you can help me?
REBTer:	Well you have told me that you have three problems. You think that your poor presentation skills and losing your temper at work are affecting your promotion prospects and the other one reflects that you feel depressed about not getting promotion.
	Let me share with you my thinking and let me know what your reaction is to my suggestion. OK?
Keith:	OK.
REBTer:	My view is that as long as you are depressed about being passed over for promotion again you are not going to be in the best frame of mind to tackle the other two problems. So my suggestion is that we start with addressing your feelings of depression about your promotion failure. Does that make sense to you?
Keith:	That makes sense.
REBTer:	Then, when you have addressed your depression, my suggestion is that we then target your anger issue before looking at ways of improving your presentation skills. Here's the reason why I suggest this. Even if you improve your presentation skills, the fact that you are still losing your temper will probably make it more difficult for you to get promotion than if you curbed your temper but still had some way to go in honing the skills at making presentations. Your displays of anger would still make you unpleasant to work with and thus less likely to get

	promotion. What do you think of this order of tackling your problems?
Keith:	That makes perfect sense. I agree.

Now let's consider how the trainee intervenes.

Keith:	So how do think you can help me?
Trainee:	Well you have one practical problem, namely your presentation skills at work and two emotional problems, your anger at work and your depression about not getting promoted. In REBT, we tackle emotional problems before practical problems because it's harder to deal with practical issues when you are emotionally disturbed. So which of your emotional problems, your anger or your depression, would you like to start with?
Keith:	. . . Um, I'm not sure, what do you suggest?
Trainee:	It's your choice.

Both the REBT therapist and the trainee have implemented the REBT principle of tacking emotional problems before practical problems in giving their rationale to the client concerning the order of addressing the client's problems. However, the trained therapist gives a clear rationale for dealing with the client's depressed feelings before his angry feelings, while the trainee wants the client to choose the order, but provides no guidelines to help the client choose. Notice also how the REBT therapist engages the client more than the trainee does in their respective interventions.

What is an unhealthy negative emotion (UNE)?

As I have discussed above REBT strongly recommends that a practitioner works with his client's emotional problems before addressing her practical problems. The rationale for this, which appears in the material presented above, is that a client is more likely to address her practical problems successfully when she is not emotionally disturbed about them than when she is so disturbed.

But what constitutes emotional disturbance or, if you dislike the term 'disturbance', an emotional problem?

From an REBT perspective, when a person is emotionally disturbed she:

- Tends to experience one or more unhealthy negative emotions that feel very painful (with the exception of unhealthy anger which can be experienced as positive).
- Tends to act in ways that are self-defeating. This means that when these tendencies are acted on her behaviour interferes with her long-term interests in one or more areas of her life. She may experience relief in the short term by taking such actions, but they will get her into greater trouble in the longer term. Even if she does not act on what are called 'action tendencies' their presence often serves to prevent her from acting in ways that will help her achieve her longer-term goals.
- Tends to have subsequent thoughts that are highly distorted and exaggerated which the person takes as reflecting reality rather than her emotional disturbance. Thinking that such cognitive distortions are real she takes action (usually self-defeating) to avoid encountering this 'reality'.
- Tends to feel stuck in that she does not see that she has plausible alternative ways of dealing with the situation that she feels disturbed about. Or if she sees these alternatives, she does not think that she can choose to take them.

Let's see how a trained REBT therapist and a trainee think when faced with a client who is unsure whether she has an emotional problem. We will then consider their respective interventions.

Cleo has been referred for counselling by her employer for 'anger management'. She recognises that she gets angry at work, but is not sure that it constitutes a problem. I will first show how a trained REBT therapist thinks about and responds to such a situation.

Cleo:	So although my employer is paying me to come for so-called 'anger management', I think they are wasting my time and their money.
REBTer:	In what way, Cleo?
Cleo:	Well I don't think I have a problem with anger.

[REBTer's thinking: There are a number of ways that I can intervene now. It's unlikely that Cleo finds her anger a painful emotion, so I will find out what her work goals are and use these as a way of helping her judge whether or not her anger is problematic. But first, I need to get her on board to do that.]

REBTer: I am not sure either but can we work together to determine whether or not your anger is a problem for you?

Cleo: Fair enough. I have to be here so why not.

REBTer: Do you like your job?

Cleo: Yes I do. It means a lot to me.

REBTer: So what are your goals at work?

Cleo: Well, I would like to manage my own department.

REBTer: And how many promotions are you away from that?

Cleo: Two.

REBTer: And from your appraisals at work, has anything been mentioned that might stand in the way of getting those promotions?

Cleo: Well, the only thing that has been mentioned is my temper.

REBTer: And in how many appraisals has that been mentioned?

Cleo: The last three.

REBTer: Your anger has been mentioned for three years running as something that may well stop you from realising your goals at work.

Cleo: I can see what you are getting at.

REBTer: What's that?

Cleo: That even though I don't regard my anger as a problem, it is a problem for me because it is stopping me from getting what I want.

REBTer: And what do you think of that analysis?

Cleo: I think you are right.

[REBTer's thinking: It is important that I attribute that insight to Cleo herself and not take any credit for it myself. I want to stress that all my questions did was to clarify her thinking for her. I want her to 'own' her problem.]

> *REBTer*: Actually, I haven't passed any opinion. All I have done is asked you some pertinent questions and you have come up with that conclusion for yourself.
>
> *Cleo*: I guess you are right.
>
> *REBTer*: So would you like to address your anger problem?
>
> *Cleo*: Yes I would.

Now let's consider a trainee's thinking and intervention in response to the same material.

> *Cleo*: So although my employer is paying me to come for so-called 'anger management', I think they are wasting my time and their money.
>
> *Trainee*: In what way, Cleo?
>
> *Cleo*: Well I don't think I have a problem with anger.
>
> *[Trainee's thinking: Well I know that anger is a disturbed emotion, so I will outline REBT's position on this and point out how painful it is.]*
>
> *Trainee*: OK, in REBT unhealthy anger is seen as an emotional disturbance.
>
> *Cleo*: So are you saying I am disturbed?
>
> *Trainee*: Not you, just your anger.
>
> *Cleo*: On what basis do you say that?
>
> *Trainee*: Well anger is a very painful emotion.
>
> *Cleo*: Not for me it isn't. I feel powerful when I experience it.
>
> *[Trainee's thinking: Help! She won't take my word for it so I will bring in the weight of authority – Dr Albert Ellis.]*
>
> *Trainee*: Well, don't take my word for it. The founder of REBT, Dr Albert Ellis, says that anger is a disturbed emotion. I am going to suggest you read his book *Anger: How to Control it Before it Controls You* so that you learn more about anger.
>
> *Cleo*: Have you had much experience dealing with people's anger?

Now let's compare the thinking and subsequent interventions of the trained REBT therapist and the trainee.

You will note that the trained REBT therapist used REBT theory without mentioning it to the client, whereas the trainee asserted an REBT principle without explanation hoping that doing so would persuade the client that anger was a disturbance. This signally failed. The trained therapist, by expert guided questioning, helped the client to see that her anger was stopping her from achieving her stated goals. In contrast, the trainee seemed to antagonise the client and called into question her expertise by appealing to the authority of Albert Ellis (probably unknown to the client) when his initial attempt to show that anger is an unhealthy emotion proved unsuccessful.

Finally, the trained therapist made no mention of the 'pain' of anger whereas the trainee did advance this point, which was denied by the client. The trained therapist knows that for clients anger often feels good and therefore does not take the risk of raising this issue with the client. Lacking the clinical experience, the trainee used the 'pain' argument', which had a rebound effect on his endeavours.

Discriminating between unhealthy negative emotions (UNEs) and healthy negative emotions (HNEs)

REBT theory is unique in advancing a distinction between unhealthy negative emotions and healthy negative emotions. Unhealthy negative emotions (UNEs) are emotions that are negative in tone and have the following features as described more fully above:

- They are generally very painful to experience (with certain exceptions; for example unhealthy anger).
- They tend to lead to self-defeating behaviour.
- They tend to lead to subsequent thinking that is highly distorted in nature.
- They tend to lead to the person 'feeling' stuck.

By contrast, healthy negative emotions (HNEs) are also negative in tone, but have the following different characteristics:

- They are generally painful to experience, but may not be as painful as UNEs.
- They tend to lead to self-enhancing behaviour.
- They tend to lead to subsequent thinking that is balanced in nature.
- They tend to lead to the person acknowledging that she has options rather than 'feeling' stuck.

While there is no generally accepted language to help clients and therapists alike to discriminate between UNEs and HNEs, the above are useful criteria to bear in mind and use when appropriate.

Let's see how a trained REBT therapist's thinking and intervention compare to those of a trainee when it is not immediately clear whether a client's negative emotion is healthy or unhealthy. Here the focus will be on the assessment of action tendencies.

HNE or UNE: the assessment of action tendencies

Patrick has been referred by his doctor for help with his anger. At the initial session, it is unclear whether Patrick's anger is healthy or unhealthy and Patrick himself is unsure whether or not it is a problem for him.

Let's start by considering how a trained REBT therapist thinks and responds while working with Patrick on this issue.

REBTer: So it's not clear to you whether or not your anger is a problem for you.

Patrick: That's right. My doctor seemed to think so but he didn't explain why.

[REBTer's thinking: I think that a concrete example of Patrick's anger may illuminate matters so I am going to ask him for that.]

REBTer: Can you come up with a good specific example of your anger so that we can work out together where your anger is healthy or unhealthy?

Patrick: A typical example of my anger occurred last night as a matter of fact. I was watching TV and my son came up and asked me a question about his homework. I very politely asked him to wait until the programme I was watching had finished and he did go away. But five minutes later he came back and asked me the same question and interrupted me watching the programme. My wife said I shouted at him and was very rude to him and certainly he started crying.

REBTer: You mentioned what your wife said about your reaction, but how did you feel when your son interrupted you the second time.

Patrick: I felt angry.

[REBTer's thinking: It is not yet clear whether Patrick's anger is healthy or unhealthy. So first I am going to see what he did and also what he felt like doing because these may be different.]

REBTer: When your son interrupted you the second time how did you think you responded to him?

Patrick: Well, I did raise my voice but I don't think I was nasty to him

[REBTer's thinking: So his report of his reaction suggests healthy anger. Let me now assess his action tendency.]

REBTer: At the moment when you were angry with your son for interrupting you, did you feel like doing something to him or saying something to him that you suppressed?

Patrick: Interesting question. I have never thought of that . . . Let me see. Well to be honest, and I am not proud of this, I felt an urge to hit him and really shout at him . . . I didn't of course, but in the moment, I really felt those urges . . .

REBTer: So if we go on what you did, it seems like your anger is healthy although it's not entirely clear. Indeed your wife seems to imply that it wasn't. But what do you think that your suppressed urges tell us about your anger in terms of whether it was healthy or unhealthy?

Patrick: Put like that, it was definitely unhealthy. I was just going on what I actually did, not what I felt like doing, but suppressed. That is very helpful. I admit it, my anger is unhealthy because as I think about other examples I am suppressing some quite destructive impulses in all of them.

REBTer: And do you think it's possible that there is some leakage of those destructive urges in that others, like your wife, may think that your anger is unhealthy while you don't?

Patrick: I think it's very possible.

Now let's see how a trainee thinks and responds to Patrick's example.

Patrick: A typical example of my anger occurred last night as a matter of fact. I was watching TV and my son came up and asked me a question about his homework. I very politely asked him to wait until the programme I was watching had finished and he did go away. But five minutes later he came back and asked me the same question and interrupted me watching the programme. My wife said I shouted at him and was very rude to him and certainly he started crying.

Trainee: But how would you describe your behaviour?

Patrick: I raised my voice, but I wasn't nasty to him.

Trainee: Raised your voice in an aggressive or an assertive way?

Patrick: I would say an assertive way.

[Trainee's thinking: Patrick says that he raised his voice, but was assertive rather than aggressive. He also said he wasn't nasty to his son. He hasn't said anything which indicates that his anger was unhealthy so I think it was healthy and will offer him this opinion.]

The major difference between the trained REBT therapist and the trainee in working with Patrick is centred on the emphasis they both give to Patrick's verbal report of his behaviour at 'C'. You will see that the trainee bases his judgement about whether Patrick's anger is healthy or unhealthy on Patrick's verbal report of his behaviour while the trained REBT therapist does not. What the trained therapist does that the trainee does not do is to assess Patrick's action tendencies, behaviours that he feels like engaging in, but suppresses. It is the assessment of these action tendencies that makes clear to the trained therapist and to Patrick himself that his anger is unhealthy. Because he failed to assess these action tendencies, the trainee concludes wrongly that Patrick's anger is healthy.

The important point to stress therefore is this. When it is not clear from a client's report that her negative feelings are healthy or unhealthy and her account of her behaviour is equivocal on this issue, then it is very important to assess her action tendencies. The same point can also be made with respect to a client's subsequent thinking as will be shown below.

HNE or UNE: the assessment of subsequent thinking

Maureen agreed to seek counselling after a suggestion from her personal tutor who thought that she was quite anxious while giving a paper in a group tutorial.

Again it was not clear from her general description whether Maureen felt anxious (UNE) or concerned (HNE) so both the trained therapist and the trainee asked for a specific example to clarify this. What follows is how a trained REBT therapist and trainee differ in their thinking and interventions in response to what Maureen says.

Maureen: Last week I had to give a paper in a group tutorial. I thought I was appropriately nervous, but my tutor thought I was anxious.

[REBTer's thinking: Let me see what subsequent thinking Maureen engaged in after she began to feel concerned or anxious. This will help me to judge whether she was anxious or concerned.]

REBTer: When you began to feel concerned or anxious what were you focusing on in your mind?

Maureen: I thought that people in the class would think I was stupid.

REBTer: How many people were in the class?

Maureen: Including me and the group tutor, 15 people.

REBTer: And when you were feeling concerned or anxious, how many of the 14 people did you think would consider you to be stupid?

Maureen: All of them.

[REBTer's thinking: In all probability Maureen was feeling anxious rather than concerned because the subsequent inference was highly distorted in that she thought all 14 people in the tutorial would consider her to be stupid. I will double check on this by outlining a scenario whereby her subsequent thinking was more balanced and I will see whether this changes her feeling.]

REBTer: Let me ask you to imagine that instead of thinking everybody in the tutorial would think that you were stupid, you thought that different people had different opinions about you. One or two thought you were stupid, one or two thought that you were clever and the others varied between these two positions. Would that change the feeling that would give rise to these thoughts?

Maureen: Yes it would.

REBTer: In what way?

Maureen: I would feel calmer.

REBTer: I wonder if the distinction between feeling anxious and feeling concerned is useful here. Focus on the feeling that gave rise to you thinking that everyone would think you were stupid and compare this feeling with the one that would give rise to you thinking that different people would have different opinions about you. Which feeling would you call anxiety and which concern?

Maureen: Oh I see. Anxiety led me to think that everyone would think I was stupid.

REBTer: So when you were giving your paper in the group were you anxious or concerned?

Maureen: Definitely anxious.

Now let's see how the trainee would think and respond to the same material.

Maureen: Last week I had to give a paper in a group tutorial. I thought I was appropriately nervous, but my tutor thought I was anxious.

[Trainee's thinking: I'm not sure what to do now, so I'll ask her more about her feelings.]

Trainee: Can you tell me more about your feelings when you were giving your paper?

Maureen: Well I had butterflies in my tummy and I felt a bit restless.

[Trainee's thinking: That sounds like healthy nervousness. So let me ask her about why her tutor thought she was anxious.]

Trainee: Why do you think your tutor thought you were anxious?

Maureen: I'm not sure, but when he suggested that I see you, I didn't want to appear ungrateful so I agreed to come.

[Trainee's thinking: I don't think Maureen has a problem. She seems appropriately nervous so I am going to tell her that I don't think she has a problem.]

The major difference between the trained REBT therapist and the trainee in working with Maureen is that the trained therapist assesses and makes use of her subsequent thinking while the trainee doesn't. Like the trainee working with Patrick (see above) this trainee takes at face value Maureen's report that she was appropriately nervous. He neither has nor uses a more sophisticated understanding that when a person experiences a negative emotion her subsequent thinking gives a clear indication concerning whether this emotion is healthy or unhealthy (Dryden and Branch, 2008).

The trained therapist knows that a healthy negative emotion tends to lead to subsequent thinking that is balanced whereas an unhealthy negative emotion leads to subsequent thinking that is highly distorted. Knowing this, the trained REBT therapist carefully assesses Maureen's actual subsequent thinking in the group tutorial situation and hypothesises that this thinking reveals that Maureen experienced anxiety in the situation. To test this further, the therapist asks Maureen to imagine thinking more balanced thoughts in the same situation and to see if these would stem from a different feeling. This strategy helped Maureen see that she would have felt concern if her subsequent thoughts were balanced and that her actual highly distorted thoughts indicated that she was anxious (rather than concerned or appropriately nervous) in the group tutorial situation.

Helping clients to discriminate between different UNEs

In my experience, clients seek help for eight major unhealthy negative emotions: anxiety, depression, guilt, shame, unhealthy anger, hurt, unhealthy jealousy and unhealthy envy (Dryden, 2009). Clients are not always accurate in describing their emotions and sometimes say that they feel one UNE when in reality they feel another.

Let me outline why I think that it is important for an REBT therapist to accurately assess a client's UNE. In REBT theory, a client tends to experience a UNE when she holds an irrational belief about 'A'. As we will see later, an 'A' is often inferential in nature and the client forms an inference at 'A' with reference to her personal domain. Beck (1976) considers that the personal domain maps out what a person has an investment in. This includes, amongst others, people, objects and principles. When a person experiences different UNEs, she forms different inferences with respect to her personal domain. Table 1 outlines the major inference(s) with respect to her personal domain that are associated with each UNE.

Table 1 Inferential themes

Emotion	Inferential themes
Anxiety	Threat; danger
Depression	Loss; loss of value; failure
Shame	Public disclosure of weakness; falling very short of one's ideal
Guilt	Moral violation (sin of commission and/or omission); hurting others
Hurt	Others treat you badly (and you consider that you do not deserve such treatment)
Anger	Frustrated; transgressed against; ego attacked
Jealousy	Threat to present relationship posed by another person
Envy	Others experience the good fortune which you lack and covet

If a therapist assesses a client's UNE wrongly, therefore, he runs the risk of looking for an inference associated with that UNE which, in fact, the client has not made. For example, if a client wrongly says that she felt unhealthily jealous in a situation where she actually felt unhealthily envious, the therapist will look for a jealousy-related inference concerning someone posing a threat to her relationship rather than an envy-related inference concerning someone else having something that the person prizes, but does not have.

It is also important for the therapist to assess accurately the client's UNE because different UNEs are associated with different actions/action tendencies and different thinking consequences (Table 2).

Thus, if a client wrongly says that she felt unhealthily jealous in a situation where she actually felt unhealthily envious, the therapist

Table 2 Unhealthy negative emotions, actions/action tendencies and thinking consequences

Unhealthy negative emotions	Action/action tendency	Thinking consequence
Anxiety	Avoiding threat; seeking reassurance even though you are not reassurable	Overestimates negative features of the threat
Depression	Prolonged withdrawal from enjoyable activities	Only sees pain and blackness in the future
Guilt	Begging for forgiveness	Assumes more personal responsibility than the situation warrants
Hurt	Sulking	Thinks that the other has to put things right of own accord first
Shame	Averting one's eyes from the gaze of others; withdrawal from others	Overestimates the 'shamefulness' of what has been revealed
Unhealthy anger	Shouting; bad mouthing another person to others	Sees malicious intent in the motives of others, whether there is evidence for this or not
Unhealthy jealousy	Prolonged suspicious questioning of the other	Tends to see threats to one's relationship when none really exists
Unhealthy envy	Spoiling the other's enjoyment of the desired possession	Tends to denigrate the value of the desired possession

will look for actions/action tendencies associated with unhealthy jealousy (e.g. looking for clues that her partner has been unfaithful) and subsequent thinking associated with that emotion (e.g. thinking that her partner is being unfaithful when he is away from her). In reality, the therapist should be looking for actions/action tendencies associated with unhealthy envy (denigrating to people what the other has if she cannot get it herself) and subsequent thinking associated with that emotion (such as plotting in her mind to destroy or damage the envied object).

In this section, I will consider how a trained REBT therapist thinks and responds when faced with a situation where the client claims to feel one UNE where in reality she experiences another and compare it with how a trainee might think and respond in the same situation.

Glenda has come to therapy because she finds it difficult to say 'no' to people's requests with the result that she rarely has time to pursue her interests. She is describing a situation when a friend asked her to babysit on an evening when Glenda wanted to see a play at the local theatre. In this first segment, she is working with a trained REBT therapist.

REBTer: So, Glenda, you wanted to go and see the play, but you agreed to babysit for your friend instead. How did you stop yourself from saying 'no' to your friend when she asked you?

Glenda: I am not sure.

REBTer: Well if you had said 'no' to her how would you have felt?

Glenda: Ashamed.

[REBTer's thinking: That doesn't quite sound right. My hypothesis would have been that she would have felt guilty. Let me keep an open mind about this and see if I can clarify this by asking Glenda what she would have felt 'ashamed' about.]

REBTer: What would you have felt ashamed about, Glenda?

Glenda: Hurting my friend's feelings if I said 'no' to her.

[REBTer's thinking: That seems more like guilt to me. I wonder if Glenda is confusing shame with guilt. I will test this

out by looking at her predicted actions or action tendencies associated with the emotion that she is calling shame if she had said 'no' to her friend.]

REBTer: And if you did feel ashamed what would you have done?

Glenda: I would have begged my friend to forgive and have implored her to let me do the babysitting for her.

[REBTer's thinking: OK, that confirms it. Glenda would have felt guilt and not shame because both her inference at 'A' and her actions at 'C' are associated with guilt rather than shame. Let me put this to Glenda and see how she responds.]

REBTer: Glenda, when someone hurts the feelings of a friend and then begs for forgiveness, then that person usually feels guilt rather than shame. So, I'm a bit confused about what you mean by shame.

Glenda: By shame, I mean what you mean by guilt.

REBTer: OK, thanks for clarifying that.

Now let's see how a trainee might deal with the same situation.

Trainee: So, Glenda, you wanted to go and see the play, but you agreed to babysit for your friend instead, How did you stop yourself from saying 'no' to your friend when she asked you?

Glenda: I am not sure.

Trainee: Well if you had said 'no' to her how would you have felt?

Glenda: Ashamed.

[Trainee's thinking: So if Glenda would feel ashamed then her inference is about falling very short of her standards. I will use that in my next question.]

Trainee: So if you were to feel ashamed what standard do you think you would fall very short of?

Glenda: I am not sure I follow you.

Trainee: Well, when a person feels ashamed she thinks she has fallen very short of one of her standards.

Glenda: I am not sure that that applies to me.

[*Trainee's thinking: Let me focus on what she would do if she did feel ashamed. Shame leads a person to avoid the other person.*]

Trainee: So if you did feel ashamed then you would want to avoid your friend.

Glenda: But I wouldn't.

Trainee: So then you wouldn't feel ashamed.

The trainee shows that he knows the inferences and actions associated with shame and has learned that he can use this information in framing questions to clarify a person's unhealthy negative emotions. However, he has not learned when to use this strategy. It would be much better if he asked open-ended questions such as:

- If you had felt ashamed what would you have been ashamed about?
- If you had felt ashamed what would you have then done?

If the trainee had asked such questions, he might have realised that Glenda was feeling guilt rather than shame, but that she calls guilt shame. By being more open-ended in his questioning than the trainee, the trained REBT therapist realised quite early on that Glenda would probably have felt guilt rather than shame, but that she refers to guilt as shame. He is also experienced enough to know that it is best to use the client's emotional language and make the appropriate translation in his head than to encourage the client to use language suggested by REBT theory but which would be alien to her.

When clients use vague language to refer to UNEs

I have often joked that assessment in REBT would be much easier if as a client entered therapy a chip was inserted into her brain with the result that she understood the REBT model of conceptualising UNEs and HNEs. Unfortunately, clients don't have such understanding and as such they will express themselves in their own way and this raises issues for the trained REBT therapist and the trainee alike.

One of these issues that occurs when assessing a client's UNE is that the client may use vague language to represent her feelings. Here are some examples of such language:

- 'I felt bad.'
- 'I felt upset.'
- 'I felt disturbed.'
- 'I felt, like, gross.'

As you can see, it is impossible to say which emotion each of these clients experienced and thus the therapist has to make use of other information.

There are, in fact, two issues raised when a client uses vague language in this context:

1 Is she experiencing a UNE or an HNE?
2 What type of emotion is she experiencing?

I will demonstrate how an REBT therapist thinks and intervenes when a client uses vague language in attempting to represent her negative emotion. As you will see this involves assessing inferences at 'A' and behaviour or action tendencies at 'C'. Furthermore, I will compare this to how a trainee might typically think and respond to the same situation.

Naomi has come to therapy because she has relationship problems with her friends. In response to a request to give an example of this difficulty, Naomi says the following:

Naomi: I found out that two of my friends went to see a movie and did not invite me.
REBTer: And how did you feel about that?
Naomi: I felt upset about that.

[REBTer's thinking: I am not sure what Naomi means by 'upset'. Given that she is talking about a situation where she was not invited to something my hunch is that she felt hurt or its healthy counterpart, sorrow. I will now try and discover

what inference she made about this situation and assess her behaviour. This should help me clarify her 'upset' feelings.]

REBTer:	Naomi, I am not sure what you mean by upset here since this could represent a number of different emotions. Would you mind if I ask you a number of questions to help me pinpoint what you were feeling more accurately?
Naomi:	That's fine.
REBTer:	When you found out that your friends had gone to the movie and had not invited you, what was particularly upsetting for you about that?
Naomi:	I thought that they had excluded me.

[REBTer's thinking: So being excluded is her 'A', now let me ask for her behaviour at 'C'.]

REBTer:	And when you felt upset about being excluded by them what did you do?
Naomi:	I withdrew into myself to lick my wounds.

[REBTer's thinking: That behaviour is typical behaviour when someone feels hurt, but it may have been her first response and she may have responded more healthily later. I need to check on this point.]

REBTer:	And after you licked your wounds what did you do?
Naomi:	Nothing.
REBTer:	So you haven't contacted them and told them how you felt about being excluded?
Naomi:	No, I haven't.

[REBTer's thinking: So my conclusion from these data is that the emotion Naomi felt about being excluded was hurt because 'being excluded' is a typical inference in hurt and when someone feels hurt she often withdraws from those who she thinks have 'hurt' her not just in the short term, but in the longer term as well. Let me put this to Naomi.]

REBTer:	So, Naomi, based on the information that you have given me, I think that the emotional upset that you were experiencing when you thought

> that your friends had excluded you was hurt.
> What do you think?
> *Naomi:*   Definitely. That's exactly it, I felt hurt.

Now let me discuss how a trainee might typically think about and respond to the same situation.

> *Naomi:*   I found out that two of my friends went to see a movie and did not invite me.
> *Trainee:*   And how did you feel about that?
> *Naomi:*   I felt upset about that.
>
> *[Trainee's thinking: Now 'upset' is a vague emotion and I know that I have to help the client to clarify this.]*
>
> *Trainee:*   That's a vague emotion. Can you specify how you felt?
> *Naomi:*   Well . . . I felt teary.
>
> *[Trainee's thinking: That's another vague emotion. I am struggling here. Let me try again.]*
>
> *Trainee:*   That's also vague. Can you try again?
> *Naomi:*   That's all that comes to mind.
>
> *[Trainee's thinking: That isn't working. I will have to go with upset and hope that it is an unhealthy negative emotion]*
>
> *Trainee:*   Don't worry. Let's stick with the term 'upset'.

Let's consider how the trained REBT therapist thought about and dealt with this situation and compare this to the thinking and intervention of the trainee.

The trainee correctly noted in his thinking that Naomi was vague in representing her feeling and that he needed to ask her to clarify it. However, when this did not bear fruit, he had no alternative strategy and kept asking her to clarify her emotion, a strategy which did not yield success. Consequently, the trainee had no 'plan B' alternative but to accept the vague 'upset' as Naomi's feeling. This would create two problems. In the first place, the trainee would not be clear that the client's emotion was negative and unhealthy. He thereby would run the risk of encouraging her to change a negative emotion that was healthy and based on rational beliefs. Then, in the second place, even if Naomi's emotion was negative and unhealthy, the trainee would not know in precise enough detail which emotion it was and thereby would run two risks. First, he would run the risk of not understanding fully what the client was 'upset' about (i.e. the theme of her 'A') and second, he would run the risk of not identifying what her subsequent behaviour and thinking would be if she was vague in describing these behavioural and thinking consequences. Knowing precisely what UNE Naomi experienced would have given the trainee clues as to what her accompanying behaviour and subsequent thinking might have been if the client was not forthcoming on these points.

By contrast, the trained REBT therapist first assesses Naomi's inference which helps him to understand that the client is experiencing either hurt or sorrow (the healthy alternative to hurt in the REBT theory of emotions). However, the therapist knows that discovering the client's inference is insufficient to help him to understand whether, in this case, the client experienced hurt (UNE) or sorrow (HNE). In order to differentiate between these linked emotions, the trained therapist investigated the client's behaviour that accompanied her 'upset' and discovered that the actions indicated that she was feeling hurt rather than sorrow. This was confirmed by the client.

When clients use events or inferences of those events to refer to UNEs

Another issue that occurs when assessing a client's UNE is that the client may use events or inferences of those events to represent her feelings. Here are some examples of such language:

- 'I felt rejected.'
- 'I felt used.'
- 'I felt trapped.'
- 'I felt criticised.'

As with the situation when a client uses vague language, when she uses events or inferences to represent feelings (as above) it is not possible to say what emotion each of these clients was experiencing and thus the therapist has to make use of other information as before.

The same issues are raised when a client uses inferences or events to represent feelings as when she uses vague language in this context, namely:

1   Is she experiencing a UNE or an HNE?
2   What type of emotion is she experiencing?

I will illustrate this by referring to a case example. As before, I will show how a trained REBT therapist thinks and responds when a client refers to her emotion as an event or inference and compare such thinking and interventions with those typical of a trainee.

Peter came to therapy because he was experiencing great difficulty at work. In response to a request to give a specific example, Peter said the following.

> *Peter:*   Well, my boss called me into his room and told me what he thought of the report I had prepared for him. I didn't think it was that bad, but he really ripped into it.
>
> *REBTer:*   And how did you feel when he did that?
> *Peter:*   I felt criticised.
>
> *[REBTer's thinking: Peter has taken his boss's response, i.e. criticism, and used that as a feeling. I need to ask him how he felt about being criticised.]*
>
> *REBTer:*   And how did you feel about being criticised?
> *Peter:*   I felt inadequate.
>
> *[REBTer's thinking: Inadequate is not really a feeling, it is more of a negative judgement. I still need to clarify Peter's feeling. I think he was experiencing shame and I will test this out by looking at his behaviour or action tendencies. If all else fails, I will go along with 'feelings of inadequacy'.]*
>
> *REBTer:*   When you were feeling inadequate what did you do?
> *Peter:*   Nothing.
>
> *[REBTer's thinking: I need to assess Peter's action tendencies – urges to act that were not converted into overt behaviour.]*

REBTer: What did you feel like doing that you didn't do?

Peter: I felt like running out of the room.

[REBTer's thinking: His responses are not helping me to identify his precise feeling since 'feeling like running out of the room' could be associated with different emotions. So I am going to test for shame more directly by asking Peter if he experienced something that is very associated with shame.]

REBTer: While you were standing there feeling inadequate, did you have the experience of wanting the ground to open and swallow you up?

Peter: Very much so. I can also remember feeling very small if that makes any sense.

[REBTer's thinking: Those two experiences: wanting the ground to open and swallow one up and feeling small are very much associated with shame. So let me put this to Peter.]

REBTer: It makes perfect sense. So when you were feeling small and hoping the ground would open and swallow you up, were you experiencing shame?

Peter: Yes very much so.

REBTer: And does shame capture what you were feeling more closely than feeling inadequate or vice versa?

Peter: No, shame is more accurate for me.

Now let's see how a trainee might deal with the same situation.

Peter: Well, my boss called me into his room and told me what he thought of the report I had prepared for him. I didn't think it was that bad, but he really ripped into it.

Trainee: And how did you feel when he did that?

Peter: I felt criticised.

[Trainee's thinking: Well, I know that 'criticised' is not a feeling. So I will explain this to my client and ask him again what his feelings were in this situation.]

> *Trainee*: 'Criticised' is not a feeling. I am interested in your feelings. So, how did you feel when your boss ripped into your report?
>
> *Peter*: Ripped apart.
>
> *[Trainee's thinking: That is still not a feeling. I will have to try again. I remember my supervisor saying that when the question 'What were you feeling?' doesn't elicit a specific response try asking 'What was your emotion?', so I will try asking that.]*
>
> *Trainee*: Ripped apart is not a feeling. Let me put it another way. What was your emotion when your boss ripped into your report?
>
> *Peter*: I thought I had answered your question. I don't know what you want me to say.

As you can see there is a world of difference between the thinking and interventions of the trained REBT therapist and the trainee. The trained therapist first takes the client's response 'I felt criticised', recognises that it is an event or an inference and asks the client how he felt about that event/inference. When the client responded with 'inadequate', the therapist noted to himself that this is also not a feeling and tried to clarify Peter's feeling by asking first about his behaviour in the situation and, when this was unrevealing, about his action tendencies. This approach was useful and confirmed the therapist's hypothesis that the client's emotion was one of shame.

In contrast, while the trainee knows that the client's statement that he felt 'criticised' was not representative of a feeling, his continued use of asking for Peter's feelings and then his emotion while declaring that Peter's responses were not feeling statements quickly led the client to show frustration and a sense that the trainee wanted a particular answer from him that he wasn't providing. In short, the trained therapist's thinking and responses were sophisticated and flexible showing a creative application of REBT theory. The trainee, on the other hand, knew that 'criticised' was not a feeling, but other than continuing to assert this fact did little to help the client along the way to identify his feelings.

Table 3 The eight UNEs and HNE alternatives

Unhealthy negative emotion	Healthy negative emotion
Anxiety	Concern
Depression	Sadness
Guilt	Remorse
Shame	Disappointment
Hurt	Sorrow
Unhealthy anger	Healthy anger
Unhealthy jealousy	Healthy jealousy
Unhealthy envy	Healthy envy

Negotiating emotional language with clients

The REBT model of emotions outlines eight unhealthy negative emotions (UNEs) and eight alternative healthy negative emotions (HNEs) (Table 3).

In the practice of REBT, this emotional language framework should preferably be used as a guide rather than as a rigid prescription.

In this section I will consider how to negotiate emotional language with a client, first when the client's emotion is unhealthy and negative and second when discussing a healthy alternative to the client's UNE.

Negotiating emotional language with a client when the client is experiencing a UNE

We have already seen that in working with Glenda (see pp. 45–47), the trained therapist discovered that Glenda used the term 'shame' when an assessment of her UNE indicated that she was really experiencing guilt. Thus:

REBTer: Glenda, often when someone hurts the feelings of a friend and then begs for forgiveness, then that person usually feels guilt rather than shame. So, I'm a bit confused about what you mean by shame.

Glenda: By shame, I mean what you mean by guilt.

REBTer: OK, thanks for clarifying that.

The REBT therapist then needs to work with the client to agree the term that they are going to use. I call this process 'negotiating emotional language with clients'.

Let's return to the trained therapist's work with Glenda.

[REBTer's thinking: I need to agree which term we are going to use, shame or guilt. Let's see which word Glenda prefers.]

REBTer: So which term would you prefer to use?
Glenda: Shame.
REBTer: OK

[REBTer's thinking: That means that when Glenda mentions 'shame' in this context I will have to remind myself that she is really talking about guilt. I will make a note of this.]

Negotiating emotional language with respect to healthy negative emotions

Table 3 showed the emotional terminology employed by REBT therapists. As we do not have agreed terms in the English language for healthy negative emotions, it is important to negotiate carefully the agreed use of such language with a client. I will again compare the thinking and interventions of a trained REBT therapist with those that might be made by a trainee.

Michele came to therapy because she often experienced hurt in her relationships. When asked to give an example of her hurt feelings she discussed feeling hurt when her husband forgot her birthday. In the following sequence we will see how a trained therapist negotiates a term with Michele for a healthy alternative to hurt.

REBTer: Instead of feeling hurt what would be a healthy emotional response to your husband forgetting your birthday.
Michele: I am not sure.

[REBTer's thinking: First, I am going to explain to Michele the concept of a healthy negative emotion and then see what happens.]

REBTer:	Let me help you identify one. OK?
Michele:	OK.
REBTer:	If I understand you, your husband forgetting your birthday is a negative event. Is that right?
Michele:	Correct.
REBTer:	So it's unrealistic to expect you to feel a positive emotion or a neutral emotion as an alternative to hurt. Do you see what I mean?
Michele:	I do.
REBTer:	So the emotion we are aiming for will need to be negative in tone in response to the negative event of your husband forgetting your birthday and it will need to be an alternative to hurt. Are you with me?
Michele:	I am.

[REBTer's thinking: In order to help Michele identify a healthy emotional alternative to hurt, I will need to discover what she did when she felt hurt. Then, I will help her to identify a healthy alternative to that behaviour. Once I have found it, I will ask her for the name of the negative emotion that goes along with that healthy behaviour.]

REBTer:	When you felt hurt about your husband forgetting your birthday, what did you do?
Michele:	Nothing.
REBTer:	Did you feel like telling him about your feelings?
Michele:	No:
REBTer:	Why not?
Michele:	I was so hurt, I did not want to talk to him.
REBTer:	In terms of your goals what would you have liked to have done instead?
Michele:	I would have liked to have told him that I felt hurt, but my hurt prevented me.
REBTer:	You would have liked to have shared your feelings with him. So you need to experience an emotion that has a number of qualities. First, it needs to be a negative emotion because him forgetting your birthday was negative. Second, it needs to help you express your feelings to him.

>   And third, it has to be a healthy alternative to
>   hurt. What would you call such a feeling?
> Michele: Disappointment.
>
> *[REBTer's thinking: REBT considers 'sorrow' to be the
> healthy alternative to hurt. However, as disappointment is close
> enough, I am in two minds raising this issue with Michele. As
> disappointment approximates to sorrow, I can easily work with
> disappointment as a goal. On the other hand, nothing ventured,
> nothing gained and there is no clear contra-indication to me
> raising this issue with Michele, so I will.]*
>
> REBTer: We call the healthy alternative to hurt sorrow in
>   REBT. But disappointment would also be good.
>   What term shall we use in our work together?
> Michele: Can we use 'disappointment'? I don't relate to
>   the word 'sorrow'.
> REBTer: Fine.

Now let's see how a trainee might deal with this situation in his
thinking and response.

> Trainee: OK, Michele, so you felt hurt when your
>   husband forgot your birthday. In your mind
>   what would be a healthy alternative feeling?
> Michele: I am not sure.
>
> *[Trainee's thinking: Well, I know that sorrow is the healthy
> alternative to hurt, so I will suggest that we use that term.]*
>
> Trainee: Well in REBT, we consider that sorrow is the
>   healthy alternative to hurt, so shall we use that
>   term?
> Michele: Well the word sorrow doesn't sound quite right.
> Trainee: But it's close enough so let's use it.
> Michele: (*hesitantly*) Well, er . . . I guess . . . OK.

The trainee knows from REBT theory that 'sorrow' is the
healthy alternative to hurt when her husband forgets her birthday.
However, he is overly simplistic in his interpretation of REBT
theory on this point. The theory does indeed outline specific HNE

alternatives to UNEs. However, the theory also notes that the words used to represent these HNE alternatives are not universally accepted in the English language and such words may not resonate with some clients. In which case alternative terms more acceptable to these clients should be sought. This is the case with Michele. It is clear that she is not happy with the term 'sorrow' as the healthy alternative to 'hurt'. However, the trainee does not pick up on her hesitancy and proceeds with 'sorrow', possibly creating problems for himself later.

By contrast, the trained REBT therapist is much more sophisticated in his thinking and in the interventions that he makes in response to Michele's initial puzzlement concerning the healthy alternative to hurt.

First of all, the trained therapist helps prepare the ground by helping Michele to see that the healthy alternative to hurt in the face of a negative response is a negative emotion. Then, by contrasting Michele's behaviour when she was feeling hurt in this situation (i.e. withdrawal) with its behavioural alternative (telling her husband how she feels) and establishing that her goal was the latter, the therapist has now fully prepared the ground for asking Michele which negative emotion would accompany such disclosure in the face of his forgetfulness. Michele responds with 'disappointment'. It is at this point that the therapist informs the client that REBT's position on the HNE alternative to hurt is sorrow, but in doing so he stresses that the term 'disappointment' is also acceptable. Michele feels free to say that she would prefer to use her term as the term 'sorrow' does not resonate with her in this context.

In the next chapter I will outline how an REBT therapist thinks about 'A' (i.e. what the client was most disturbed about in an emotional episode) once he has assessed 'C' and how that thinking influences his interventions. I will then discuss the thinking and interventions of a trainee.

Chapter 4

Thinking and intervening related to 'A'

Typically 'A' in the 'ABC' framework of REBT stands for activating event. But what does the term 'activating event' mean? If we take the term 'activating' first, it is clear that something is serving as the 'activator' and that something is being activated. It is perhaps easier to deal with the latter question first. When we are thinking about an episode of emotional disturbance, what are being activated are the irrational beliefs at 'B' that underpin the emotional disturbance at 'C'. I will discuss these irrational beliefs presently.

But what is activating these irrational beliefs? When an REBT therapist is assessing a specific example of his client's problem, he is particularly interested in what has activated the person's irrational beliefs that underpin her disturbed emotions and behaviour at 'C'.

Before returning to the issue of the 'activator', let me discuss the term 'event'. This word conjures up something that has actually happened, but this is only partly what is meant by the term. For an event can be something that the person has imagined or it can be an inference about what has happened. For example, a future event is, by definition, an inference about something happening in the future.

I prefer to think about 'A' as the aspect of a situation that the person is most disturbed about. This can be something that has actually happened or more frequently, it is inferential in nature. An inference is a hunch about reality which goes beyond the data at hand and needs to be tested against the available information

Critical 'A' vs. non-critical 'A'

I distinguish between a critical 'A' and a non-critical 'A'. In any situation, a person can disturb herself about many aspects. The aspect of the situation about which the person most disturbs herself is known as the critical 'A'. The other aspects (i.e. those about which the client could, but in fact does not, disturb herself) can be regarded as non-critical 'As'. Since the critical 'A' is the key to understanding what the person is most disturbed about, it can be equated with 'A' when discussing specific episodes of client disturbance.

Let me illustrate how the REBT therapist thinks about 'A' by discussing the case of Keith, a postgraduate student.

> *REBTer*:   OK, Keith so what are you anxious about?
> *Keith*:   Well, my Head of Department has asked me to run an undergraduate seminar and I am anxious about doing so.
>
> *[REBTer's thinking: Well, this is a description of the situation, but it provides no clue about what Keith is anxious about so it is likely that Keith's 'A' (or critical 'A') is inferential in nature. I need to investigate further.]*

In the course of the therapy session, the following emerged as candidates for Keith's 'A':

- He would think he ran a poor seminar.
- The students would think he ran a poor seminar.
- He would sweat in the seminar, but the students would not notice.
- The students would notice him sweating and would think that there was something wrong with him.

As can be seen below, helped by the careful questioning of his therapist, Keith realised that what he was most anxious about was this: that running a poor seminar would have an adverse effect on his career. Here is the thinking that the trained REBT therapist engaged in at this point.

> *REBTer*:   So of all these situations what one are you most anxious about?
> *Keith*:   The students thinking I have run a poor seminar.
>
> *[REBTer's thinking: It is not clear to me why he would be anxious about this. There appears to be something missing. Is*

he scared of developing a bad reputation among undergraduates or is the role of his Head of Department important here? I need to ask.]

REBTer: You mentioned your Head of Department before. Is he relevant here?
Keith: Oh yes!
REBTer: In what way?
Keith: Well, I am scared that if I do a lousy seminar they will tell my Head of Department.

[REBTer's thinking: OK so now I know it has more to do with Keith's Head of Department than with the students, but I don't know what it is about the Head hearing that he has done a lousy job that Keith fears. So I need to ask.]

REBTer: If you do a lousy job and the Head of Department hears of it, what are you particularly anxious about?
Keith: It may adversely affect my career.

[REBTer's thinking: That seems nearer to the mark, but I just need to check if there is anything else more anxiety-provoking for Keith.]

REBTer: And if it does?
Keith: That would be terrible.

[REBTer's thinking: Well, as Keith has spontaneously revealed an irrational belief it seems like his critical 'A' is 'doing a lousy job in the seminar adversely affects my career'. I just need to double check on that.]

REBTer: So, it sounds like the reason that you're anxious about doing a lousy seminar is because you think that it might adversely affect your career. But what if you knew it wouldn't, would that change things for you?
Keith: Definitely. I wouldn't be anxious.
REBTer: Even if your Head of Department found out about it?
Keith: As long as it did not adversely affect my career, no.

Comment on REBTer's thinking and interventions

Here the REBT therapist's thinking reflects a number of REBT-based points. First, as I will discuss later in this book, the therapist knows that Keith is anxious about something that he finds personally threatening to his personal domain. Second, although Keith reveals a number of things that could serve as threats, the REBT therapist does not assume that any of them are Keith's critical 'A' until he has evidence to support this. He is guided by the notion that the critical 'A' is the aspect of the situation that the client is most disturbed about. Even when the client spontaneously reveals an irrational belief (i.e. 'That would be terrible) in relation to the inference 'Doing a lousy seminar may adversely affect my career', the REBT therapist double checks this by subtracting this inference from the client's inferential field to see the effect of doing so. When the client reveals that this subtraction would have a significant effect on his target emotion (in this case, anxiety), the therapist has even more evidence that he has found the client's critical 'A'.

In summary, the REBT therapist discovered that Keith's critical 'A' was 'Doing a lousy seminar may adversely affect my career' and the other events he mentioned can be best thought of as non-critical 'As' in that, potentially, Keith could have disturbed himself about them, but did not do so.

It is worth noting that when a person disturbs herself about a critical 'A', the nature of her disturbed emotion gives a clue to the inferential theme implicit in her critical 'A', as I pointed out in Chapter 3.

Assuming temporarily that 'A' is true

One of the most common errors that participants on the Primary Practicum make is challenging 'A' before helping clients to identify and dispute their irrational beliefs at 'B'. The kind of thinking that informs this 'challenge "A" before "B" strategy' is based on the idea that if the client has made an obvious cognitive distortion at 'A', then this needs to be challenged as soon as it is expressed, particularly if it seems to account for the person's disturbed emotion at 'C'.

Let me give an example. In the course of a peer counselling session, Arthur was counselling Maureen. Maureen had identified guilt as a problem and Arthur was doing a good job at working with a specific example of Maureen's guilt. Maureen felt guilty about saying that she would not visit her mother the following weekend because she had been asked out on a date by a man that she was interested in. When Arthur correctly enquired what she was most guilty about, Maureen replied that she felt most guilty about being selfish. At this point, Arthur spotting an obvious cognitive distortion challenged Maureen's notion that she would be selfish if she put her mother off for a week. During supervision, it emerged that Arthur thought that Maureen's inference 'I am being selfish' accounted for her guilt and was obviously distorted and thus constituted a good target for intervention.

An REBT therapist would have engaged in a different type of thinking.

Let me construct a dialogue between Maureen and an REBT therapist and highlight the therapist's thinking at important junctures, showing particularly how this therapist's thinking would differ from Arthur's.

REBTer: So, Maureen, can you give me an example of your guilt?

Maureen: Well, last night I spoke to my mother and she wants me to stay next weekend. Ordinarily, I would have been happy to visit her, but next weekend this guy I'm interested in has asked me out.

REBTer: So what did you do?

Maureen: I didn't say anything to her because I would have felt guilty.

REBTer: Guilty about what?

Maureen: About being selfish.

[REBTer's thinking: Maureen's idea that she would be selfish if she put her mother off is clearly an inference at 'A' and therefore I am not going to challenge this idea here even though it seems quite distorted. I am going to use it to help us both identify the irrational beliefs that underpin her guilt.]

REBTer: Well, let's assume that you would have been selfish if you put your mother off. What were you demanding about being selfish that led you to feel guilty and not say anything to her?

Note how the REBT therapist's thinking differs from Arthur's.

- The therapist's thinking is properly informed by REBT's theory of disturbed emotions which states that a client's disturbed feelings are based on her irrational beliefs about 'A' and not on 'A' even if this 'A' may be obviously distorted.
- Arthur appears to be thinking more like a general CBT therapist in that he thinks that Maureen's distorted 'A' (i.e. her selfish behaviour) accounts for her guilt at 'C'.

It is interesting to note that both Arthur and the therapist agree that Maureen's 'A' is distorted, but because the latter is thinking like an REBT therapist, he uses this to identify Maureen's irrational beliefs at 'B', while Arthur's non-REBT thinking leads him to make a very different intervention.

I turn now to the heart of the REBT 'ABC' model of emotions, i.e. the beliefs at 'B', and will discuss the thinking and interventions related to 'B' carried out by both trained therapist and trainee.

Chapter 5

Thinking and intervening related to 'B'

Beliefs are at the very heart of the REBT model of emotions. This model has two parts:

- Part 1: People disturb themselves about life's adversities by holding rigid and extreme beliefs about these adversities.
- Part 2: People respond healthily to life's adversities by holding flexible and non-extreme beliefs about these adversities.

So what largely explains why one person may handle an adversity well and another may respond to the same adversity with disturbance is the different beliefs that these two people hold about the adversity in question. In REBT parlance, rigid and extreme beliefs are known as irrational beliefs and flexible and non-extreme beliefs are known as rational beliefs.

Classical REBT theory has it that there are four irrational beliefs and four rational beliefs. Of the four irrational beliefs the demand is regarded as primary and the other three irrational beliefs as secondary in that they are derived from the primary irrational belief. Similarly, of the four rational beliefs, the non-dogmatic preference is regarded as primary and the other three rational beliefs as secondary in that they are derived from the primary rational belief. This is shown in Table 4.

I can best show how to think like an REBT therapist by taking one irrational belief at a time and discussing how these differ from their rational belief alternative.

Table 4 Irrational and rational beliefs

Irrational beliefs	Rational beliefs
Demands	Non-dogmatic preferences
↓	↓
Awfulising beliefs	Non-awfulising beliefs
Low frustration tolerance (LFT) beliefs	High frustration tolerance (HFT) beliefs
Self-/other-/life-depreciation beliefs	Self-/other-/life-acceptance beliefs

Demands vs. non-dogmatic (or full) preferences

To grasp fully the difference between demands and non-dogmatic (or full) preferences, it is important to understand that both are usually based on what are called 'partial preferences'. A partial preference is a statement of preference. Here the person states what she would like to happen or what she would like not to happen.

Here is how an REBT therapist's thinking differs from a trainee's when both hear a client's partial preference.

> *Henry*:   So I would like my boss to approve of my work.
>
> *[REBTer's thinking: I don't know at the moment whether this statement is an example of a demand or a non-dogmatic (full) preference, I need to find this out.]*
>
> *[Trainee's thinking: The client has articulated a preference. In REBT, preferences are rational beliefs so the client's belief is rational.]*

The REBT therapist knows REBT theory better than the trainee. He knows that the client has only provided half the story and for a preference statement to be an example of a rational belief it needs to be expressed in its full or non-dogmatic form as shown below:

Henry: So I would like my boss to approve of my work, but he does not have to do so.

The REBT therapist knows, therefore that in a primary rational belief (i.e. a non-dogmatic or full preference), the client needs to assert her preference and negate the possible demand. This knowledge leads him to ask a question that the trainee does not ask:

Henry: So I would like my boss to approve of my work.
REBTer: And are you saying that she has to do so or that she does not have to do so?

By not asking this question, the trainee leaves open the possibility that the client will implicitly transform her partial preference into a demand as in the following:

Henry: So I would like my boss to approve of my work and therefore he has to do so.

Here the client asserts his preference and makes explicit his implicit demand.

In REBT theory and practice it is usual for a demand to be expressed just as that – a demand. For example, the client might say: 'My boss must approve of my work'. It is useful, though, to remember that this demand is often based on a partial preference and thus the therapeutic task is to help the client to formulate and increase conviction in the negated demand component rather than convert her partial preference into a demand. These two different routes are shown below:

- Common pathway: I would like my boss to approve of my work . . .
- Rational route: . . . but he does not have to do so.
- Irrational route: . . . and therefore he has to do so.

The problematic nature of language I: distinguishing between demands and non-dogmatic preferences

When it comes to distinguishing between demands and non-dogmatic (full) preferences, language can sometimes clarify and sometimes confuse. Therefore, it is important that the REBT therapist keep in mind the actual differences between these two as summarised below:

- Demand = Assertion of preference transformed into a demand. For example: 'I want my boss to approve of my work and therefore he has to do so.'
- Non-dogmatic preference = Assertion of preference and negation of demand.
  For example: 'I want my boss to approve of my work, but he does not have to do so.'

The word 'should'

Because he keeps firmly in mind the distinction between a demand and a non-dogmatic preference, the REBT therapist engages in a particular type of thinking when faced with ambiguous client language. One of the most ambiguous words that clients use when referring to their beliefs is the word 'should'. The word 'should' has several different meanings in the English language which makes it particularly problematic for REBT therapists. The different meanings of the word 'should' that are particularly relevant to REBT therapists are as follows:

The recommendatory 'should'

This means 'I recommend that . . .' or 'It would be a good idea if . . .' (e.g. 'As a boss, you should praise me for my work').

The ideal 'should'

This means that it would be good if an ideal situation were to happen (e.g. 'People should all love one another and live in peace and harmony').

The empirical 'should'

This means that if all the conditions are in place for 'x' to happen, then 'x' will happen (e.g. after his boss disapproved of his work, Henry's friends argued, using the 'ideal' should (see above), that his boss 'should' not have done so. Henry replied, using the empirical should, 'No, my boss should have disapproved of my work because all the conditions were in place for him to do so').

The preferential 'should'

This means that you would prefer it if certain things would happen or not happen. It can either be a partial preference as when Henry states: 'My boss should not disapprove of my work' or it can be a full or non-dogmatic preference as when Henry states: 'My boss should not disapprove of my work, but it does not follow that he must not do so'. Only in the latter sense is 'should' an indicator of a rational belief.

The absolute 'should'

When a 'should' is used in its absolute sense, it indicates an irrational belief. Since there are so many different meanings of the word 'should', the REBT therapist either avoids using the word altogether, preferring to use the less ambiguous term 'must' or uses it with the qualifier 'absolutely'. What the REBT does refrain from doing is using the word 'should' without qualification since doing so creates confusion for the client.

Here is an example of an REBT therapist's thinking in response to a client using the word 'should' ambiguously. Then compare it with a trainee's thinking.

Henry: My boss should not disapprove of my work.

[REBTer's thinking: Henry's use of the word 'should' without any qualifier is ambiguous. It is just not clear whether he is being demanding or not. So, I need to ask him a question to clarify this.]

REBTer: OK, Henry, I am not sure what you mean here. Do you mean that your boss ideally should not disapprove of your work, or that you would prefer him not to do so, but he doesn't have to do what you want? Or do you mean that he absolutely should or must not disapprove of your work?

Henry: I mean that he absolutely should or must not disapprove of my work.

Now here is the trainee's thinking:

Henry: My boss should not disapprove of my work.

[Trainee's thinking: Henry used the word 'should'. I have learned that shoulds are irrational so this is an irrational belief which I will now dispute.]

Trainee: Why should he not disapprove of your work?

Note that both the REBT therapist and the trainee are correct in identifying Henry's belief as irrational. However, the trainee is fortunate in the sense that if Henry's belief was not irrational, the trainee would have proceeded as if it was (without checking the meaning of Henry's 'should') and would have run into a therapeutic obstacle later.

By contrast, the REBT therapist proceeded only on the basis of evidence after carefully checking the meaning of Henry's 'should'. If Henry's 'should' was not absolute in nature, the therapist would have discovered this, but the trainee would not have done so.

Must: conditional or unconditional?

I pointed out above that the word 'must' captures the rigid nature of a demand much better than the unqualified 'should' does. However, not all 'musts' are indicators of an irrational belief. The criterion that needs to be met for a 'must' to be an irrational belief is unconditionality. However, some 'musts' as expressed by clients are conditional and this can be the source of much confusion among trainees.

When a 'must' is unconditional, it does not stipulate why the person believes that the condition has to be met. Thus, when Lorna says, 'My colleagues must like me', and her 'must' is unconditional, she means that they have to like her and that is that.

However, when a 'must' is conditional, the person believes that the condition has to be met for a reason or purpose. Thus, when Sarah says 'My colleagues must like me' and her 'must' is conditional, then in her mind there is a reason why her colleagues must like her (e.g. 'My colleagues must like me in order to help me with my work when I get stuck' or 'My colleagues must like me for me to get promotion'). The point is that conditional 'musts' are not irrational beliefs and, thus, are not at the core of disturbance.

When conditional 'musts' are expressed in their full form, it is clear that they are inferences that are either accurate or inaccurate.

Thus, when Sarah says that 'My colleagues must like me for me to get promotion' she is inferring one of two things.

First, she is inferring that being liked by her colleagues is a necessary, but not sufficient condition for her to be promoted. This means that in her mind, she won't get promoted unless she is liked by her colleagues, but that being liked is not a sufficient condition for her promotion. In other words, she may think that there are a number of conditions that have to be met for her to be promoted of which being liked by her colleagues is one such condition. It is difficult for Sarah to know if her 'conditional must' inference relating to being liked and getting promoted is correct in advance unless she is told specifically so by those who are in charge of granting promotions. However, if she has evidence that she is disliked by her colleagues and still is promoted then her inference is disconfirmed.

Second, when Sarah is inferring that she must be liked by her colleagues in order to be promoted, she may think that being liked is both a necessary and a sufficient condition for her to be promoted. This means that being liked has to be present for Sarah to receive promotion and that no other conditions are necessary. Again, this inference may be accurate or inaccurate and it is again difficult for Sarah to know in advance whether it is accurate, although it is unlikely for a single criterion to be put forward by promotion panels.

Finally, the reason or purpose behind a person's conditional 'must' may be an unconditional 'must' in its own right. Thus, when Sarah says 'My colleagues must like me for me to get promotion' she may then hold an unconditional 'must' about promotion (e.g. 'I must be promoted'). However, this 'must' about promotion may itself be conditional (e.g. 'I must be promoted in order to have equal status with my friends').

The main point I want to make here is that the word 'must' like the word 'should' is not always indicative of an irrational belief and this needs to be explored with the client.

Here is how an REBT therapist thinks when a client reveals a 'must'.

REBTer:	So what were you demanding at that point?
Hilary:	That I must impress my brother.

[REBTer's thinking: I am not sure if this 'must' is conditional or unconditional so I need to clarify this. I need to discover if there is a reason behind her 'must'.]

REBTer: Why do you think that you have to impress your brother?

[Note that this is not a question designed to dispute an irrational belief, but a question designed to assess a possible reason for the client's demand.]

Hilary: Because if I do he will give me a job and I am desperate for a job.

[REBTer's thinking: I want to double check to see if Hilary is demanding to impress her brother or if she is demanding a job so I will ask about that.]

REBTer: So if you weren't desperate for a job, would you still have to impress your brother?
Hilary: No.

Compare the above with how a trainee thinks when a client reveals a 'must'.

Trainee: So what were you demanding at that point?
Hilary: That I must impress my brother.

[Trainee's thinking: That is the client's irrational belief.]

Trainee: Why must you impress your brother?

[Here, the trainee is disputing what he sees as the client's irrational belief.]

Finally, as with other irrational beliefs, what provides the most reliable clue to whether or not the person holds a demand is the person's 'C'. If the person's emotional 'C' is unhealthy, his behavioural 'C' is dysfunctional and his cognitive 'C' is highly distorted then he is more likely to hold a demand than a non-dogmatic (full) preference.

Extreme vs. non-extreme beliefs

According to REBT theory, extreme and non-extreme beliefs are derived from rigid and flexible beliefs respectively. As such, they are regarded as secondary irrational beliefs.

In REBT theory, there are three sets of extreme and non-extreme beliefs which are seen as derivatives of demands and non-dogmatic preferences respectively. These are:

- awfulising beliefs vs. non-awfulising beliefs
- low frustration tolerance (LFT) beliefs vs. high frustration tolerance (HFT) beliefs
- depreciation beliefs vs. acceptance beliefs.

I will consider these one at a time.

Awfulising beliefs vs. non-awfulising beliefs

To grasp fully the difference between awfulising beliefs and non-awfulising beliefs, it is important to understand that both are usually based on what are called partial non-awfulising beliefs. A partial non-awfulising belief is an evaluation of badness when a person's preference is not met. Here, the person states that it would be bad if what she would like to happen does not happen or if what she would like not to happen happens.

Here is an example of what I mean:

Henry: It would be bad if my boss does not approve of my work.

Here is how an REBT therapist's thinking differs from a trainee's when both hear this client statement.

Henry: It would be bad if my boss does not approve of my work.

[REBTer's thinking: I don't know at the moment whether this statement is an example of a non-awfulising belief or not. I need to find this out.]

[Trainee's thinking: The client has articulated a non-awfulising belief. In REBT, non-awfulising beliefs are rational beliefs so the client's belief is rational.]

Again, the REBT therapist knows REBT theory better than the trainee. He knows that the client has only provided half the story and for a non-awfulising belief to be an example of a rational belief it needs to be expressed in its full or non-extreme form as shown below:

Henry: So it would be bad if my boss did not approve of my work, but it would not be the end of the world.

The REBT therapist knows, therefore, that in a secondary, non-awfulising, rational belief, the client needs to assert her evaluation of badness and negate the awfulising component. This knowledge leads him to ask a question that the trainee does not ask:

Henry: So, it would be bad if my boss does not approve of my work.
REBTer: And are you saying that it would be terrible if she doesn't or that it would be bad, but not terrible?

By not asking this question, the trainee leaves open the possibility that Henry will implicitly transform his partial non-awfulising belief into an awfulising belief as in the following:

Henry: It would be bad if my boss did not approve of my work and therefore it would be terrible if she does not do so.

Here the client asserts his evaluation of badness and makes explicit his implicit awfulising belief.

In REBT theory and practice it is again usual for an awfulising belief to be expressed just as that – an awfulising belief. For example, the client might say: 'It would be terrible if my boss does not approve of my work.'

It is useful, though, to remember that this awfulising belief is often based on a partial non-awfulising belief (or evaluation of badness) and thus the therapeutic task is to help the client to formulate and increase conviction in the negated awfulising component rather than convert her partial non-awfulising belief into an awfulising belief. These two different routes are shown below:

- Common pathway: It would be bad if my boss did not approve of my work . . .
- Rational route: . . . but it would not be terrible if he does not do so.
- Irrational route: . . . and therefore it would be terrible if he does not do so.

'Very, very bad' is not necessarily awfulising

In REBT theory, it is possible for a person to hold a belief to the effect that 'It would be very, very bad if "x" happened' and for that belief to be rational even though it seems extreme and thus irrational. The way to determine this is, as before, to see if the person has negated the awfulising component or not. Here is how an REBT therapist thinks when faced with this situation as contrasted with the thinking of a trainee.

> *Henry*: So it would be very, very bad if my boss did not approve of my work, but it would not be the end of the world.
>
> *[REBTer's thinking: Even though the client has used the term 'very, very bad', I am not sure if this is a rational or an irrational belief. So I need to ask about this.]*
>
> *REBTer*: And are you saying that it would be terrible if she doesn't or that it would be very, very bad, but not terrible?

Here is how the trainee thinks about the same client statement.

> *Henry*: So, it would be very, very bad if my boss does not approve of my work

[Trainee's thinking: Very, very bad sounds like awfulising to me so I have found the client's irrational belief.]

By accepting 'very, very bad' as an awfulising belief, the trainee does not help himself or his client to discover whether this statement represents an irrational belief or a rational belief. The trainee needs to be guided by the following:

- Common pathway: It would be very, very bad if my boss did not approve of my work . . .
- Rational route: . . . but it would not be terrible if he does not do so.
- Irrational route: . . . and therefore it would be terrible if he does not do so.

The important thing to remember here is that the mark of an awfulising belief is its extreme nature. While a statement like 'very, very bad' sounds extreme, it may not be and the way to determine this is to check further. As noted above, if the belief has a partial non-awfulising component and a negated awfulising component, it is a non-awfulising belief. However, if it has a partial non-awfulising component and an awfulising component, it is an awfulising belief.

The problematic nature of language II: distinguishing between awfulising beliefs and non-awfulising beliefs

As I argued in the section on the problematic nature of language with respect to demands and non-dogmatic preferences, it is important to distinguish between language and meaning in REBT (Dryden, 1986b). This issue is also salient when we consider the meaning of words that are often used to represent awfulising and non-awfulising beliefs. Let's start with the word 'awful'.

The meaning of awful

In REBT, an awfulising belief occurs in the form 'It would be awful if "x" happens'. It is an extreme belief which indicates that the person believes at the time that if 'x' happens:

1   nothing could be worse;
2   'x' is worse than 100% bad; and
3   no good could possibly come from this bad event.

However, the term 'awful' can mean different things in different contexts. Thus, it is often a synonym for 'bad' or 'very bad'. For example, if the weather is poor and I say that the weather is awful, I mean that the weather is bad and not that nothing worse could possibly happen to me.

As with other irrational beliefs, what provides the most reliable clue to whether or not the person holds an awfulising belief is the person's 'C'. If the person's emotional 'C' is unhealthy, his behavioural 'C' is dysfunctional and his cognitive 'C' is highly distorted then he is more likely to hold an awfulising belief than a non-awfulising belief.

Catastrophising vs. awfulising

REBT tends to distinguish between the terms 'catastrophe' and 'tragedy' on the one hand and the term 'awful' on the other. At first sight this may seem like splitting hairs, but it is not. Let me consider the terms 'catastrophe' and 'tragedy' first. A catastrophe normally affects a large number of people (like a tsunami, 9/11 or an earthquake), while a tragedy normally affects one person or a close-knit group of people (like the premature death of a loved one or a serious illness). Whatever language is employed, they both are usually seen as a great adversity that has a very significant impact on people's lives, an event that people would struggle to come to terms with and transcend, even if they thought rationally about it. However, it is possible for people to transcend the catastrophe or tragedy and go on to live healthily and happily in the future.

The term 'awful', however, when it is used in an episode of personal disturbance implies, as stated above, that something is worse than it absolutely should be, an event so bad that it cannot be transcended. Thus, if a person believes that it is awful that a tragedy or catastrophe has occurred then she is adding disturbance to the distress that she would naturally and healthily experience in the face of the great adversity.

You may see the terms 'awfulising' and 'catastrophising' used interchangeably in the CBT literature, but these should not be regarded as synonymous. The former means that the person is holding an awfulising belief which in REBT is defined as an extreme belief stemming from a demand. It is thus seen as a secondary irrational belief stemming from a primary irrational belief.

The latter, on the other hand, is often seen in REBT as a cognitive distortion, which exaggerates the negativity of possible events without it reaching extreme proportions and without implying that the events cannot be transcended. Such distorted catastrophes are best regarded as consequences of irrational beliefs, both primary and secondary, and are inferences rather than beliefs.

Low frustration tolerance (LFT) beliefs vs. high frustration tolerance (HFT) beliefs

As with demands vs. non-dogmatic preferences and awfulising beliefs vs. non-awfulising beliefs, LFT beliefs and HFT beliefs are both usually based on what are called partial HFT beliefs. A partial HFT belief involves an acknowledgement that it is a struggle to put up with the adversity at 'A'. This is known as the struggle component and occurs when a person's preference is not met. Here, the person states that it would be a struggle to tolerate it if what she would like to happen does not happen or if what she would like not to happen happens.

Here is an example of what I mean:

Henry: It would be a struggle to put up with my boss not approving of my work

Here is how an REBT therapist's thinking differs from a trainee's when both hear the above client statement.

Henry: It would be a struggle to put up with my boss not approving of my work.

[REBTer's thinking: I don't know at the moment whether this statement is an example of an HFT belief or not. I need to find this out.]

[Trainee's thinking: The client has articulated an HFT belief since he hasn't said that he can't tolerate his 'A'.]

Once again, the REBT therapist knows REBT theory better than the trainee. He knows that the client has only provided half of the belief and for an HFT belief to be an example of a rational belief it needs to be expressed in its full, non-extreme form as shown below:

Henry: It would be a struggle to put up with my boss not approving of my work, but I could bear it.

The REBT therapist knows, therefore, that in a secondary, HFT, rational belief, the client needs to assert the struggle component and negate what I call the unbearability component. This knowledge leads him to ask a question that the trainee does not ask:

Henry: It would be a struggle to put up with my boss not approving of my work.

REBTer: And are you saying that it would be bearable or unbearable if she doesn't?

By not asking this question, the trainee leaves open the possibility that Henry will implicitly transform his partial HFT belief into an LFT belief as in the following:

Henry: It would be a struggle to put up with my boss not approving of my work and therefore it would be unbearable.

Here the client asserts the idea that it would be a struggle for him to deal with his boss's disapproval and makes explicit his implicit LFT belief.

In REBT theory and practice it is again usual for an LFT belief to be expressed as just that – an LFT belief. For example, the client might say: 'I could not bear it if my boss does not approve of my work.'

It is useful, though, to remember that this LFT belief is often based on a partial HFT belief and thus the therapeutic task is to help the client to formulate and increase conviction in the negated LFT component rather than convert the partial HFT belief into an LFT belief. These two different routes are shown below:

•   Common pathway: It would be a struggle to put up with my boss not approving of my work . . .

- Rational route: . . . but I could tolerate it if she does not do so.
- Irrational route: . . . and therefore I could not tolerate it if she does not do so.

The 'worth it' component

So far I have outlined two components of an HFT belief: (i) the struggle component and (ii) the negated LFT component. In addition, there is a third component of an HFT belief and this is what I call the 'worth it' component. In this component, the person acknowledges that it is worth it to her to tolerate the adversity in question. Applying this to Henry's case, we have:

Henry: It would be a struggle to put up with my boss not approving of my work, but I could bear it and it is worth it to me to do so.

The REBT therapist knows that an HFT belief has three components, but the trainee, in all probability doesn't. This difference is reflected in their thinking as shown below.

Henry: It would be a struggle to put up with my boss not approving of my work, but I could bear it.

[REBTer's thinking: Henry has two of the three components of an HFT belief, but I wonder if he has the third. Although he states that he can bear his boss's disapproval, I don't know if he thinks it is worth bearing. So I need to ask him about this.]

REBTer: So, Henry, you say that you can bear your boss's disapproval, but do you think that it is worth bearing or not?
Henry: How do you mean?
REBTer: Well, you said that you wanted to be concerned but not anxious about the prospect of your work being disapproved by your boss; will believing that you can bear this disapproval help you to achieve this goal?
Henry: Yes, it will.
REBTer: So is it worth it to you to bear her disapproval?
Henry: Putting it that way, yes.

> *[REBTer helps Henry to link the third component of his HFT belief to the latter's goal for change.]*

Compare REBTer's thinking and the interventions that it spawns with the trainee's thinking.

> *Henry:*   It would be a struggle to put up with my boss not approving of my work, but I could bear it.
>
> *[Trainee's thinking: That is definitely a rational belief. Henry says that he can bear his boss's disapproval and this is good enough for me.]*

Note that the trainee's thinking does not lead to a further intervention, while the trained therapist's does. The problem with the trainee's thinking is that it does not enable him to deal with the case that Henry may believe that it is not worth it to him to tolerate his boss's disapproval even though he believes that he can do so.

The problematic nature of language III: LFT beliefs vs. HFT beliefs

As I have already argued, it is important to distinguish between language and meaning in REBT. This issue is relevant when we consider the meaning of words that are often used to represent LFT and HFT, particularly with the phrase 'I can't stand it'.

'I can't stand it'

In common parlance, when someone says 'I can't stand it', that person often means that the 'it' in question is difficult to tolerate and not that it's unbearable. However, in REBT terms when someone says 'I can't stand it!' and this represents an LFT belief, the person is deemed to mean the following:

1   I will die or disintegrate if the frustration or discomfort continues to exist.

2   I will lose the capacity to experience happiness if the frustration or discomfort continues to exist.

As with other irrational beliefs, what provides the most reliable clue to whether or not the person holds an LFT is the person's 'C'. If the person's emotional 'C' is unhealthy, his behavioural 'C' is dysfunctional and his cognitive 'C' is highly distorted then he is more likely to hold an LFT belief than an HFT belief.

However, let's see how an REBT therapist and a trainee think and intervene when they both hear a client articulate the phrase 'I can't stand it'. First, here is the REBT therapist.

> *Henry*:   My boss did not approve of my work and I can't stand it.
>
> *[REBTer's thinking: OK, Henry has said that he can't stand his boss not approving of his work, but I am not sure what he means by this so I need to clarify it with him.]*
>
> *REBTer*:   OK, when you say that you can't stand your boss not approving of your work, do you mean at the time that it's hard to tolerate but you could still be happy, or do you mean at the time that you couldn't be happy again?
> *Henry*:   At the time it feels like I couldn't be happy again so I guess that's what I mean.

Compare this with the how the trainee thinks.

> *Henry*:   My boss did not approve of my work and I can't stand it.
>
> *[Trainee's thinking: Henry says that when his boss did not approve of his work that he can't stand it. This is clearly an LFT belief.]*

Because the trainee considers that Henry's statement 'I can't stand it' represents an LFT belief, he does not think he needs to clarify this statement further. By failing to clarify this, he may assume wrongly that the statement 'I can't stand it' is an LFT belief whereas it may not be, as shown in the following dialogue:

Henry: My boss did not approve of my work and I can't stand it.

[REBTer's thinking: OK, Henry has said that he can't stand his boss not approving of his work, but I am not sure what he means by this so I need to clarify it with him.]

REBTer: OK, when you say that you can't stand your boss not approving of your work, do you mean at the time that it's hard to tolerate but you could still be happy, or do you mean at the time that you couldn't be happy again?

Henry: At the time and now I meant that it's hard to tolerate but I can certainly be happy again.

While I have focused on the phrase 'I can't stand it', similar points can be made with respect to the terms 'I can't bear it', 'I can't tolerate it', etc.

In this section, I hope I have shown clearly the difference between an REBT therapist's and a trainee's thinking and interventions. The REBT therapist clearly recognises that words may have different meanings when it comes to rational and irrational beliefs and does not take at face value clients' statements when they seem to indicate the presence of these beliefs. The trainee, on the other hand, is much more likely to think that the words a client uses are a reliable guide to the presence of rational or irrational beliefs.

Depreciation beliefs vs. acceptance beliefs

Depreciation beliefs and acceptance beliefs share one idea: that when a person has acted badly or something bad has happened to him then it is possible and realistic for him to evaluate a part of himself or what has happened to him as shown in the underlined section below:

- When I am not approved of that is bad.
- When you don't treat me fairly that is very regrettable.
- If life is uncomfortable it is only uncomfortable in this respect.

Depreciation beliefs

Depreciation beliefs differ from acceptance beliefs in the following respect.

In depreciation beliefs, the person believes that he and others can be rated on the basis of one of their aspects and the world can be rated on the basis of one of its aspects as shown in the underlined material below:

- When I am not approved that is bad <u>and proves that I am an unlikeable person</u>.
- When you don't treat me fairly that is very regrettable <u>and proves that you are a bad person</u>.
- If life is uncomfortable it is not only uncomfortable in this respect, <u>life is bad</u>.

Acceptance beliefs

In acceptance beliefs, on the other hand, the person believes that he and others cannot be rated on the basis of one of their aspects and the world cannot be rated on the basis of one of its aspects. Here, the depreciation of the person or life is negated as shown in the underlined material below:

- When I am not approved of that is bad, <u>but it does not prove that I am unlikeable person</u>.
- When you don't treat me fairly that is very regrettable, <u>but it does not prove that you are a bad person</u>.
- If life is uncomfortable it is only uncomfortable in this respect; <u>life is not bad</u>.

In addition, in acceptance beliefs the person holds that when a person acts badly or something bad happens to him, this does not affect the fallibility of the people involved or the complexity of life. This is what I call the 'assertion of acceptance' component. These are shown in the underlined material below:

- When I am not approved of that is bad, but it does not prove that I am an unlikeable person. <u>Rather, I am a fallible human being whether I am approved or not</u>.

- When you don't treat me fairly that is very regrettable, but it does not prove that you are a bad person. <u>You are the same fallible person whether you treat me well or badly</u>.
- If life is uncomfortable it is only uncomfortable in this respect, life is not bad. <u>It is a complex mixture of the good, the bad and the neutral whether or not it is uncomfortable in this respect</u>.

Distinguishing between a depreciation belief and an acceptance belief

In distinguishing between a depreciation belief and an acceptance belief, it is important to ensure that the acceptance belief has all three components:

- The evaluation of part of oneself or of what happened to one
- The negation of depreciation component
- The assertion of acceptance component.

The trained REBT therapist is more likely to ensure this than the trainee as shown in the following two sections. In these two sections I will analyse a case where the focus is on self-depreciation and self-acceptance. The arguments provided, however, are equally applicable to other-depreciation and other-acceptance on the one hand and to life-depreciation and life-acceptance on the other.

The absence of depreciation is not necessarily acceptance

If a client refers to something that has happened to her as being bad, she is evaluating that happening. On its own, we have no idea whether or not she is also evaluating herself on the basis of that initial evaluation. Let's first consider the thinking of the trained REBT therapist and then that of a trainee on this point and the effects of their thinking on their interventions or lack of interventions.

> *Kathy*:   Being disapproved of is bad.
>
> *[REBTer's thinking: Kathy has made no reference to the implications that this occurrence has for her belief about herself so I need to ask her.]*

REBTer: And are you judging yourself for being dis-approved of or not?

Kathy: Yes, I think I am unlikeable.

Kathy: Being disapproved of is bad.

[Trainee's thinking: Kathy hasn't said that she is depreciating herself so she isn't. She seems to have a rational belief about being disapproved of.]

The trainee's thinking leads to no further enquiry on his part concerning whether or not Kathy has a self-depreciation belief. As shown above, she has, so the trainee's assumption that the lack of a stated depreciation belief signifies acceptance led to him making an error which the trained REBT therapist did not make.

The negation of depreciation is not necessarily acceptance

When the client states that she is not a worthless person, for example, this is known as negating her self-depreciation. Let's consider the thinking and subsequent response (or lack of response) from the REBT therapist and the trainee.

Kathy: Being disapproved of is bad, <u>but it does not prove that I am an unlikeable person</u>.

[REBTer's thinking: I know that a self-acceptance belief has three components: (i) an evaluation of an aspect of self or of what has happened to the person; (ii) negation of the self-depreciation component and (iii) assertion of the self-acceptance component. Kathy has provided the first two, but she has not yet asserted the self-acceptance component. So I need to ask her about this for it is still possible for her to negate the self-depreciation component and still hold a more subtle form of a self-depreciation.]

REBTer: So if it does not make you an unlikeable person, what does it make you?

Kathy:	Well, I'm not sure . . .
REBTer:	Well, would your attitude toward yourself change if the person approved of you rather than disapproved of you?
Kathy:	Yes.
REBTer:	In what way?
Kathy:	Well, I would regard myself as more likeable if I were approved of.
REBTer:	And therefore less likeable if you are disapproved of?
Kathy:	Yes.

Comment on the trained therapist's thinking and interventions

Here the trained therapist keeps in mind the three components of a self-acceptance belief and by matching this concept with what the client actually says realises that the client has not asserted the self-acceptance component of a self-acceptance belief. This leads the REBT therapist to investigate further to see if the assertion of a self-acceptance component is present, but not expressed, or not present. As can be seen above, the client was still holding a self-depreciation belief albeit a more subtle form of this belief. I will discuss the different forms that a self-depreciation belief can take in the following section. But first let's see how a trainee would tend to think and the effect of that thinking on what he does or does not do subsequently.

Kathy:	Being disapproved of is bad, but it does not prove that I am unlikeable person.

[Trainee's thinking: I think that the client is expressing a self-acceptance belief. She has said that she is not an unlikeable person and there is no indication that she is depreciating herself. So the client's belief is rational.]

Comment on the trainee's thinking and interventions

It is apparent that the trainee is holding a different, less sophisticated conceptualisation of a self-acceptance belief than the trained REBT therapist. The trainee thinks that because the client has negated self-depreciation then it follows that she is holding a self-acceptance belief. The trainee believes therefore that a self-acceptance belief has two components, while the trained REBT therapist correctly believes that it has three. While the absence of a self-depreciation component may indicate that the client is holding a self-acceptance belief, this is not necessarily the case, as the trained REBT therapist revealed when he investigated Kathy's belief further. The point to bear in mind, as is amply demonstrated by the trained REBT therapist, is that when a client reveals two of the three components of a self-acceptance belief, then the therapist (trained or trainee) needs to investigate further to see if she also holds the third or whether (as was the case with Kathy) she holds a more subtle form of a self-depreciation belief.

The problematic nature of language IV: depreciation vs. acceptance beliefs

While the term 'depreciation' is readily understandable by clients sometimes what they mean by depreciation is less easily understood by their therapists.

I am worthless vs. I am less worthy

If one thinks of a scale of negative evaluation ranging from 1 per cent to 100 per cent, it is clear that when a client evaluates herself negatively, she does not always mean that she is worthless. Sometimes she means that she is less worthy, but not worthless.

Let's compare the thinking and interventions of a trained REBT therapist with those of a trainee when a client who is depreciating herself resists the idea that she thinks she is worthless because in reality she thinks she is less worthy. First, let's see how the trained therapist responds to this situation.

Fay:	I felt depressed when my boyfriend left me for my best friend.
REBTer:	Did you judge yourself when you felt depressed?
Fay:	Yes.
REBTer:	What judgement did you make of yourself?
Fay:	I am not sure.

[REBTer's thinking: I will suggest that she thought that she was worthless and see how she responds.]

REBTer: Did you think you were worthless when your boyfriend left you for your best friend?

Fay: Well, it was a matter of my worthiness but worthless sounds a little extreme.

[REBTer's thinking: OK, I will see if she thought of herself as less worthy rather than worthless.]

REBTer: So were you saying that you were less worthy than you would be if it didn't happen?

Fay: Yes, less worthy is much more accurate.

Now let's see how a trainee might have thought and intervened in response to the same situation.

Fay: I felt depressed when my boyfriend left me for my best friend.

Trainee: Did you judge yourself when you felt depressed?

Fay: Yes.

Trainee: What judgement did you make of yourself?

Fay: I am not sure.

[Trainee's thinking: I will suggest that she thought that she was worthless since I am sure that was her self-depreciation belief.]

Trainee: Did you think you were worthless when your boyfriend left you for your best friend?

Fay: Well, it was a matter of my worthiness but worthless sounds a little extreme.

[Trainee's thinking: I will have to show her that if she held a self-depreciation belief this is extreme.]

Trainee: But, Fay, a self-depreciation is extreme so you did think of yourself as worthless.

Fay: Well, if you say so, although I don't really connect with that belief.

Because the trained therapist is aware that a self-depreciation belief in the 'worth' domain can be of the 'I'm worthless' type or the 'I'm less worthy' type, he can put the second type to Fay when she does not connect with the first type. However, since the trainee does not make this distinction, he can only do one thing – try to persuade Fay that she held an 'I'm worthless' belief when she held an 'I'm less worthy' belief.

Problems with the term 'acceptance'

When encouraging a client to accept herself, the REBT therapist knows what he means by this term. He means that he wants his client to regard herself as:

- unique
- fallible
- unrateable.

He also wants her to hold this attitude towards herself unconditionally, which means that she can accept herself no matter what.

However, when a client hears the term 'acceptance' in the term self-acceptance, she may think that this means something very different. She may think that it means:

- resign yourself to who you are because you cannot change
- self-satisfaction or complacency.

Neither of these meanings is part of the REBT view of self-acceptance since an attitude of self-acceptance encourages a person to change aspects of herself that she can change.

Let's consider how a trained REBT therapist and a trainee think and intervene when faced with a client who misunderstands the meaning of self-acceptance, beginning with the trained therapist. The client, June, depreciates herself for performing poorly at work.

June: So the alternative to me thinking that I am worthless when I perform poorly at work is to accept myself for doing poorly?

REBTer: That's right.

June: I'm not sure that I like the sound of that

[REBTer's thinking: June probably misunderstands what I mean by self-acceptance, but first let's see what she thinks I mean by it.]

REBTer: What don't you like about it?

June: Well, if I accept myself then I won't try to improve my work performance.

[REBTer's thinking: OK, so June equates acceptance with resignation. I need to correct this misconception straight away.]

REBTer: Would you be interested in an attitude towards yourself that would enable you to improve your performance while allowing you not to be disturbed when you don't?

June: Yes I would.

REBTer: Are you willing to be open-minded about the concept of self-acceptance?

June: OK.

REBTer: First let's take the situation where you do poorly at work. What you said earlier is that when this happens you think you are worthless. When you think that way about yourself how do you feel?

June: Depressed.

REBTer: And when you think that way does it help you to improve your performance?

June: No because I am depressed.

REBTer: Correct. Now let's take self-acceptance. If you were to do poorly at work and instead of regarding yourself as worthless you think of yourself as a unique, fallible human would you feel depressed?

June: No.

REBTer: How would you feel?

June: Disappointed.

REBTer: Now if you think of yourself as unique and fallible why would that mean that you would not try to improve your performance given that you want to do well at work?

June: I guess it wouldn't.

[REBTer's thinking: Now I am going to encourage June to put into her own words why self-acceptance can help her.]

REBTer: Can you put into your own words what you now think of the idea of self-acceptance?

June: I thought it meant resignation, but it doesn't mean that. It's a realistic way of viewing yourself which helps you not disturb yourself when you do poorly and helps you have the state of mind to improve.

REBTer: That's a great summary.

Now let's consider how a trainee might think and intervene in response to the same situation.

June: So the alternative to me thinking that I am worthless when I perform poorly at work is to accept myself for doing poorly?

Trainee: That's right.

June: I'm not sure that I like the sound of that.

[Trainee's thinking: I need to ask why.]

Trainee: Why?

June: Well, if I accept myself then I won't try to improve my work performance.

[Trainee's thinking: That's a misconception and I am going to disabuse June of this idea.]

Trainee: That's not true. Self-acceptance doesn't mean resignation. It helps you to improve.

June: Well, if you say so.

In the first segment, the trained therapist carefully elicits June's misconception about self-acceptance and then corrects this misconception by carefully deconstructing the concept of self-acceptance and showing June that it helps her (a) not to disturb herself about poor performance and (b) to improve her poor performance. He also shows her that self-depreciation leads to both negative consequences. The therapist then encourages June to put her learning into her own words to check that she has understood the points that he has been making.

Although the trainee also elicits June's misconception about self-acceptance, he tries to correct this misconception basically by assertion. He repeats REBT theory in a bald manner and makes no attempt to deconstruct the concept of self-acceptance as the trained therapist did. It is clear that June is not convinced by the trainee's assertions and indicates that she is willing to comply with him, albeit with reluctance. In short, the trained therapist promotes true client understanding, while the trainee elicits client compliance.

Other important issues

One of the difficulties that an REBT therapist has with identifying and working with a client's self-depreciation belief is to make sure that the belief that the client has articulated is really a self-depreciation belief. There are usually two areas of confusion here: self-depreciation vs. trait-depreciation and self-depreciation vs. role-depreciation.

Self-depreciation vs. trait-depreciation

When a client confuses trait-depreciation with self-depreciation, she takes a particular negative trait that she is focusing on and then uses this trait to make what appears to her to be a self-depreciation belief. Here the person is equating her 'self' with the trait. Here are a few examples that are common in clinical practice:

- 'I am selfish.'
- 'I am lazy.'
- 'I am weak.'

Let us see how a trained REBT therapist and a trainee think and intervene in response to a client's trait-depreciation statement masquerading as a self-depreciation belief.

Mary:	I felt guilty because I put myself first and hurt my friend's feelings as a result.
REBTer:	What did you think about yourself when you felt guilty about hurting her feelings?

> *Mary*:   I thought that I was a selfish person.
>
> *[REBTer's thinking: That is a trait-depreciation statement. Let's see if I can help Mary to articulate her self-depreciation belief.]*
>
> *REBTer*:   And when you thought you were selfish did you think less of yourself?
>
> *Mary*:   Yes, I did. I thought that I was a bad person.

Now let's see how a trainee might respond to the same situation

> *Mary*:   I felt guilty because I put myself first and hurt my friend's feelings as a result.
>
> *Trainee*:   What did you think about yourself when you felt guilty about hurting her feelings?
>
> *Mary*:   I thought that I was a selfish person.
>
> *[Trainee's thinking: That sounds like a self-depreciation belief to me. The person is evaluating herself. I will dispute that now.]*

The main difference here is that the trained REBT therapist knows that there is a difference between a trait-depreciation statement and a self-depreciation belief and intervenes accordingly whereas the trainee does not see this difference and treats the trait-depreciation statement as a self-depreciation belief.

Self-depreciation vs. role-depreciation

When a client confuses role-depreciation with self-depreciation, she takes a particular role in which she is performing badly in some respect and then equates herself with this poor role performance. Here are a few examples that are common in clinical practice:

- 'I am a bad mother.'
- 'I am a poor therapist.'
- 'I am a bad son.'

Let us see how a trained REBT therapist and a trainee think and intervene in response to a client's role-depreciation statement masquerading as a self-depreciation belief.

> *Judy:* I felt depressed because my daughter's teacher told me that she was regularly misbehaving in class.
>
> *REBTer:* What did you think about yourself when you felt depressed about being told this?
>
> *Judy:* I thought that I was a bad mother.
>
> *[REBTer's thinking: That is a trait-depreciation statement. Let's see if I can help Judy to articulate her self-depreciation belief.]*
>
> *REBTer:* And when you thought you were a bad mother did you think less of yourself?
>
> *Judy:* Yes, I did. I thought that I was worthless.

Now let's see how a trainee might respond to the same situation.

> *Judy:* I felt depressed because my daughter's teacher told me that she was regularly misbehaving in class.
>
> *Trainee:* What did you think about yourself when you felt depressed about being told this?
>
> *Judy:* I thought that I was a bad mother.
>
> *[Trainee's thinking: That is an overgeneralisation since Judy is jumping from an aspect of mothering which she may be doing badly at to being a bad mother. I am going to challenge this overgeneralisation.]*

The main difference here is that the trained REBT therapist knows that there is a difference between a role-depreciation statement and a self-depreciation belief and intervenes accordingly whereas the trainee does not see this difference. Rather, he treats Judy's role-depreciation statement as an overgeneralisation and plans to challenge this cognitive distortion. While this is not incorrect, it is not a classical REBT strategy. What the trained therapist did, on the other hand, is.

In the following chapter I will discuss how an REBT therapist thinks about two key aspects of psychological disturbance and show how this thinking affects his interventions. I will then compare these with the thinking and interventions of a trainee in response to the same material.

Chapter 6

Thinking and intervening related to disturbance

In the previous four chapters I have considered how an REBT therapist thinks about the individual components of the 'ABC' framework as it is used within a situational context and how this affects the therapist's interventions. I also looked at how a trainee might think and intervene in the same examples.

In this chapter, I am going to consider how an REBT therapist thinks and intervenes in two key aspects of disturbance. First, I will consider how an REBT therapist thinks and intervenes when helping a client to see the relationship between her feelings and her beliefs. This is known in REBT circles as the 'B'–'C' connection. Second, I will consider how an REBT therapist thinks and intervenes when a client has a meta-disturbance (which occurs when a person disturbs herself about her original disturbance).

I will not cover the REBT conceptualisation of different emotional disorders because this is covered in detail elsewhere (Dryden, 2009). Nor will I consider the complex interaction between ego disturbance and non-ego disturbance since this is an advanced topic and beyond the scope of the present work.

Helping clients to make the 'B'–'C' connection

REBT's basic model of disturbance stresses that irrational beliefs are at the core of a disturbed response to an adversity and that if a person is to deal healthily with that adversity, then she needs to change her irrational beliefs to rational beliefs. Initially, this is done by a process called disputing where the therapist helps the client to reflect on the empirical, logical and pragmatic status of both her irrational and rational beliefs.

However, before this is done it is important that the client is helped to see the relationship between her disturbed responses at 'C' to the adversity at 'A' and her irrational beliefs about this adversity at 'B'. Technically, this is known as the 'iB'–'C' connection.

It is useful at the same time if the therapist also helps the client understand the relationship between her healthy responses at 'C' to the same adversity at 'A' and her rational beliefs about this adversity at 'B'. Technically, this is known as the 'rB'–'C' connection.

Helping clients to make the 'B'–'C' connection: an example

In this section, I will discuss Penny, who came for counselling for help with feelings of shame. The therapist asked her for a specific example and she chose to discuss a situation where she felt ashamed about making what she considered to be a silly mistake on a PowerPoint presentation at work. Thus, Penny's 'A' was making a silly mistake and her emotional 'C' was shame. Let's pick up the dialogue at this point.

REBTer: So you felt ashamed about making what was in your mind a silly mistake?

Penny: Yes.

[REBTer's thinking: My task is now to help Penny understand that her 'silly mistake' at 'A' did not cause her feelings of shame at 'C'. Rather her shame was largely determined by her irrational belief at 'B'.]

REBTer: OK, Penny, now there are two major explanations of your shameful feelings. One says that your silly mistake caused your shame while the other one says that it is the belief you hold about your silly mistake that is more important in explaining why you felt ashamed. Which do you think explains why you felt ashamed?

Penny: That the belief I held about my silly mistake led to me feeling ashamed about it.

[REBTer's thinking: OK, now I am going to help Penny to identify the belief that underpinned her shame. I am going to do

this by outlining her rational belief and her irrational belief and ask her which belief accounted for her shame.]

REBTer: Now, Penny, you obviously would have preferred not to have made what you considered a silly mistake. Is that right?

Penny: Quite right.

REBTer: Now that desire can be the first part of a belief known as a non-dogmatic preference or the first part of a belief known as a demand. Your non-dogmatic preference in this situation would be something like: 'I would have preferred not to have made that silly mistake, but that does not mean that I have to be exempt from making it'. Your demand in this situation would be something like: 'I absolutely should not have made that silly mistake'.

            Now, when you felt ashamed about making what you called that silly mistake in the PowerPoint presentation, which of these two beliefs led to your feelings of shame?

Penny: I believed that I absolutely should not have made that stupid mistake.

[REBTer's thinking: That's the 'iB'–'C' connection. Let's see if I can also help Penny see the 'rB'–'C' connection.]

REBTer: Right, and if you believed instead: 'I would have preferred not to have made that silly mistake, but that does not mean that I have to be exempt from making it', how would you have felt about making the mistake?

Penny: I would have felt disappointed.

REBTer: But not ashamed?

Penny: No, not ashamed.

[REBTer's thinking: I am going to ask Penny to put these two connections into her own words.]

REBTer: Can you put into your own words which of the two beliefs I outlined underlies shame and which underlies disappointment?

Penny: When I feel ashamed I held a demand and if I held the other one I would feel disappointment.

[REBTer's thinking: Penny gets the main point about the two 'B'–'C' connections even though she doesn't articulate the beliefs. That's good enough for the present.]

Now let's consider how a trainee might think about and respond to the same situation.

Trainee: So you felt ashamed about making what was in your mind a silly mistake?
Penny: Yes.

[Trainee's thinking: I need to help Penny make the 'B'–'C' connection.]

Trainee: So what were you telling yourself about making the silly mistake that led you to feel ashamed?
Penny: That everyone will look down at me for making such a silly mistake.

[Trainee's thinking: I am supposed to help her identify her demand. Let me try again.]

Trainee: And if everyone looks down on you for making such a silly mistake, what would you be telling yourself about that?
Penny: That I would not be able to face them again.
Trainee: And if you couldn't face them again, what would you be telling yourself about that?
Penny: That I would have to leave my job, but then I would still be anxious about giving presentations at my next job.

[Trainee's thinking: I'm stuck. I'm not helping Penny to identify her irrational beliefs and thus, I can't teach her the 'B'–'C' connection.]

Let me compare the thinking and interventions of the trained REBT therapist with those of the trainee.

The trainee tries to help Penny to identify her irrational belief prior to getting her to see the relationship between this irrational belief and her feelings of shame. However, as can be seen, Penny does not articulate an irrational belief in response to the trainee's questions. The problem here is rooted in the open-ended questions asked by the trainee. By using the question : 'What were you telling yourself?', the trainee increases the risk of not identifying Penny's irrational belief. Because the question is open-ended, the client scans her memory for thoughts she had at the time. Unless the client is specifically directed to her irrational belief after being helped to understand that the core of such a belief is a demand, then she will focus on thoughts that were more at the forefront of her mind; for an irrational belief is usually an attitude that underpins more surface cognitions. Using such surface cognitions as a way of encouraging a client to identify an underlying irrational belief requires a high level of skill from an REBT therapist. While a trained REBT therapist is likely to have this level of skill, it is unlikely that a trainee will. And in Penny's example, the trainee in question does not have such skill.

What happens when the trainee asks his first open-ended question: 'So what were you telling yourself about making the silly mistake [i.e. 'A1'] that led you to feel ashamed?', Penny responds not with an irrational belief which is what the trainee is hoping for, but with a second inference or 'A2' (i.e. 'Everyone will look down at me for making such a silly mistake'). This inference is most probably a thinking consequence of Penny's as yet undisclosed irrational belief, but the trainee does not appreciate this and treats this inference as another 'A' and asks a similar ('What would you be telling yourself about that?') question directed at this second inference ('A2'). Rather than coming up with an irrational belief, Penny responds with a third inference ('A3') concerning how she would act in the face of 'A2' (i.e. 'That I would not be able to face them again'). This is probably a behavioural consequence ('C') of an irrational belief about 'A2'.

Again the trainee takes this response and asks Penny to treat this as a further 'A' (i.e. 'A3') . He then asks the 'What would you be telling yourself about that?' question again, but still does not get an irrational belief. He then is stuck and recognises this, but does not know why. The reason is largely that he asked an open-ended question about Penny's original 'A' ('A1') – i.e. making a silly mistake in the PowerPoint presentation – rather than helping

Penny to understand what constitutes an irrational belief and to judge, using this information, whether she held such a belief when she felt ashamed about making the silly mistake.

Now let's consider the thinking and interventions of the trained therapist in comparison.

The trained therapist begins his intervention by outlining the 'event causes feelings' model and the REBT model and asks the client which model best explains why she felt ashamed.

Once the client indicates that the REBT model best explains her shame, the therapist outlines the difference between a demand (irrational belief) and a non-dogmatic preference (rational belief) and asks Penny which of the two best accounts for her feelings of shame. Penny can see that her shame is underpinned by her irrational belief. The therapist then capitalises on this by helping Penny to see the connection between the healthy alternative to shame (i.e. disappointment) and her rational belief. He will refer to this later in the therapeutic process when setting goals with Penny and disputing her beliefs.

Having done a lot of focused work on the two 'B'–'C' connections in a short period of work, the therapist wants to assess the extent to which the client has processed this work. He thus asks Penny to put into her own words what she understands about the points he has been making. He notes that her understanding is less than full, but recognises that it is good enough to enable them to proceed to the next phase of therapy.

Perhaps the biggest difference between the trained REBT therapist and the trainee in their respective thinking and interventions in helping the client understand the connections between (a) her feelings of shame and the irrational belief that underpins them and (b) her potential feelings of disappointment and its underpinning rational belief lies in the use of REBT theory to inform their thinking and interventions. The trained therapist uses REBT theory quite precisely in two ways. First, he uses REBT theory to contrast the 'event causes feelings' model with the REBT model where a belief about events is the central determining factor of the client's feelings. Second, he uses REBT theory to contrast a demand (irrational belief) with a non-dogmatic preference (rational belief) and uses this contrast to help the client understand which belief underpins shame and which underpins disappointment. It is important to note that the trained REBT therapist's use of REBT theory is clearly present in both his thinking and his interventions.

By contrast, the trainee uses REBT theory in a much more general, imprecise manner and, as already discussed, runs into trouble quite quickly because he asks the general 'What were you telling yourself?' question and does not know how to deal with the answers he is given. So the trainee needs to use REBT theory more precisely in the way demonstrated by the trained therapist if he is to help the client understand the 'B'–'C' connection.

Dealing with meta-disturbance

Once a client has disturbed herself at 'C' then it is important for the therapist to check whether she further disturbs herself about this original emotional problem. When this happens, the person:

- disturbs herself at 'C1' about 'A1';
- focuses on this 'C1', which then becomes 'A2';
- disturbs herself about 'A2' at 'C2' (this is the level of meta-disturbance).

REBT theory suggests that the therapist works with a client's meta-disturbance before her original disturbance under the following conditions:

1 When the presence of the client's meta-disturbance interferes with both therapist and client focusing on the client's original problem in the session.
2 When the presence of the client's meta-disturbance interferes with her working on her original problem outside therapy sessions.
3 When the meta-disturbance is the most important of the two from a clinical perspective. For example, in some forms of anxiety, the client's anxiety about her anxiety is the real clinical issue to be addressed first.
4 When the client can see the sense of, and agrees to, working on her meta-disturbance before her original problem.

Such judgements concerning which client problem to target for change first, her original problem or her meta-disturbance, are often complex and one would expect the trained therapist to be more sophisticated in this area than the trainee. It is important to stress that there are no absolutely correct decisions to be made about this matter and what is perhaps most important is that both therapist and client adopt an experimental attitude towards the issue at hand. This means that they both make an agreement about which problem to start with, begin the work and see the effects of such work. If it turns out they have chosen incorrectly at that point they can decide together to change the therapeutic focus.

Dealing with meta-disturbance: an example

Let's see how a trained therapist thinks and intervenes when the client reveals meta-disturbance and compare this with the thinking and interventions of a trainee.

Rose came to therapy because she found it difficult to say 'no' to people. This meant that she rarely did what she wanted to do and often considered that her friends and work colleagues took advantage of her good nature. She wanted to learn to say 'no' even though she recognised that she would find this difficult. As is typical in REBT, the therapist has asked Rose for an example.

Rose: Yesterday, at about 4.30pm, one of my colleagues at work asked me to help her with a report which she had to finish before she went home. I had planned to go home at 5pm, have a bath, watch TV and have an early night and I was really looking to having a relaxing evening. I really needed one. Anyway, I could see that if I said 'yes' to helping her it would mean that we would both stay quite late. She often asks for my help and like an idiot I always say 'yes'.

[REBTer's thinking: Rose clearly has an emotional problem about saying 'no', but by saying 'and like an idiot I always say yes' she has just revealed the possible presence of meta-disturbance. I will keep this in mind and check this out when the time is right. But, first, I will summarise her original problem.]

REBTer: So you wanted to say 'no', but didn't. Is that right?

Rose: Yes.

REBTer: Why do you think that you didn't?

Rose: I was scared that she wouldn't like me.

REBTer: So you wanted to say 'no' to her request, but you were scared that she would not like you if you did, so you didn't say 'no'. Is that right?

Rose: Yes.

[*REBTer: Now I will check whether Rose has meta-disturbance about her lack of assertion.*]

REBTer: Rose, I noticed earlier you said that this work colleague often asks for your help and like an idiot you always say 'yes'. Did you think you were an idiot for not saying 'no' on this occasion?

Rose: Yes, I did.

REBTer: And how did you feel when you thought that you were an idiot for once again saying 'yes' when you wanted to say 'no'?

Rose: I felt really angry with myself.

REBTer: And did your self-anger help you?

Rose: No, it increased my misery.

[*REBTer's thinking: So there is the client's meta-disturbance. Let me summarise these two problems for the client and then I will discuss with her which of her problems – her original problem or her meta-disturbance – we should target for change first.*]

REBTer: So, Rose, it seems that this episode shows that you have two problems. First, you are anxious about saying 'no' to your colleague so you don't say 'no', and second, you are angry with yourself for not saying 'no' and this adds to your misery. Have I understood you correctly?

Rose: Very much so.

REBTer: Let's talk about which of these two problems we should start with. If we target your unassertive-ness and the anxiety that underpins it first, do you think that your self-anger will get in the way of us doing work on this problem here in the session?

Rose: I don't think so.

REBTer: And would this self-anger interfere with you working on your unassertiveness outside of the therapy session?

Rose: It might. I often berate myself when I agree to do things that I don't want to do.

[REBTer's thinking: Rose's answers on the first two criteria do not suggest a clear way forward. It's also not clear that either problem has the greater significance from a clinical perspective, so let me ask her which problem she thinks we should start with.]

REBTer: From what you have said so far, it is not clear which problem we should start with. In the session, you think that your self-anger would not interfere with us focusing on your unassertiveness, but outside you think that it may very well do so. Based on that, which problem do you think we should start with?

Rose: When I think about it, I think we should start with my anger towards myself because when I get angry with myself, I find it difficult to think about how to assert myself.

Now let me consider how a trainee might think and intervene in the same situation. Here is Rose again:

Rose: Yesterday, at about 4.30pm one of my colleagues at work asked me to help her with a report which she had to finish before she went home. I had planned to go home at 5pm, have a bath, watch TV and have an early night and I was really looking to having a relaxing evening. I really needed one. Anyway, I could see that if I said 'yes' to helping her it would mean that we would both stay quite late. She often asks for my help and like an idiot I always say 'yes'.

[Trainee's thinking: So Rose is unassertive. I need to ask how she feels about her unassertiveness to see if she has meta-disturbance.]

Trainee: So you did not assert yourself with your work colleague. How did you feel about not asserting yourself with her?

Rose: I felt bad about that.

[Trainee's thinking: I am not sure from Rose's response whether or not she has meta-disturbance. So let me ask again.]

Trainee: When you agreed to help your colleague against your better judgement, how did you feel about doing so?

Rose: I felt badly about not asserting myself.

[Trainee's thinking: Rose is too vague about her emotional 'C', so I need to be more active in helping her to clarify it.]

Trainee: Rose, what was that bad feeling?

Rose: I was annoyed that I did not assert myself.

[Trainee: I am really struggling here. I don't think from her responses that Rose has meta-disturbance about her unassertiveness.]

Notice how the trained REBT therapist and the trainee end up coming to different conclusions as a consequence of the differences in their thinking and subsequent interventions.

While they both accurately identify the client's original problem, the trained therapist succeeds in identifying her meta-disturbance because he does the following. He picks up on a statement that Rose made which indicates the possible presence of meta-disturbance (i.e. 'She often asks for my help and like an idiot I always say "yes"'). Using this statement, the trained therapist discovers that Rose is angry with herself for being unassertive and that this self-anger adds to her misery. The trained therapist then clarifies with Rose that both problems needs addressing.

By contrast, the trainee does not use Rose's reference to being an idiot for being unassertive with her work colleague. He asks her a general question about her feelings and when she gives unclear responses fails to help her to clarify these. Because Rose's emotion seems healthy, the trainee assumes, wrongly, that she does not have meta-disturbance.

Having accurately identified Rose's meta-disturbance, the trained therapist uses three of the four criteria discussed above for deciding which problem to work with first, Rose's original problem or her meta-disturbance. As a result of the therapist's skilful interventions on this issue, Rose opts to target her meta-disturbance for change first.

Avoid switching focus back and forth

As I have just discussed, in the situation where a client has an emotional problem and meta-disturbance, it is important that therapist and client agree which to target for change first. Once the REBT therapist has made such an agreement with his client, then it is important that both keep the therapeutic focus on this agreed target problem. It often happens, however, that the client may switch focus back and forth from her target problem to the other one (and indeed to and from other issues) and sometimes she may do so several times. It is important for the REBT therapist to appreciate that such switches are commonplace in ordinary conversation and that the client needs help to keep the focus on the agreed target problem. Let's see how a trained REBT therapist responds to focus switching in his thinking and intervention and compare these to how a trainee might think and intervene in the same situation.

Lionel has come to therapy for help with being depressed about losing his job. He is also anxious about blushing. He is also ashamed about being depressed and this meta-disturbance is the problem that Lionel and the therapist have agreed to work on first. I will first consider the trained REBT therapist's thinking and interventions in this situation.

REBTer: So, Lionel, what is shameful for you about feeling depressed?

Lionel: Well I need to be in employment and having a job will help me stop feeling ashamed.

[REBTer's thinking: Immediately, Lionel has switched his focus from his shame about his depression to how he feels about not having a job. I need to intervene quickly to point this out to him and encourage him to go back to his meta-disturbance and to focus on this agreed target problem.]

REBTer:	We need to discuss your employment situation and we will do this. However, as we just agreed, as long as you are feeling ashamed of being depressed about your lack of employment, these feelings will interfere with us dealing with your depression and your lack of employment. So let's focus on your shame about feeling depressed. OK?
Lionel:	Yes, OK.
REBTer:	So when we focus on your shame what are you particularly ashamed about with respect to feeling depressed?
Lionel:	Well I feel weak when I feel depressed.
REBTer:	Apart from feeling weak, do you think you are a weak person?
Lionel:	Yes I do. It reminds me about how I used to feel when I was at school and I used to get low about not having friends. I wasn't very popular you know.

[REBTer's thinking: Lionel seems to have a style more akin to free association. I am going to have to be far more structured and give a rationale for doing so. I am also going to suggest that we use the whiteboard here to do an 'ABC' on his shame. If I point to the relevant parts of the framework this may help. I will also ask him for permission to interrupt him whenever he deviates from this 'ABC' framework.]

REBTer:	Lionel, may I help to keep you focused on your shame problem, since twice now you have started to discuss other issues?
Lionel:	But aren't I supposed to go with whatever thought comes into my mind?
REBTer:	Not in this kind of therapy. In REBT, it's important to focus on one problem at a time. Would you like me to help you to keep focused?
Lionel:	That would be helpful because I do tend to go all over the place.
REBTer:	Well, what I suggest is that we use the white-board here and I will help you to use the

	'ABC' framework to keep focused. Would you mind if I interrupt you if you depart from this framework?
Lionel:	No, I would find that helpful.
REBTer:	OK. So let's do that. So, 'C' is your feelings of shame and you feel ashamed about feeling depressed. What is particularly shameful about feeling depressed?
Lionel:	Well I see depression as a weakness. But I would not be in this situation if I had a job.

[REBTer's thinking: I am going to interrupt Lionel since he has switched focus.]

REBTer:	OK, Lionel, you are moving away from your shame problem. Let's go back. You see depression as a weakness. Is that what you are most ashamed of, having a weakness?
Lionel:	Yes.
REBTer:	What are you demanding about having this weakness that leads to you feeling depressed?
Lionel:	I must not be weak.
REBTer:	So your 'A' is having a weakness known as depression, your 'B' is your belief that you must not be weak, and your 'C' is your feelings of shame. Can you see the relationship between your belief that you must not be weak and your feelings of shame?

As you can see, after a struggle, the trained REBT therapist helped Lionel to stay focused on his shame problem. Let's now see how a trainee might think and intervene in the same situation.

Trainee:	So, Lionel, what is shameful for you about feeling depressed?
Lionel:	Well I need to be in employment and having a job will help me stop feeling ashamed.
Trainee:	But why must you be in employment?

[Comment: The trainee correctly begins with the agreed focus which is Lionel's feelings of shame about being depressed about

not having a job. However, Lionel immediately changes the focus to not having a job and the trainee follows Lionel's lead.]

Lionel: Well if I am not, I won't be able to afford to pay the mortgage.

Trainee: How would you feel about that?

Lionel: That would be terrible?

Trainee: Why would that be terrible?

Lionel: The bank will foreclose on the house and my family and I will be homeless.

[Comment: By following the client, the trainee unwittingly encourages the client to switch focus. What he needs to do is what the trained therapist did, keep the focus on the client's meta-disturbance and retain that focus in the face of the client's attempts to switch away from it. The therapist gives the client a rationale for using the 'ABC' framework and asks for permission to interrupt him should he switch focus. By interrupting Lionel as soon as he changes the subject and using the 'ABC' framework to maintain the focus, eventually the trained therapist helps the client to keep to the agreed focus.]

To switch focus or not: that is the question

It is generally good practice to keep to a therapeutic focus once one has been established, and therefore when a client begins to switch focus she should be discouraged from doing so. However, REBT theory advocates flexibility and therefore there may be times when you may go along with a client's wish to switch focus after agreeing to work on a specific problem. The following are instances when a therapist should go with a switch in therapeutic focus initiated by a client.

* When the switch in focus is accompanied by significant affect and the client will not be able to concentrate on the original focus if encouraged to return to that focus.
* When the client keeps switching focus to a particular issue which seems to have more resonance for the person than the original agreed focus.
* When the client switches focus to a problem which both therapist and client agree is more clinically significant for the

person. The switch in focus should be allowed if work on the original problem has not progressed very far. However, if significant progress has been made on the original target problem then the therapist should suggest that they finish the work on the original problem before switching to the more clinically significant problem.

• If failing to go with the switch in focus constitutes a significant threat to the therapeutic alliance.

In the following vignette, Edwina and the therapist have agreed to target Edwina's problem with social anxiety. In the course of discussing a specific example of this problem Edwina becomes distressed. I will first discuss how a trained REBT therapist thinks and intervenes when this happens and I will then consider how a trainee might think and intervene in identical circumstances.

Edwina:	I went to a party over the weekend and could only go once I had a few stiff drinks.
REBTer:	What would have happened if you hadn't had those drinks?
Edwina:	I would have gotten very anxious.
REBTer:	About what?
Edwina:	About people there thinking what an ugly cow I am.
REBTer:	So in order to deal with that anxiety, you drank . . . how much?
Edwina:	(*getting very distressed*) Er . . . I'm not . . . er . . .

[REBTer's thinking: Edwina is becoming very distressed, I need to understand what's going on here.]

REBTer:	You seem to be becoming very distressed. What are you experiencing now, Edwina?
Edwina:	I just had an image of my mother who was an alcoholic. It just occurred to me that I may be turning into her. Oh, God!!

[REBTer's thinking: This seems like it has great resonance for Edwina. I will decide with her if we need to switch focus. We haven't gone far with her social anxiety so we could switch if the new problem is more clinically significant.]

REBTer:	Should we stay with your anxiety about going to the party or switch to your idea that you are turning into your mother?
Edwina:	Well, I have always wondered why I have an ambivalent attitude to drink, but I am not sure we need to switch.
REBTer:	So while this sudden realisation is accompanied by distress, it is not more important to you than your social anxiety.
Edwina:	No.
REBTer:	And do you think that you can focus on the work that we need to do on your anxiety about the party even though you have just recognised the similarity between you and your mother with respect to drink?
Edwina:	Yes I can concentrate on the party situation.
REBTer:	So let's go back to my original question. It sounds like you would have gotten anxious if you hadn't had those drinks.
Edwina:	That's right.
REBTer:	So let's assume that you hadn't drunk. What would you have been anxious about with respect to being at the party?

Now let's consider the thinking and responses of a trainee to the same scenario.

Edwina:	I went to a party over the weekend and could only go once I had a few stiff drinks.
Trainee:	What would have happened if you hadn't had those drinks?
Edwina:	I would have gotten very anxious.
Trainee:	About what?
Edwina:	About people there thinking what an ugly cow I am.
Trainee:	So in order to deal with that anxiety, you drank . . . how much?
Edwina:	(*getting very distressed*) Er . . . I'm not . . . er . . .

[Trainee's thinking: Edwina is getting very distressed and seems not able to concentrate on the target problem. So that is a good reason to switch focus.]

Trainee: Edwina, you seem to be very distressed right now. What's going on for you?

Edwina: I just had an image of my mother who was an alcoholic. It just occurred to me that I may be turning into her. Oh, God!!

[Trainee's thinking: Edwina's exclamation, 'Oh, God', indicates the presence of an irrational belief. I need to pursue this.]

Trainee: And how would you feel if you were turning into your mother?

Edwina: Well, I don't want to be like her.

Trainee: But if you are?

Edwina: It would piss me off.

Trainee: In what way?

As you can see, the session with Edwina proceeds in one way with the trained REBT therapist and in a different way with the trainee. Let's compare their thinking and interventions to see how this happened.

Both the trained REBT therapist and the trainee notice that Edwina became distressed. In response, the trained REBT therapist's thinking demonstrates flexible use of the criteria REBT therapists employ to judge whether or not to switch focus:

- Whether Edwina can still focus on the target problem.
- How far the two have reached on the target problem.
- The clinical significance of the issue Edwina is switching to.
- What Edwina wishes to focus on.

Notice how the trained therapist intervened on the basis of his thinking and how he involved Edwina in the decision concerning whether to switch focus or not. By contrast, the trainee seems to use only one criterion – the presence of the client's distress – and decides to switch focus without even explaining his rationale for doing so and without involving the client in his decision. The trainee's lack of sophistication and failure to attend to the working alliance are again in evidence.

In the next chapter, I will discuss the important issue of eliciting and working with a client's goals, concentrating again on the thinking and interventions of both trained REBT therapist and trainee.

Chapter 7

Thinking and intervening related to goals

When a client comes for psychotherapeutic help, she is in a disturbed frame of mind. Her main goal, if she is asked, is to gain relief from her disturbed feelings. She will often say, therefore, that she wants to eliminate or rid herself of her disturbance.

Unfortunately, the REBT therapist cannot help her to achieve these disturbance-elimination goals. These goals are problematic for two main reasons;

1   They are unrealistic.
2   They do not specify healthy responses to adversities at 'A'.

Elimination of disturbance is unrealistic

A person who has never disturbed herself about anything or who has eliminated such disturbance once she has experienced it has probably never existed. Therefore to go along with a client's goal that she wants to eliminate a disturbed emotion so that she will never experience such an emotion again is unrealistic. No matter how psychologically healthy a person is, that person will, on occasion, disturb herself about some adversity or other. It is unrealistic for a person to completely eliminate a disturbed feeling. The best one can hope for is that the person in question minimises the experience of psychological disturbance and maximises the experience of a psychologically healthy response.

Non-specification of healthy responses to adversity

When asked what her goals are for therapy, the client will rarely articulate what REBT theory would see as a healthy negative emotional response at 'C' to an adversity at 'A'. She will either say that she wants to achieve a neutral response to the adversity (e.g. 'I want to be calm when people criticise me') or she will put forward a vague positive response to an unspecified set of circumstances (e.g. 'I want to be happy').

Healthy negative emotions as goals in the face of adversity

REBT theory argues that when a person disturbs herself or experiences an unhealthy negative emotion (UNE) about an adversity, then a healthy goal would be for that person to experience instead a healthy negative emotion about that adversity. This position follows logically from REBT's view that disturbance is based on irrational beliefs about adversity and that healthy negative emotions are based on rational beliefs about the same adversity.

The main task of the REBT therapist is to help the client to see what constitutes a healthy response to an adversity and to encourage the client to set these as goals.

Here I will discuss how a trained REBT therapist thinks and intervenes when the issue of helping the client to set HNEs as appropriate goals becomes salient. I will then discuss how a trainee might think and respond to the same material.

Jan came to therapy because she responds angrily to rudeness in others. In response to a request from the therapist, Jan provided a specific example of her anger problem. The therapist helped Jan to identify the following 'ABC' of this specific episode, which he wrote on the whiteboard.

Situation: The girl at the check-out did not say 'thank you' to me when I gave her the money to pay for the shopping.

'A': The check-out girl was rude to me.

'B': She must be polite to me.

'C': Emotional: unhealthy anger.
　　　Behavioural:
　　　– felt like punching her in the mouth
　　　– asked to see her supervisor and wanted her to be sacked.
　　　Thinking: ruminated on the episode and imagined punching her.

Let me begin by considering how a trained REBT therapist helped Jan to set goals. As before I will focus on the therapist's thinking and the impact that this has on his interventions.

REBTer: When you stand back and think about the way you responded in this situation, let's see what you want to change, if anything. OK?

Jan: OK.

[REBTer's thinking: I first need to discover if Jan sees her angry response as healthy or unhealthy.]

REBTer: As you look back at this situation do you think that your anger was healthy or unhealthy?

Jan: Unhealthy.

REBTer: Why?

Jan: Because I felt violence and wanted to do the person harm either physically or with respect to her job.

[REBTer's thinking: Jan has focused on her violent action tendencies in outlining why her anger is problematic for her. I will use this now and suggest non-violent anger as a healthy goal.]

REBTer: So the troublesome nature of your anger was the violent tendencies that accompanied it. Is that right?

Jan: Yes.

REBTer: So how would you respond to the offer of help to feel angry about the way you were treated without the accompanying violent tendencies?

Jan: That would be really good.

REBTer: So let's look carefully at your 'ABC' in light of your response. Rather than feeling as if you wanted to punch the check-out girl, what would you have liked to have done or felt like doing instead?

Jan: I would have like to have pointed out to her that she needed to say 'thank you' to me.

REBTer:	So you would like to have been assertive rather than suppress your aggression.
Jan:	Yes.
REBTer:	And would you have liked to have done anything instead of asking to see her supervisor and wanting her sacked?
Jan:	Well, that would have depended on how she responded to my assertion. If she took my point, I would have let it go. If not, I would still have wanted to see her supervisor, but it would have been to point out what I considered to be an unacceptable response on the girl's part, but not to get her sacked.
REBTer:	So, if I have got this right, if she had acknowledged your point you would have let it go, but if not, with her supervisor you would have sought an assertive outcome rather than an aggressive outcome. Is that right?
Jan:	Well that is a really good way of putting it.

[REBTer's thinking: Now let me see if I can help Jan come up with an alternative to her angry and violent ruminations.]

REBTer:	If your anger was healthy, instead of ruminating on the episode and imagining punching the check-out girl what would you have thought and imagined?
Jan:	I would not ruminate if she apologised, but if she didn't, I would think that her rudeness was an unfortunate reflection of society and let it go.

[REBTer's thinking: I think it would be useful if I write her new 'ABC' on the board with her new emotional, behavioural and thinking goals stated. This will then help me to reiterate the 'rB'–'C' connection.]

REBTer:	Let me summarise your goals by putting up on the board a second 'ABC'.

Situation: The girl at the check-out did not say 'thank you' to me when I gave her the money to pay for the shopping.

'A': The check-out girl was rude to me.

'B': To be specified.

'C': Emotional: healthy anger.
Behavioural: assert myself with the girl. If she did not apologise or acknowledge my point I would have asked to see her supervisor and made a complaint but without asking for her to be sacked.
Thinking: thinking her rudeness was a reflection of society but no violent ruminations or fantasies.

Now I will consider how a trainee might think and intervene in the same scenario.

Trainee: So how would you like to have responded in this situation?

Jan: Well I am not prepared to tolerate rudeness of that nature. So I am not prepared to turn the other cheek or take it in my stride.

[Trainee's thinking: Jan is telling me how she doesn't want to respond rather than how she does want to respond.]

Trainee: Jan, you are telling me how you don't want to respond rather than how you do.

Jan: I don't know then.

[Trainee's thinking: Let me start by helping her to see that annoyance is a healthy alternative to anger here.]

Trainee: Well in REBT we see annoyance as a healthy alternative to anger. How about working towards feeling annoyed rather than angry in this situation?

Jan: Annoyance sounds too wishy-washy to me.

Trainee: Well it can be strong annoyance.

Jan: I still am not convinced.

Let's compare the thinking and interventions of the trained therapist with those of the trainee in this scenario.

The trained therapist begins by asking Jan to stand back and consider whether her anger was healthy or unhealthy in this situation. Asking Jan to stand back helps her to adopt an observer role and to see that her anger was unhealthy. By contrast, the trainee does not invite Jan to adopt this observer role with the result that she answers his questions from the experiencer role and either defends her position or is confused about the trainee's points.

Once the trained REBT therapist has elicited from Jan that her anger is unhealthy, he asks her to specify her reasons. In reply, Jan lists her destructive action tendencies. The REBT therapist uses this response and asks Jan if she is interested in feeling angry without experiencing the accompanying violent action tendencies. She says that she is and so the therapist worked carefully with Jan to specify healthy alternatives to her unhealthy action tendencies and her problematic thinking consequences. Having done this he summarises this work using the whiteboard. This prepares Jan to see that the way she can achieve healthy anger is by changing her irrational belief to an alternative rational belief.

By contrast, the trainee begins by asking Jan a vague open-ended question about how she would have liked to have responded differently. Jan replies by telling him how she would not have wanted to respond. Reacting to this, the trainee refers to REBT theory as a way forward and invites Jan to consider annoyance as a goal, but because he does not explain what he means by this and because he does not refer to Jan's behavioural and thinking consequences as a way of engaging her, his interventions are not effective. What happens is that Jan does not understand what the trainee means by annoyance and is not convinced by his point that annoyance can be strong.

Setting overcoming disturbance goals before personal development goals

Having a client specify what she wants to achieve from counselling is important in that it helps to give a direction to the counselling process. Bordin (1979) has argued that when the client and counsellor are working towards the same goal, then this strengthens the working alliance between them.

However, often when the therapist asks the client what she wants to achieve from counselling she says that she wants a positive goal which does not take into account the negative 'As' that she is facing and about which she is currently disturbing herself. The task of the therapist here is to help the client see that working on goals that tackle successfully her disturbance (i.e. 'overcoming disturbance' goals) which involve experiencing a healthy negative emotion at 'C' in the face of an adversity at 'A' has to be done before working towards goals that reflect personal development (i.e. 'personal development' goals).

Taking this perspective, the achievement of HNEs (at 'C') in the face of adversity at 'A' is a kind of half-way house towards the client's more positive, personal development goals. Let me give you an example of what I mean.

Stuart came to counselling because he was anxious about meeting women. I will first outline a trained REBT therapist's thinking and interventions in the context of goal-setting with Stuart and compare these with the thinking and interventions of a trainee.

REBTer: So, Stuart, you are anxious about meeting women. What would you like to achieve from counselling with respect to this problem?

Stuart: I want to be confident when meeting women.

[REBTer's thinking: Obviously, I have to help Stuart understand that I will have to help him over his anxiety first.]

REBTer: Do you think you can go from being anxious about meeting women to feeling confident in one jump?

Stuart: I guess not.

REBTer: Why not?

Stuart: Because it is too much of a leap.

REBTer: What would be more realistic?

Stuart: I guess more of a step-by-step approach towards feeling confident about meeting women.

[REBTer's thinking: Now that Stuart has accepted that there will be at least one step between where he is now and where he wants to be, I will introduce the idea that he needs to address

his anxiety about meeting women before working on becoming more confident.]

REBTer: How does this sound? At the moment, you are anxious about meeting women. So, let's address your anxiety first and then we can help you become more confident.

Stuart: That sounds reasonable.

[REBTer's thinking: Now that Stuart has accepted targeting his anxiety first before working on improving his confidence, I can discuss with him what would be a healthy negative emotional alternative to anxiety about whatever he is anxious about.]

The trained therapist then helped Stuart to find out what he found threatening about meeting women and then proceeded to help him to aim towards feeling healthily concerned, but not anxious about this threat should it happen. Once Stuart had become thus concerned, he would in a better frame of mind to work towards improving his confidence when meeting women.

Now let's see how a trainee might think and intervene with Stuart.

Trainee: So, Stuart, you are anxious about meeting women. What would you like to achieve from counselling with respect to this problem?

Stuart: I want to be confident when meeting women.

[Trainee's thinking: I need to help Stuart to see that first we have to address his anxiety.]

Trainee: Before I help you to do that, I need to help you address your anxiety.

Stuart: But if I was more confident, I wouldn't be anxious. Why can't you help me develop confidence?

[Trainee's thinking: Let's see if I can help him see that anxiety impedes the development of confidence.]

Trainee: Well when you are anxious you can't really concentrate on your strengths which you need to do when you are confident.

Stuart: But what I had in mind is that you or someone like you would train me to the point where I could go out and believe that I can have any woman that I wanted and if I believed that then I wouldn't get anxious.

[Trainee's thinking: Stuart has a model of change that is unrealistic since it is unlikely that he can bypass his anxiety. Let's see if I can come up with a metaphor to help him see this.]

Trainee: But you are trying to bypass your anxiety which I believe can't be done. It's like trying to learn to drive when you are anxious about driving. You can develop confidence about driving under controlled conditions like with a driving instructor with you, but if you are anxious about driving on the roads on your own then you need to deal with your anxiety before you can develop driving confidence.

Stuart: But I would still like to try it my way.

Let me now compare the trained REBT therapist's thinking and interventions with those of the trainee. By asking open-ended questions, the trained therapist helps Stuart to see that there is an intermediate step between his being anxious about meeting women and being confident about meeting them. The important ingredient here is that Stuart is helped to come to his own conclusion. By contrast, the trainee's attempt to persuade Stuart that he needs to address his anxiety about women before working towards becoming more confident about meeting them seems to fail. This seems largely due to the persuasive approach of the trainee entrenching Stuart in his position. The more the trainee tries to get Stuart to accept targeting his anxiety first, the more Stuart resists this persuasion and reiterates his wish to work on developing.

Because the trained therapist was successful at helping Stuart to target his anxiety first he was then able to help Stuart to set the 'half-way house' goal of feeling concerned, but not anxious about what he found threatening about meeting women. The trainee was unable to do this primarily because he failed to help Stuart to target his anxiety problem before his confidence problem.

Helping the client to set emotional goals at 'C' before changing 'A'

When clients come to counselling, it is often because they are disturbing themselves about an adversity at 'A'. At the outset of REBT, clients often do not understand the REBT model of emotions which holds that people disturb themselves about adversities because they hold rigid and extreme beliefs about these adversities. Rather, they hold an 'event causes feelings' model.

Even when a client understands REBT's 'ABC' model of the emotions, she will still be inclined to change 'A' if it can be changed before changing 'C'. While REBT is certainly not against a client changing an adversity at 'A', it argues that as long as the client is disturbed at 'C' about 'A' then any attempts to change this 'A' will be disrupted by this disturbance. Once the client has successfully addressed her emotional disturbance about 'A' then her attempts to change this 'A' will be more likely to be successful.

Let's see how a trained therapist thinks about and responds to a situation when a client wishes to change 'A' before changing 'C'. I will then show how a trainee might think and respond to the same situation.

Thelma has come to counselling because she is experiencing problems in her relationship with her boyfriend. She is angry towards him because he is a poor timekeeper and often lets her down at the last minute. She comes into her second counselling session particularly furious about her boyfriend's behaviour.

Thelma:	That's it! I have had it with him. I am ending the relationship.
REBTer:	What happened?
Thelma:	He let me down again last night.
REBTer:	And how do you feel?
Thelma:	Mad as hell.

REBTer: And you want to end the relationship?
Thelma: Yes. I'm going to tell him right after this session.

[REBTer's thinking: Thelma told me in the first session how much she loves her boyfriend, so her decision to end her relationship seems coloured by her unhealthy anger. I need to help her to address her anger before making a decision concerning whether or not to end the relationship.]

REBTer: In our first session, you told me that while you got angry with your boyfriend from time to time that you loved him a lot. Is that right?
Thelma: Yes.
REBTer: Well you are bound to be angry about him letting you down yet again. But is the best time to judge whether or not you should end the relationship when you are furious with him or when you are angry at his behaviour but not furious at him?
Thelma: I guess the second.
REBTer: And which type of anger are you experiencing now?
Thelma: The first.
REBTer: So can I help you develop the kind of anger that will allow you stand back and put this latest episode in context before I help you decide whether or not to end the relationship?
Thelma: OK. That makes sense.

Now let's see how a trainee might think and respond to the same material.

Thelma: That's it! I have had it with him. I am ending the relationship.
Trainee: What happened?
Thelma: He let me down again last night.
Trainee: And how do you feel?
Thelma: Mad as hell.
Trainee: And you want to end the relationship?
Thelma: Yes. I'm going to tell him right after this session.

[Trainee's thinking: I'm supposed to get her to work on her disturbed emotion at 'C' before she changes 'A', so let me do that.]

Trainee: Let's work on your anger problem first, shall we?

Thelma: I don't have an anger problem, I have a boy-friend problem and the bastard has let me down for the last time.

Let me compare the thinking and intervention of the trained therapist with those of the trainee. They both acknowledge in their thinking the REBT principle of helping the client work on a disturbed 'C' before changing 'A', but they communicate this in very different ways to Thelma with the result that the client accepts this 'C' before 'A' order when put to her by the trained therapist, but not when put to her by the trainee. On closer inspection, the trained therapist does six things that the trained therapist does not do.

First, he puts Thelma's episode of her anger and wish to terminate the relationship in context by reminding her that she loves her boyfriend a lot. Second, he validates anger as an understandable response to Thelma being let down by her boyfriend, but helps her to distinguish between two types of anger, one person-focused and the other behaviour-focused. Third, he helps Thelma to see that her person-focused anger will lead her to make an impulsive decision about the relationship while behaviour-focused anger will help her to stand back and make a decision based on the episode and the wider context of the relationship. Fourth, he helps Thelma to see that she is experiencing person-focused anger. Fifth, he helps her to commit herself to work on her anger before coming to a decision about the relationship. Finally, throughout this sequence, the trained therapist enables Thelma to take an observer role and moves her away from an experiencer role with the result that she can distance herself from her unhealthy anger feelings long enough to engage productively with his interventions.

By contrast, in one poorly executed intervention, the trainee asserts the REBT principle of targeting a disturbed 'C' before changing 'A' without explanation and informs Thelma that she has an anger problem to which she strongly objects. It is not that the trainee is wrong on either count, but he implements REBT theory without due regard to engaging the client in a productive dialogue on both points. It is as if the trainee is proceeding on the idea that because he is doing the right thing from the perspective of REBT theory then the client is bound to accept and go along with it.

The trained therapist, on the other hand, skilfully engages Thelma in a dialogue on both points: (a) that her anger is problematic and (b) that they need to target her 'C' before deciding whether or not to change 'A'. Notice particularly how he encourages her to stand back and reflect on her feelings in the wider context of her relationship with her boyfriend.

Helping the client to set emotional goals at 'C' in the face of an 'A' that can't be changed

The final issue with respect to helping clients to set goals that I want to discuss here concerns goal-setting in situations where clients are disturbing themselves about adversities at 'A' that cannot be changed. In effect, in these situations the client's choice is simple, but not an easy one to digest. To paraphrase Shakespeare it is: 'To disturb oneself or not to disturb oneself? That is the question.'

Let me discuss how a trained REBT therapist deals with this situation in his thinking and intervention and compare these with those of a trainee facing the same scenario.

Leonard has been referred to counselling because he has recently been diagnosed with type 1 diabetes and isn't handling his illness well at all. Let's start with how the trained therapist thinks and responds at various junctures.

REBTer:	So you have just been diagnosed with type 1 diabetes, how do you feel about this diagnosis?
Leonard:	Depressed and angry.
REBTer:	And what impact have these feelings had on your behaviour with respect to the condition?
Leonard:	Honestly?

REBTer:　Sure.

Leonard:　I tend to be erratic with injecting myself with insulin and sometimes I go out on a drinking binge.

[REBTer's thinking: Let me see if Leonard thinks that he can change 'A' and get rid of his diabetes.]

REBTer:　What have you been told about the prognosis of your diabetes?

Leonard:　That if I inject regularly and keep to a particular diet then I can manage it.

REBTer:　And if you don't do these things?

Leonard:　Then I will endanger my health and eventually my life.

REBTer:　Is there a part of you that finds it difficult to accept the reality of your condition?

Leonard:　I guess there is.

REBTer:　And when you miss your injections and go out drinking, are these behaviours stemming from the part of you that is finding it difficult to accept having type 1 diabetes?

Leonard:　I think so, yes.

REBTer:　This may sound strange, and it is only a hunch so correct me if I am wrong, but at those times do you think, at some level, that if you act as if you don't have diabetes, then you don't have it?

Leonard:　Well, put like that it sounds as if I do think like that, as you say at some level.

REBTer:　Now this also may sound stupid, but is acting as if you don't have diabetes a good way of getting rid of it?

Leonard:　(*laughing*) Well that would be nice, but no it's not. It will only make me worse.

[REBTer's thinking: Now Leonard is ready to tell me how he would like me to help him.]

REBTer:　So, Leonard, how would like me to help you?

Leonard:　I guess I need help at disciplining myself at those times when I go off the rails.

REBTer: So that you are more disciplined at injecting yourself and don't act on the urge to go out drinking?

Leonard: Yes.

[REBTer's thinking: I need to help Leonard make explicit the purpose of such discipline since self-discipline is rarely a goal in itself for people, but a means to an end.]

REBTer: Bear with me for asking another stupid question, Leonard. But, why do you want to be more self-disciplined in these areas?

Leonard: Because I want to be healthy and prolong my life.

REBTer: You see, I told you it was a stupid question, but it's good sometimes to make this explicit, don't you think?

Leonard: Yes, it is.

[REBTer's thinking: Now I am going to suggest that we focus on Leonard's feelings of anger and depression as targets for change since these seem to underpin his lack of self-discipline.]

REBTer: Leonard, from what you were saying earlier, your acts of self-discipline seem to be based on your feelings of depression and anger related to your diabetes. Have I understood that correctly?

Leonard: Yes, it seems that when I feel low and angry about being diabetic, I do tend to go off the rails.

REBTer: So would it make sense if we look at what your feelings of depression and anger are about so that I can help you to deal with these issues more effectively so that you don't go 'off the rails' as you put it?

Leonard: That would be great.

The trained therapist has now succeeded in helping Leonard to target his disturbed 'C's' for change in the face of an 'A' (i.e. his diabetes) that cannot be changed. Now let's see how a trainee might think and intervene in the same scenario.

Trainee: So you have just been diagnosed with type 1 diabetes, how do you feel about this diagnosis?

Leonard: Depressed and angry.

[Trainee's thinking: Well since Leonard can't do anything about his diabetes the only thing that he can do is to undisturb himself about it. Let me discuss this with him.]

Trainee: As you know, Leonard, once you have type 1 diabetes, you have it for life. But you do have a choice between having diabetes with depression and anger and having diabetes without depression and anger. Which option would you like?

Leonard: Well, for me it's quite natural to be depressed and angry about having diabetes. You don't expect me to feel nothing about having a life-changing illness do you?

[Trainee's thinking: I need to explain to Leonard the difference between healthy and unhealthy negative emotions.]

Trainee: Well, it's not a question of choosing diabetes with depression and anger or diabetes with no feelings. It's possible to have diabetes and experience healthy alternatives to depression and anger.

Leonard: What are these alternatives?

Trainee: Sadness and healthy anger.

Leonard: I think you are just playing with words. How would you feel if you had type 1 diabetes?

Let me now compare and contrast the thinking and interventions of the trained therapist and the trainee. The trained therapist identifies that Leonard feels depressed and angry about having type 1 diabetes and then links these emotions with his destructive behaviour (without labelling them as such). He then carefully discovers that Leonard acknowledges, at one level, that he can't change his diabetes, but skilfully elicits from the client that there is a part of him that can't accept this and acts as if it wasn't true. The trained therapist then helps Leonard to articulate the fact that his self-undisciplined behaviour will not help to rid him of diabetes, but will only make his health worse.

At this point, the therapist asks Leonard how he would like to be helped and in response, Leonard says to be more self-disciplined. The therapist helps Leonard to see that self-discipline is a means to his goals, which Leonard states are health maintenance and prolonging his life expectancy.

Once he has done this, the therapist helps Leonard to understand that he 'goes off the rails' as he calls it when he feels depressed and angry about his condition and invites the client to deal with these disturbed emotions as a way of achieving his goals with respect to his health and life expectancy through better self-discipline.

By contrast, the trainee thinks and intervenes like an REBT textbook, but without sufficiently engaging the client. He asserts quite baldly and unfeelingly that type 1 diabetes cannot be changed and correctly but unclearly points out that Leonard has the option of disturbing himself or not about this. Leonard responds as if his choice is to be depressed and angry or to have no feelings and defends the legitimacy of his depressed and angry reactions if these are the only alternatives to feeling nothing about having diabetes. It is not the only alternative, but when the trainee introduces the idea of sadness and healthy anger as healthy alternatives, done again in a declarative way without any sensitive explanation and without linking this to healthy behaviour, his intervention is dismissed as 'playing with words' and Leonard challenges the trainee to say how he, the trainee, would cope with his condition in a way that suggests that Leonard does not feel at all understood by the trainee.

In contrast, Leonard does seem to experience the trained therapist as empathic and this helps him to be open to the idea that he needs to target his UNEs for change as a way of achieving his health maintenance and life expectancy goals through the medium of better self-discipline.

In the following chapter I will consider the importance of explaining the nature of the change process to a client. This serves to structure the client's expectations about change as well as helping her to make sense of what she and her therapist will do to help her to achieve her therapeutic goals. As before I will focus on both the trained therapist's and the trainee's thinking and interventions in contrasting what to do and what not to do in carrying out this important therapeutic task.

Chapter 8

Thinking and intervening related to explaining the process of change

So far in this book I have discussed the following therapist and client tasks that are relevant to the REBT change process:

- The client has outlined the problems she would like to discuss during therapy.
- The client has targeted one such problem to focus on first and has discussed one or more specific examples of this problem with her therapist.
- The therapist has helped the client to use REBT's 'ABC' model to assess these specific examples.
- The therapist has helped the client understand the two 'B'–'C' connections: the relationship between irrational beliefs ('iBs') and disturbed responses (emotional, behavioural and cognitive) at 'C' and the relationship between rational beliefs ('rBs') and constructive responses (emotional, behavioural and cognitive) at 'C'.
- The therapist has helped the client to set appropriate goals with respect to the context of the target problem.

At some point in the counselling process, it is useful to discuss the nature of the change process with a client. While there is no definite point at which to raise this as an issue with a client, I have included it in this book after a discussion of client goals since this latter discussion gives the counselling process a direction for change and it is useful for a client to have a realistic idea of the nature of the journey before she embarks on it. This discussion also helps the client to understand the scope and purpose of some of the techniques that the therapist may use in the service of the client's goals.

Intellectual insight vs. emotional insight

An important feature of the change process in REBT that needs explaining is the difference between intellectual and emotional insight.

Intellectual insight

In an early paper, Albert Ellis (1963) argued that intellectual insight is basically a cognitive or intellectual acknowledgment that one's irrational beliefs are irrational and that one's rational beliefs are rational. Having intellectual insight does not yet impact on one's feelings, behaviour or subsequent thinking in any sustained way. It may be thought of as a platform for significant later change, a platform without which change consistent with rational beliefs would not be maintained. However, on its own intellectual insight usually does not facilitate such change.

Some REBT trainees may think that intellectual insight is sufficient for therapeutic change to occur and these trainees tend to favour cognitive techniques both within therapy sessions and between these sessions. Some clients also share this view and they think that all they need to do is to acquire or remind themselves of important rational principles (often by reading and re-reading REBT-based self-help books), insight into which will be curative in itself.

Ellis (1963) also said that intellectual insight is a conviction that is held lightly and occasionally about the irrationality of irrational beliefs and the rationality of rational beliefs.

From both perspectives, Ellis's view is that intellectual insight is an important stage in the change process without which clients would not develop the foundations for later emotional change. However, on its own such insight will only facilitate knowledge about rational principles but will not facilitate therapeutic change.

Emotional insight

In that same early paper, Ellis (1963) argued that emotional insight is basically a full, emotionally-felt and deep understanding that one's irrational beliefs are irrational and that one's rational beliefs are rational. Having emotional insight does impact on one's feelings, behaviour and subsequent thinking in an ongoing way. It may be thought of as a marker of significant change.

Ellis (1963) also said that emotional insight is an often held, strong conviction about the irrationality of irrational beliefs and the rationality of rational beliefs.

From both perspectives, Ellis's view is that emotional insight is a crucial stage in the change process without which any change that occurs would be knowledge based rather than experientially based.

Thinking and intervening related to explaining the change process: an example

Let me discuss how a trained REBT therapist discusses the change process with a client with particular emphasis on the difference between intellectual and emotional insight. As before I will focus on the therapist's thinking as well as his interventions with the client. Then, I will discuss how a trainee might think and respond to the same material.

Ruth has come to therapy for help with her chronic jealousy problem. Her therapist has helped her to do an 'ABC' assessment on a typical, specific example of her jealousy problem. Before moving on to the questioning or disputing stage with respect to the client's irrational and rational beliefs, the therapist raised the issue of the change process with Ruth.

REBTer: So, Ruth, we now understand the irrational beliefs that underpin your unhealthy jealousy in this situation and you can see that if you hold the alternative rational beliefs that we developed you would act differently and feel concerned, but not unhealthily jealous about your partner in the episode we have talked about. Is that right?

Ruth: Yes.

REBTer: Before I help you to stand back and examine both your irrational beliefs and your rational beliefs with the hope that you might internalise and act in accordance with your rational beliefs, I want to ask you one thing. OK?

Ruth: OK.

REBTer: At the moment your conviction in your irrational beliefs is strong. Right?

Ruth: Very strong.

REBTer: What do you think has to happen for you to weaken your conviction in your irrational beliefs and strengthen your conviction in your rational beliefs?

Ruth: That's a good question. Whatever it is it sounds very daunting.

[REBTer: I have to tread carefully here. On the one hand, I want to be realistic about the change process, but on the other hand, I don't want her to think that the change process is very daunting. I also want to see if Ruth has had a life experience that mirrors the process of change.]

REBTer: Ruth, let me see if we can look together at the change process and hopefully you will see it as challenging to be sure, but not overly daunting. OK?

Ruth: OK.

REBTer: Let me ask you a question that may seem irrelevant, but isn't. OK?

Ruth: OK.

REBTer: Have you ever had the experience of changing a well-ingrained habit or behaviour?

Ruth: Well, I managed to give up smoking, but it was a struggle.

[REBTer's thinking: Since she found it a struggle to stop smoking, I will use that. (Author's note: The trained therapist knows that if Ruth gave up smoking effortlessly then this would not be a good example of the nature of therapeutic change in REBT.)]

REBTer: So let me ask you some questions about how you changed to see if there are parallels with changing your beliefs. OK?

Ruth: OK.

REBTer: Why did you decide to give up smoking?

Ruth: Because it was bad for me and it was costing me a lot of money.

REBTer: Was that knowledge on its own sufficient for you to give up smoking?

Ruth: Not at all, but it gave me the motivation to do what I had to do to stop.

[REBTer's thinking: I am going to draw a parallel between this and gaining intellectual insight into rational beliefs.]

REBTer: So seeing clearly that smoking is bad for you gave you the incentive to change, but it did not lead to change in and of itself. In the same way, knowing that your jealousy-related irrational beliefs are irrational gives you the incentive to do the things that you need to do to change them and knowing why your alternative rational beliefs are rational helps you to see what you need to change your irrational beliefs to. However, such intellectual insight on its own is insufficient to lead to belief change. Can you see the parallel?

Ruth: Yes, in both cases knowledge on its own is motivational but does not lead to meaningful change.

REBTer: Very well put. Now what did you do to give up smoking?

Ruth: I monitored my urges to smoke and when I felt an urge I reminded myself why I wanted to give up smoking and rode the urge. I then did something incompatible with smoking like a brief period of exercise until the urge to smoke went away.

[REBTer's thinking: There is a lot here that I can use: monitoring, acting against an urge to do something, doing something that is incompatible with what one wants to give up.]

REBTer: So monitoring your urges to smoke is like being aware when you feel like acting in ways that are consistent with your jealousy-related irrational belief like questioning your partner when he comes home from work about who he talked to at work and what they talked about. Then reminding yourself why you wanted to give up smoking is like challenging your jealousy-related irrational belief and doing something incompatible with smoking is very similar to acting in ways that are consistent with the rational belief that you want to develop like talking about what your partner did at work as opposed to who he talked to and what they talked about.

[REBTer's thinking: I now need to find out what Ruth struggled with when giving up smoking and use that information if it is relevant.]

REBTer: Ruth, you mentioned earlier that it was a struggle for you to give up smoking.

Ruth: It sure was.

REBTer: What did you struggle with?

Ruth: Well I had been smoking for such a long time that it felt natural to do it, and refraining from smoking felt very unnatural.

[REBTer's thinking: I can certainly use this.]

REBTer: Going against your jealousy-related irrational belief in your thinking and your behaviour certainly feels unnatural as does acting and thinking in ways that are consistent with your developing rational beliefs.

[REBTer's thinking: Now I want to find out how Ruth dealt with the struggle to see if I can use this information.]

REBTer: And how did you deal with that struggle?

Ruth: Well, I found that the more I persisted with my plan to monitor, ride and go against the urges to smoke, the more natural it became over time.

REBTer: And that is exactly the same with what could be your plan to monitor, challenge and act against your jealousy-related irrational beliefs and to act in ways that are consistent with your developing rational beliefs. The more you do that the more natural it will become and the greater emotionally-based conviction you will have in these rational beliefs. Can you see that?

Ruth: Yes, so I can do what I did with giving up smoking to really change my irrational beliefs?

REBTer: Yes you can.

[REBTer's thinking: The final point that I want to get across is that change isn't smooth and in all probability the client may experience lapses.]

REBTer: Let me ask you one last question about your experience of quitting smoking. Was the process of change smooth or did you experience times when you went back to smoking for a while?

Ruth: Oh there were definitely times when I acted on my urge to smoke and had a cigarette.

REBTer: So what did you do when that happened?

Ruth: I looked at the circumstances I was in when it happened and learned from the experience. So, I discovered that I was more likely to smoke when I was with friends who smoked and I was more likely to smoke when I was having a coffee at home.

REBTer: And what did you do with that information?

Ruth: I used it to be more assertive at saying 'no' to my smoking friends when they offered me a cigarette. And I drank tea for a while until I felt stronger to not have a cigarette when I drank coffee at home.

REBTer: So it's similar to belief change. You can notice the factors that seem to explain why you go back to your jealousy-related irrational belief and act in accordance with it and you can learn from these factors. The purpose of such learning is to re-orient yourself to the task of responding rationally to your irrational beliefs and to act in ways that are consistent with your developing rational beliefs. Can you see the parallel between giving up smoking and getting real conviction in your rational beliefs, conviction that will lead to changing your feelings as well as your behaviour?

Ruth: Yes I can see the link.

[REBTer's thinking: It would be a good idea if I summarise the steps that help explain the process of REBT.]

REBTer: Would it be useful if we developed a summary of the steps towards belief change?

Ruth: Yes it would so I can write it down and remind myself of these steps later.

REBTer: Well the first stage is understanding exactly why your irrational beliefs are irrational and why your rational beliefs are rational. Knowing this gives you the incentive to do the things that you need to do later to change your irrational beliefs to rational beliefs.

           This process is called disputing or examining your beliefs and this is what we will do next in therapy. OK?

Ruth: So that's the understanding stage.

REBTer: Or to be more accurate, the intellectual understanding stage.

Ruth: OK, let me make a note of that.

REBTer: The next stage is becoming aware that you are thinking irrationally in your life, challenging this belief in the situation, refraining from acting in the way you would normally act and instead acting in ways that are consistent with your new rational belief while rehearsing this belief. And throughout recognising that doing this will feel quite unnatural to you. Shall we break this down a bit?

Ruth: Please. Let me try. You said the following:

           1 Becoming aware that I am thinking irrationally in my life.
           2 Challenging this irrational belief at the time.
           3 Not acting according to the irrational belief.
           4 Instead, acting in ways that are consistent with my new rational belief while rehearsing this belief.
           5 Accepting the unnaturalness of doing all this.

REBTer: What would you like to call this stage?

Ruth: Let me see . . . I'll call it: Changing beliefs and
            behaviour in the situation and accepting that
            this will feel unnatural.

REBTer: The next stage is what might be called the
            persistence stage. The more you do change
            beliefs and behaviour in the situation, the more
            natural these will feel and the more your
            developing rational beliefs will affect your
            feelings and behaviour.

Ruth: I'll call this the persistence stage.

REBTer: Finally, you need to appreciate that this process
            of change is not smooth and that you will
            experience lapses in your progress, but if you
            learn from these lapses you can keep going
            without relapsing.

Ruth: I called this lapsing and learning when I was
            giving up smoking and it seems to fit here too.

*[REBTer's thinking: Ruth seems to get a lot out of sum-
marising the stages so I am going to suggest that she write
these stages down on a card and get this laminated so she can
carry it around with her and consult it as needed.]*

REBTer: Would it help if you wrote your summary points
            on a card and then got it laminated so that you
            can carry it with you and consult whenever you
            needed to?

Ruth: That is a great idea. Give me a moment and I
            will rewrite my summary points down.

REBTer: Here is a 3×5 card if that helps.

Ruth: Thanks . . . (writes summary points on the 3×5
            card) . . . OK here it is:
            Stage 1: The intellectual understanding stage of
            understanding why my irrational belief is
            irrational and why my rational belief is rational.
            Stage 2: Changing beliefs and behaviour in the
            situation and accepting that this will feel
            unnatural:
            • Becoming aware that I am thinking
              irrationally in my life

- Challenging this irrational belief at the time
- Not acting according to the irrational belief
- Instead, acting in ways that are consistent with my new rational belief while rehearsing this belief
- Accepting the unnaturalness of doing all this.

Stage 3: Persistence

Stage 4: Lapsing and learning

Now let's see how a trainee might think and intervene in the same situation. We pick up the dialogue where the trainee is about to explain the change process to Ruth.

Trainee: So in order to weaken your conviction in your irrational beliefs and strengthen your conviction in your rational beliefs, what do you think you need to do?

Ruth: I don't know.

[Trainee's thinking: I am going to have explain to Ruth what she needs to do to change.]

Trainee: Well, first I will help you to question your irrational beliefs and show you that they are false, illogical and unhelpful and then I will help you to question your rational beliefs and show you that they are true, logical and helpful. Then you will do this for yourself outside therapy. You will also need to act in ways that are inconsistent with your irrational beliefs and consistent with your rational beliefs. You need to implement these cognitive and behavioural strategies many times before you believe your rational beliefs and disbelieve your irrational beliefs. Is that clear?

Ruth: Well, you have given me a lot of information there and I'm confused.

[Trainee's thinking: The proof of the pudding is in the eating so Ruth will probably understand the change process as we proceed.]

> *Trainee*:   Well, it will become clear as we proceed in therapy, so let's start to dispute your irrational and rational beliefs.

Let me now compare the thinking and interventions of the trained therapist when explaining the nature of the change process in REBT with those of the trainee.

Both the trained therapist and the trainee display in their thinking that they know what they need to cover with respect to helping Ruth understand the change process in REBT. There the similarity ends and the best way that I can outline the differences between them is to use an analogy of preparing and digesting a meal. The trained therapist is like a cook who carefully prepares ingredients, explaining to his guest what those ingredients are as he proceeds, and then makes sure that the guest digests each course before he is ready to serve the next course. Then, after his guest has eaten, the cook asks for feedback on the entire meal.

Likewise the therapist breaks down the points he needs to convey to Ruth, ensures that she understands these points, gives her sufficient time to digest the meaning of the points and then helps her to summarise these points in her own words. Ruth then takes away a written reminder of the nature of the REBT change process for later review.

By contrast, the trainee is like a cook who prepares an entire meal for his guest and force-feeds her the food in one go without giving her an opportunity to digest anything properly. This results in the guest suffering indigestion. Thus, the trainee explains the nature of the change process in REBT in one go without breaking this down into its important elements. This results in Ruth becoming confused because she has not been helped to digest the points made along the way.

Another major difference between the trained therapist and the trainee in explaining the nature of the change process to Ruth is that the trained therapist uses an example from Ruth's life where she changed an ingrained behaviour (i.e. cigarette smoking) and drew parallels between the process of change that she experienced in this personal example and the process of change in REBT. This made the therapist's points personally meaningful for Ruth and engendered hope in that she was helped to see that she had had a successful experience of going through a similar change process to the one that she was now about to embark on in REBT.

By contrast, the trainee did not try to elicit a personal example of change from Ruth that he could use in his explanation of the change process in REBT. Thus, not only did the trainee confuse Ruth in presenting too much material at once, he failed to engage her in his intervention by keeping the dialogue overly theoretical.

In the next chapter, I will consider how a trained therapist differs from the trainee in his thinking and interventions related to the process of disputing irrational and rational beliefs.

Chapter 9

Thinking and intervening related to disputing

Disputing involves helping the client to stand back and consider whether or not her irrational belief and alternative rational belief are true, logical and helpful. As mentioned in the previous chapter, the major purpose of disputing is to help the client understand that her irrational belief is irrational (i.e. false, illogical and unhelpful) and that her rational belief is rational (i.e. true, logical and helpful).

The process commonly known as disputing involves the therapist using a variety of styles including Socratic questioning, didactic explanations, the use of stories and metaphors and the use of humour all designed to help the client gain intellectual insight into the irrationality of her irrational beliefs and the rationality of her rational beliefs.

There are many issues that could be discussed when the topic of disputing comes centre stage. In this chapter, I will concentrate on three such issues:

1 the order in which beliefs are disputed with respect to the arguments used;
2 how these arguments are made in disputing beliefs;
3 the use of Socratic questioning and didactic explanations when making these arguments.

Albert Ellis (1994) argued that rigid beliefs are at the very core of psychological disturbance in the face of adversity and flexible beliefs are at the very core of psychological health in the face of the same adversity. I discussed these two beliefs in Chapter 5. He further argued that a set of extreme and non-extreme beliefs are derived from these rigid and flexible beliefs respectively. Since this is the classic REBT position and I only have the space to discuss a trained therapist's and a trainee's thinking and interventions with one set of irrational and rational beliefs, I will focus on the disputing of a rigid belief and its flexible alternative belief.

The issue of order in disputing a rigid belief and its flexible alternative belief

The therapist can use three different orders when disputing a client's rigid belief and alternative flexible belief. I will discuss these one at a time. Let me make clear at the outset that although when discussing these three orders I state that the therapist uses empirical arguments first, then logical arguments and finally pragmatic arguments, this order is not fixed and can be varied according to the practitioner's clinical judgement.

Order 1: Using the three arguments in disputing the rigid belief and the flexible belief in turn

Traditionally, disputing has involved the therapist targeting the client's rigid belief first and asking the client to assess the empirical, logical and pragmatic status of this belief. Then the therapist helps the client to construct a rational alternative to this rigid belief (known as a non-dogmatic preference) before asking her to assess the empirical, logical and pragmatic status of this rational belief.

Thus, if the client held the following rigid belief: 'I must stand up for myself with my older sister when she puts me down', the therapist, using this order, would dispute as follows:

Rigid belief:
    Empirical argument
    Logical argument
    Pragmatic argument

Then, the therapist would help the client to develop the following non-dogmatic preference: 'I would like to stand up for myself with my older sister when she puts me down, but unfortunately there is no law of nature that states that I have to do so'. Then, employing this order he would dispute as follows:

Flexible belief:
   Empirical argument
   Logical argument
   Pragmatic argument

Order 2: Using each argument in turn with the rigid belief and flexible belief taken separately

Here the therapist helps the client to develop a non-dogmatic preference alternative to her rational belief and then he applies each argument in turn with the client's rigid belief and flexible belief taken separately.

Thus, if the client held the following rigid belief: 'I must stand up for myself with my older sister when she puts me down', the therapist would first help the client to develop the following non-dogmatic preference: 'I would like to stand up for myself with my older sister when she puts me down, but unfortunately there is no law of nature that states that I have to do so'. Then, employing this order, the therapist would dispute as follows:

Empirical argument:
   Rigid belief
   Flexible belief

Logical argument:
   Rigid belief
   Flexible belief

Pragmatic argument:
   Rigid belief
   Flexible belief

Order 3: Using each argument in turn with the rigid belief and flexible belief taken together

Here the therapist helps the client to develop a non-dogmatic preference alternative to her rational belief and then he applies each argument in turn with the client's rigid belief and flexible belief taken together.

Thus, if the client held the following rigid belief: 'I must stand up for myself with my older sister when she puts me down', the therapist would first help the client to develop the following non-dogmatic preference: 'I would like to stand up for myself with my older sister when she puts me down, but unfortunately there is no law of nature that states that I have to do so'. Then, employing this order, the therapist would dispute as follows:

Rigid belief vs. flexible belief:
    Empirical argument
    Logical argument
    Pragmatic argument

Although REBT theory does not put forward a particular order in disputing beliefs, my own experience is that the third order is the most effective (Dryden, 1999a). This is because the client is being asked to consider her rigid belief and flexible alternative belief at the same time when thinking about the empirical, logical and pragmatic status of these beliefs. It is the comparative nature of this task that facilitates the disputing process in my experience. As will be discussed below, the trained therapist is more likely to use this order, while the trainee is more likely to use the first order, which again in my experience is not only the most cumbersome, but the one which leads to most practitioner errors.

How arguments are employed in the disputing process

As mentioned at the beginning of this chapter, REBT therapists tend to use three main arguments when disputing their clients' beliefs (both irrational and rational): These are:

1   The empirical argument where the therapist encourages his client to stand back and reflect on whether her belief (rigid and flexible) is true or false.
2   The logical argument where the therapist encourages his client to stand back and reflect on whether her belief (rigid and flexible) is logical or illogical.
3   The pragmatic argument where the therapist encourages his client to stand back and reflect on whether her belief (rigid and flexible) is helpful or unhelpful.

How arguments are employed in the disputing process: an example where the therapist is trained

In this section, I am going to tease out the thinking of a trained therapist when it comes to disputing a client's beliefs and show how this thinking impacts on his interventions. In the next section, I will show how a trainee might think about and intervene in response to the same material.

The client that the trained therapist is working with is called Edith and we encountered her rigid belief in the material above. Thus, Edith held the following rigid belief:

'I must stand up for myself with my older sister when she puts me down.'

In the following excerpt the trained therapist uses the third order discussed above where he uses each argument in turn against Edith's rigid belief and her alternative flexible belief taken together. In order to do this he helps Edith to construct a non-dogmatic preference (i.e. flexible belief) as follows:

'I would like to stand up for myself with my older sister when she puts me down, but unfortunately there is no law of nature that states that I have to do so.'

Having done this the trained therapist uses the following order in his disputing work with Edith:

Rigid belief vs. flexible belief:
    Empirical argument
    Logical argument
    Pragmatic argument

Let's pick up on the dialogue between the two. Remember that the therapist has helped Edith to understand the nature of belief change (as discussed in the previous chapter) and thus Edith knows that the purpose of disputing is intellectual insight (see p. 135).

The empirical argument

REBTer: So, Edith, let's take your rigid belief and flexible belief together and see which is true and which is false, which is logical and which is illogical and which is helpful to you and which is not. OK?

Edith: OK.

REBTer: I will deal with these points one at a time.

[REBTer's thinking: I am going to suggest to Edith that I write her rigid and flexible beliefs next to one another on the whiteboard so that she can have a constant visual reminder of these beliefs during the disputing process.]

REBTer: Edith, would it be useful if I write on this whiteboard the two beliefs that we are going to stand back and evaluate?

Edith: That would be useful.

Edith's rigid belief (demand):
'I must stand up for myself with my older sister when she puts me down.'

Edith's flexible belief (non-dogmatic preference):
'I would like to stand up for myself with my older sister when she puts me down, but unfortunately there is no law of nature that states that I have to do so.'

REBTer: OK, looking at these beliefs together which do you think is true and which is false?

Edith: The flexible belief is true and the rigid belief is false.

[REBTer's thinking: Edith has given the right answer, but it is important that I assess the reasoning behind her answer.]

REBTer: That's right, but why is it right?

Edith: Well, it intuitively feels right.

[REBTer's thinking: That answer won't do because Edith is not giving any reasons that inform her intuitive 'feel', so I am going to encourage her to give reasons for her intuitive response.]

REBTer:　Your intuitive feeling is probably based on an underlying reason. Let's see if I can help to identify that. When you look at the two beliefs does the rigid belief seem more false to you than the flexible belief seems true or vice versa?

Edith:　The flexible belief seems more true.

REBTer:　Why is that?

Edith:　Well it is true that I want to stand up to my older sister when she puts me down, but it is also true that there is no law of nature that states that I have to do so. I wish there was, but there isn't.

[REBTer's thinking: This is a good answer, I am going to use it to help Edith to see why her rigid belief is false.]

REBTer:　If there were a law of nature that said you had to stand up to your older sister when she put you down, what would you have to do?

Edith:　I would have to stand up to her.

REBTer:　That is right, you would have no choice but to stand up to her. But we know that you are not standing up to her even though you want to. That is why your rigid belief is false because it states a law of nature that does not exist.

[REBTer's thinking: I am going to ask Edith to summarise what she has learned about the empirical status of her rigid and flexible beliefs. The more active she is in the process, the more she will learn.]

REBTer:　Can you summarise what you have learned about the truth and falsity of both beliefs?

Edith:　Well my rigid belief is false because if it were true, I would stand up for myself, no question. But I don't, so that is not true. My flexible belief is true because it is a fact that I want to stand up to my older sister and it is a fact that I don't

> have to do so. If that were true, I would stand
> up for myself when she puts me down no matter
> what was going on and that is not the case.
> *REBTer*:   Excellent.

The logical argument

*[REBTer's thinking: Now I am going to ask Edith to consider
the logic of each of her beliefs. In order to do this effectively, I
am going to use a diagram which will help her understand that
both her demand and her non-dogmatic preference have a
common component and two different conclusions from that
component. In the non-dogmatic preference the conclusion is
logically derived from the common component while in the rigid
demand it isn't.]*

The trained therapist then puts the diagram shown in Figure 1
on the whiteboard.

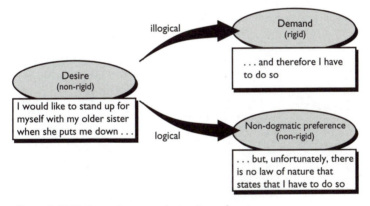

Figure 1 Rigid demand vs. non-dogmatic preference

> *REBTer*:   Edith, this diagram shows that both your rigid
> demand and your non-dogmatic preference are
> based on the same partial preference statement,
> which is:

'I would like to stand up for myself with my older sister when she puts me down . . .'

Now when your belief is in the form of a rigid demand, you add the following to the partial preference:

'. . . and therefore I have to do so.'

This is shown in the top right-hand box in the diagram. *[REBTer points to the relevant box in Figure 1.]*

On the other hand, when your belief is in the form of a non-dogmatic preference you add the following to the partial preference:

'. . . but unfortunately there is no law of nature that states that I have to do so.'

This is shown in the bottom right-hand box in the diagram. *[REBTer points to the relevant box in Figure 1.]* Is this clear so far?

Edith: Yes, it is.

REBTer: Now just considering the partial preference in the left-hand box here *[REBTer points to the relevant box]*, namely:

'I would like to stand up for myself with my older sister when she puts me down . . .'

Is this belief rigid or non-rigid?

Edith: It is non-rigid.

REBTer: Correct. Let me write down 'non-rigid' next to that component on the board *[writes it down]*. Now let's consider the second component in the non-dogmatic preference *[REBTer points to the appropriate box]*. Is this statement rigid or non-rigid?

Edith: Definitely non-rigid.

REBTer: Right, so let me write down 'non-rigid' next to that component on the board *[writes it down]*. Now, does the second part follow logically from the first?

Edith: Yes . . . I guess . . . since they are both non-rigid.

[REBTer's thinking: Edith seems a little hesitant here. I am going to make a short didactic point to underscore the idea that Edith's non-dogmatic preference is logical.]

REBTer: You are right. Your non-dogmatic preference is logical because its second non-rigid component is logically derived from its first non-rigid component. Are you with me?

Edith: Yes.

REBTer: Now again if you look at the box on the left here, you can see as we have already established that it is non-rigid. Right?

Edith: Right.

REBTer: Now let's consider the second component in your rigid demand *[REBTer points to the appropriate box]*. Is this statement rigid or non-rigid?

Edith: It is obviously rigid.

REBTer: Right so let me write down 'rigid' next to that component on the board *[writes it down]*. Now, does the second part follow logically from the first?

Edith: No, it doesn't.

REBTer: Why not?

Edith: Because the first part is non-rigid and the second part is rigid.

[REBTer's thinking: Another opportunity for a short didactic point.]

REBTer: And in logic you cannot logically derive something that is rigid from something that is non-rigid.

Edith: I see.

The pragmatic argument

[REBTer's thinking: Now I am going to ask Edith to consider each of her beliefs in terms of how helpful they are to her.]

REBTer: Now let's consider your two beliefs in terms of how helpful they are to you. Which of the two beliefs is helpful and which unhelpful?

Edith: My rigid demand is unhelpful and my flexible belief is helpful.

[REBTer's thinking: Once again, Edith is correct, but I want her to provide reasons.]

REBTer: Why?

Edith: My rigid demand does not help me to assert myself. In fact, I feel so bad about myself when I hold this belief that I start to think that I deserve to be put down.

REBTer: So you get a kind of triple whammy. First, your rigid demand does not help you to stand up for yourself with your sister. Second, it leads you to feel badly about yourself. What would you call that feeling by the way?

Edith: Depressed.

REBTer: OK, so second, your rigid demand leads you to feel depressed. And third, it affects your subsequent thinking in the sense that you start to think that you even deserve the put-downs that you get from your sister. Is that right?

Edith: Absolutely.

REBTer: Now let's consider the consequences of holding your non-dogmatic preference and let's compare the effects one at a time. What effect would holding your flexible belief have on your assertion?

Edith: Well, It would help me to stand back and consider how I stop myself from asserting myself with my older sister.

REBTer: And if you feel depressed about not asserting yourself with your older sister when you hold your rigid belief, how would you feel about not asserting yourself with her when you hold your non-dogmatic preference?

Edith: I would feel disappointed rather than depressed.

REBTer:	OK, and finally, if you hold your flexible belief about not asserting yourself with your older sister would you still think that you deserve her put-downs?
Edith:	Not at all. I would think that I don't deserve them and that I am determined to tell her that.

[REBTer's thinking: Edith seems to grasp the points that I have been helping her to see concerning the irrationality of her irrational beliefs and the rationality of her rational beliefs. Let me see if she can summarise what she has learned.]

REBTer:	Edith, I wonder if you could summarise what we have discussed concerning your rigid demand and its flexible alternative.
Edith:	Well, my rigid demand is false, illogical and unhelpful and my flexible belief is true, sensible and helpful to me.

[REBTer's thinking: Edith has summarised the main point well here, but I am not sure if she has any doubts, reservations and objections to it. So I am going to ask her about that.]

REBTer:	That's a good summary, Edith. Do you have any doubts, reservations or objections to it?
Edith:	Only, how I am going to get myself to believe it.
REBTer:	That's a common concern, but if you recall what we said about the change process, you need intellectual insight before you do the things that will lead you to develop emotional conviction in your flexible belief. Do you remember?
Edith:	Oh yes.
REBTer:	Leaving aside your concern about getting yourself to believe your non-dogmatic preference, do you have any doubts, reservations or objections to the idea that your rigid demand is false, illogical and unhelpful and your flexible belief is true, logical and helpful?
Edith:	No. I agree with all that.

How arguments are employed in the disputing process: an example where the therapist is a trainee

In this section, Edith is working with a trainee. If you recall, Edith held the following rigid belief:

'I must stand up for myself with my older sister when she puts me down.'

In the following excerpt the trainee employs the first order discussed above (see pp. 147–148) where he uses each argument in turn against Edith's rigid belief. He starts with the empirical argument.

> *Trainee*: Where is the evidence that you have to stand up to your older sister when she puts you down?
> *Edith*: Well if I don't then she will continue to put me down.
>
> *[Trainee's thinking: Edith hasn't answered my question so I will ask it again.]*
>
> *Trainee*: But why do you have to stand up to her?
> *Edith*: I thought I told you, because if I don't she will keep putting me down.

The trainee is running into trouble here because he is not showing Edith that her answer to his question 'where is the evidence that you have to stand up to your sister?' is evidence not for the existence of her demand but for the existence of her preference about asserting herself with her sister.

> *[Trainee's thinking: I am not getting through to Edith, so I am going to explain what I mean.]*
>
> *Trainee*: Well, Edith, if there was a law of the universe that states that you must assert yourself with your sister then you would do so. Do you see?
> *Edith*: I think so . . .
>
> *[Trainee's thinking: That's the best I can do so I will move on to the logical belief.]*

From her response, Edith is indicating that she does not really understand the trainee's point. But, rather than asking Edith to put her understanding in her own words, he moves on to logical disputing.

> *Trainee*: Is it logical for you to believe that you have to stand up to your older sister when she puts you down?
>
> *Edith*: Well again, if I don't then she will continue to put me down.
>
> *[Trainee's thinking: Edith is again not answering the question. Let me try again.]*
>
> *Trainee*: But is it sensible to demand that you have to assert yourself with her when the reality is you are not doing so?
>
> *Edith*: I guess not.

As frequently occurs with novice REBT therapists, this trainee is really using an empirical argument here when he thinks he is using a logical argument. The trained therapist shows how to use logical arguments when questioning beliefs (rigid and flexible). The clue to the fact that the trainee is really employing an empirical argument and not a logical one is in the word 'reality' that he employs. If you compare the trainee's question here with the trained therapist's questions as outlined on pp. 153–155, you will see the difference.

The trainee then moves on to the pragmatic argument.

> *Trainee*: Does it help you to believe that you have to assert yourself with your older sister when she puts you down?
>
> *Edith*: Well, it helps to keep the importance of asserting myself with her in my mind.
>
> *[Trainee's thinking: I am going to show her that this is not helpful to her.]*
>
> *Trainee*: But does keeping the importance of asserting yourself in mind help you to assert yourself?

Edith: Not entirely, but if I don't keep it in mind, then I definitely won't assert myself.

[Trainee's thinking: I can't seem to persuade Edith that her rigid demand is not helpful to her. I will quote Ellis.]

Trainee: Well, Dr Albert Ellis, the founder of REBT, said that rigid demands are false and illogical which you can now see, but he also said that such beliefs are also unhelpful and thus you need to surrender them.

Edith: I have never heard of Dr Albert Ellis and I am sure he is a very clever man, but my demand does help me to keep the importance of asserting myself with my sister in mind and you are not going to convince me otherwise.

The trainee is beginning to argue with Edith in a non-productive way which should be avoided and which the trained therapist in his work with Edith does successfully avoid. The reason why this is happening is that the trainee has made an error in implementing REBT theory. The trainee correctly notes that Edith's rigid demand is unhelpful to her and (in desperation it must be said) quotes Ellis to support his point. However, he seems to work on the assumption that Edith's rigid demand is not helpful to her in any way. This leads the trainee into attempting to show Edith is misguided in thinking that her demand has some helpful features. In taking that position, ironically the trainee is interpreting REBT theory in a rigid manner! In reality, while REBT theory says that rigid demands largely lead to unhelpful consequences for the individual, it does not say that such demands lead to no helpful consequences for the person. What the trainee needed to do with Edith is to acknowledge that her rigid demand does help her to keep the importance of asserting herself with her sister in her mind, but to help her to see that her non-dogmatic preference also does this, but without the other unhelpful consequences that stem from her rigid demand. By clinging to the idea that he has to convince Edith that no helpful consequence of her rigid demand is possible, he does not help her to understand the other largely unhelpful consequences that stem from her demand.

At this point the trainee thinks that he has completed his disputing work with Edith on this belief and he is preparing to move to the next stage, which is to negotiate a suitable homework assignment with Edith. In doing so, the trainee makes an error often made by novice REBT therapists and one that is commonly associated with the disputing order that the trainee employed. If you recall, the trainee used 'Order 1', which when used properly would involve the trainee using the three arguments in disputing Edith's rigid belief and the flexible belief in turn. What the trainee actually did was to use the three arguments to dispute Edith's rigid demand, but he does not help Edith to construct a rational alternative to this rigid demand (i.e. a non-dogmatic preference) and thus he cannot use the three arguments to dispute her flexible belief. Even if the trainee demonstrated a high level of skill in using the three arguments to dispute Edith's rigid demand, by not helping her to construct a feasible alternative belief and thus not using the three arguments to dispute this flexible belief, he would have left her in a belief vacuum. Thus, although Edith would have seen that her rigid demand was false, illogical and unhelpful, she would not have known what to change this belief to and the benefits to be gained by making such a change. Faced with operating in a belief vacuum, it would be very likely that Edith would go back to her rigid demand since she would perceive this to be her only option.

This is the reason that I personally favour disputing 'Order 3', the one employed by the trained REBT therapist in his work with Edith since one cannot dispute a client's beliefs without disputing both her rigid demand and her flexible non-dogmatic preference at the same time. Consequently, the risk of encouraging the client to operate in a belief vacuum is minimised.

Comparing the thinking and interventions of the trained therapist with those of the trainee

Although I have made some observations about the disputing work carried out by both the trained therapist and the trainee, let me here compare and contrast their thinking and interventions as they help Edith to dispute her beliefs.

The main difference between the two in their thinking and interventions with Edith is that the trained therapist is very much concerned with structuring the work so that Edith understands why her rigid demand is false, illogical and unhelpful to her and why her flexible alternative belief is true, logical and helpful to her, whereas the trainee seems more concerned with doing the right thing. Thus, the trained therapist makes use of visual aids by writing Edith's rigid demand and non-dogmatic preference on the whiteboard and drawing a diagram on the board to best convey the logical argument. He asks Edith to summarise the points made and elicits and responds productively to any doubts, reservations and objections that she may have concerning the information that he has presented.

By contrast, the trainee does not use visual aids to convey rational principles, does not ask Edith to summarise these principles and does not attempt to elicit her apparent doubts, reservations and objections concerning these principles. He interprets REBT theory incorrectly with respect to the logical argument and too rigidly and therefore incorrectly with respect to the pragmatic argument. Finally, when he gets stuck he appeals to the authority of Albert Ellis to get him out of trouble but does so in an unhelpful and clearly unsuccessful manner. In short, the trainee's work is characterised by being overly concerned with the client giving the right answers whereas the trained therapist's work is characterised by a strong desire to facilitate Edith's learning.

The use of Socratic questioning and didactic explanations in the disputing process

So far in this chapter, I have discussed the order in which REBT therapists can dispute their clients' beliefs and the three major arguments that they tend to use when disputing these beliefs. In this section I will discuss the two main styles that REBT therapists use in helping their clients to dispute their irrational beliefs. These involve the use of Socratic questioning and didactic explanations (DiGiuseppe, 1991). I will discuss these styles one at a time and as usual I will consider the thinking and interventions engaged in by both a trained REBT therapist and a trainee.

Socratic questioning

When a therapist uses Socratic questions, his purpose is to encourage his client to think for herself about matters to do with the irrationality of her irrational beliefs and the rationality of her rational beliefs. While the questions are largely open questions in nature, they are informed by REBT theory. In the same way as Socrates guided his students to knowledge through the thought-provoking questions he asked them (now known as Socratic questions), so an REBT therapist, when using Socratic questioning, guides his client to knowledge about the empirical, logical and pragmatic status of her rigid demand and non-dogmatic preference.

Socratic questioning: the thinking and interventions of a trained therapist

In the following exchange, a trained REBT therapist is working with Jenny, who is seeking help for depression. The therapist is using the second disputing order discussed above (see p. 148) with respect to the following two beliefs:

- Rigid demand: 'I must be approved of by my friend, Helen'.
- Non-dogmatic preference: 'I would like to be approved of by my friend, Helen, but she does not have to approve of me'.

REBTer: So, is it true that you have to be approved of by Helen?

Jenny: Well, if she does not approve of me, it will make life much more difficult for me.

[REBTer's thinking: Jenny hasn't answered the question that I asked her. Rather, she has answered a question that I did not ask her. If I had asked her: 'Is it true that it would preferable but not necessary for you to be approved of by Helen?', then her response would have been a good one. I need to help her to see that point.]

REBTer: Is your response a good answer to my question: 'Is it true that you have to be approved of by Helen' or a good answer to a different question, namely: 'Is it true that it would preferable but not necessary for you to be approved of by Helen?'

Jenny: I guess it's a good answer to the latter question.

[REBTer's thinking: Jenny is correct, but I need to be sure that she understands why she is correct.]

REBTer: Why do you say that?

Jenny: Well, because, if it were true that I have to be approved of by Helen then that is what has to happen. And it doesn't have to happen like that.

[REBTer's thinking: I will now ask her to reflect on her original answer and see if she knows why it was wrong.]

REBTer: So when I originally asked you; 'Is it true that you have to be approved of by Helen?' and you replied because if she does not approve of me, it will make life much more difficult for me, what error were you making?

Jenny: Well as I can see clearly now, I was giving you an answer as to why it was desirable for me to be approved of by Helen, not why I have to be approved of by Helen. The only correct answer to the question: 'Is it true that I have to be approved of by Helen?' is 'no'.

Let's now consider how the REBT therapist used Socratic questioning to help Jenny consider the pragmatic consequences of her rigid demand.

REBTer: How helpful to you is your demand that you must be approved of by Helen?

Jenny: Well, it helps me to think about what I can do to please her.

[REBTer's thinking: I know that her demand will have some good consequences for her such as the one she mentioned, but I also know that depression and/or anxiety is likely to accompany this advantage. Also, REBT theory argues that the same consequence can be achieved from her flexible belief but without the underlying anxiety/depression. Let's see if I can help her to see that.]

REBTer: And when you think about what you can do to please Helen while holding the rigid demand that you must have her approval, are you feeling anxious or concerned, but not anxious about having her approval?

Jenny: I would be anxious about having her approval.

REBTer: And if you thought that Helen disapproved of you and you believed that you had to have her approval would you feel depressed or would you feel sad, but not depressed?

Jenny: I would feel depressed.

[REBTer's thinking: I am going to follow up on this by asking her if her rigid belief does all that she wants it to do for her or if not, whether she would be interested in a belief that helps her to think about how to please Helen, but without the accompanying anxiety and depression if she thinks that Helen actually does disapprove of her.]

REBTer: So your demand that you must have approval from Helen does help you to think about how to please her and from your perspective that is a good consequence. Is that right?

Jenny: Correct.

REBTer: However, this is accompanied by feelings of anxiety when you think that she might not approve of you and you demand that she has to. Have I got that right?

Jenny: Yes.

REBTer: Also, if Helen were to disapprove of you, your demand that she has to approve of you would lead to depression. Correct?

Jenny: Yes.

[REBTer's thinking: I am now going to capitalise on her answers to these questions and ask if her she would be interested in developing a belief that would have the advantage of her rigid demand without its identified disadvantages.]

REBTer: So would you be interested in developing an alternative belief that enabled you to keep the advantage of thinking how you might please Helen, but without the disadvantages of anxiety

> and depression? A belief that would lead you to feel concerned, but not anxious about the prospect of Jenny not approving of you and one that would lead you to feel sad, but not depressed if it turned out that she doesn't approve of you. Would developing that belief interest you?
>
> *Jenny*:   Very much so.

The trained REBT therapist would then help Jenny to develop her non-dogmatic preference alternative to her rigid belief and then employ Socratic questioning in the same way as he did in helping her to question this rigid demand.

Socratic questioning: the thinking and interventions of a trainee

In this section, I will outline the thinking and interventions of a trainee responding Socratically to Jenny, beginning with his use of the empirical argument and followed by the pragmatic argument.

> *Trainee*:   So, why do you have to be approved of by Helen?
> *Jenny*:   Well, if she does not approve of me, it will make life much more difficult for me.
>
> *[Trainee's thinking: Jenny's answer shows that I need to take her response and dispute her implied rigid belief about this 'A': 'Life will be much more difficult for me'.]*
>
> *Trainee*:   And why must life not be more difficult for you?
> *Jenny*:   Well nobody likes life to be more difficult, do they?
> *Trainee*:   But we are talking about you. Why must life not be difficult for you?
> *Jenny*:   Because it gets me away from what's important in my life.
>
> *[Trainee's thinking: OK, I need to do the same thing here; take Jenny's answer, treat it as an 'A' and dispute the implicit rigid belief that underpins it.]*

> *Trainee*:   And why must you not get away from what is important in your life?
>
> *Jenny*:   I'm sorry. I am getting confused. I don't know what you are trying to get at.

What the trainee is doing is taking every response from Jenny and treating it as an 'A', assuming that there is a rigid demand that underpins this new 'A' and disputing this new rigid demand. It appears that the trainee is using a technique called inference chaining (see Neenan and Dryden, 1999), a difficult skill for trainees to master and one which this trainee is misusing. As a result, the trainee is taking Jenny further and further away from her original and specific 'A' about which she is disturbing herself. As Jenny is asked to dispute rigid demands about distant and general 'As' she gets increasingly confused.

Let's now consider how the trainee might use Socratic questioning to help Jenny consider the pragmatic consequences of her rigid demand.

> *REBTer*:   How helpful to you is your demand that you must be approved of by Helen?
>
> *Jenny*:   Well, it helps me to think about what I can do to please her.
>
> *[Trainee's thinking: I need to help Jenny to focus on the unhelpful aspects of her demand.]*
>
> *Trainee*:   Is your demand unhelpful to you?
>
> *Jenny*:   I guess so. I get nervous when I am around Helen in case she disapproves of me, but that is the price I have to pay, I guess.
>
> *Trainee*:   Price you have to pay?
>
> *Jenny*:   For having strong feelings about Helen.
>
> *Trainee*:   You make it sound like it's an advantage?
>
> *Jenny*:   Well, I am a woman of strong feelings.
>
> *[Trainee's thinking: I am getting lost here. I need to back up.]*
>
> *Trainee*:   But where does it get you to believe that you have to have Helen's approval?
>
> *Jenny*:   I thought that I'd answered that already.

In the above exchange, it is clear that the trainee has lost focus and is getting caught up with Jenny's replies which his poor questions have elicited. What he needs to do is to take a leaf out of the trained therapist's book and help Jenny understand (through Socratic questioning) that her demand has some advantages which are also achieved by her flexible alternative belief (i.e. her non-dogmatic preference). But that it has mainly disadvantages which are avoided by her flexible belief.

Socratic questioning: a comparison of the thinking and interventions of the trained therapist and the trainee

Let me more formally compare the thinking and interventions of the trained therapist and the trainee in their respective disputing work with Jenny.

While both trained therapist and trainee do use questions in the service of their disputing work, their respective thinking shows that the trained therapist uses such questions in the service of a planned strategy which is flexible enough to take into account and incorporate the client's responses. By contrast, the trainee does not have a sophisticated strategy in mind and is too easily blown off course by Jenny's responses. Understandably, the trainee does not have a well-honed ability to think on his feet characteristic of the trained REBT therapist. For example, when employing Socratic questioning disputing Jenny's demand pragmatically, the trainee does know that her demand can have helpful as well as unhelpful consequences (unlike the trainee in the excerpt on p. 160 who incorrectly thinks that a demand can only have unhelpful consequences). Thus, when Jenny provides what is for her a helpful consequence of her demand, the trainee nicely follows up by asking whether it has any unhelpful consequences: Thus:

Trainee:	Is your demand unhelpful to you?
Jenny:	I guess so. I get nervous when I am around Helen in case she disapproves of me, but that is the price I have to pay, I guess.
Trainee:	Price you have to pay?

By asking 'Price you have to pay?', the trainee is responding to the last thing that the client says and gets caught up in Jenny's subsequent response and in doing so, moves away from the topic in question, i.e. the pragmatic nature of Jenny's demand. The trained therapist, by contrast, shows that he is very aware of the focus of his interventions i.e. the empirical and pragmatic consequences of Jenny's demand and does not allow himself to move away from this focus. He deals with Jenny's responses in a way that incorporates these into his overall strategy. For example:

REBTer:	So, is it true that you have to be approved of by Helen?
Jenny:	Well, if she does not approve of me, it will make life much more difficult for me.
REBTer:	Is your response a good answer to my question: 'Is it true that you have to be approved of by Helen' or a good answer to a different question, namely: 'Is it true that it would preferable but not necessary for you to be approved of by Helen?'

In summary, the purpose of Socratic questioning in the disputing process is to encourage the client to think for herself in response to questions that are informed by REBT theory. While both the trained therapist and the trainee know the REBT position on the empirical, logical and pragmatic status of Jenny's beliefs, it is the trained therapist who uses such knowledge to guide Jenny successfully to the correct conclusion. He could have told her the conclusion at the outset, but if he had done so he would have deprived Jenny of an opportunity to think for herself.

Didactic explanations

While the use of Socratic questioning is perhaps the preferred style in disputing a client's beliefs in REBT, there are times when a client cannot engage in a productive Socratic dialogue with the REBT therapist or a client may favour the therapist being more didactic. In such cases the therapist will impart REBT-based information using didactic explanations.

In doing so, the therapist needs to be guided by the following points:

1   Any points made didactically should be as short as possible.
2   Didactic explanations of longer points should be broken down into manageable chunks.
3   Material should be presented visually, for example on a whiteboard, whenever appropriate.
4   Didactic explanations should be made with the client very much in mind. Thus, explanations should be given at a pace and using language to facilitate client comprehension.
5   The therapist is strongly advised to check the client's understanding of points presented didactically. In doing so, the client should be advised to put her understanding into her own words.
6   If the client understands the point made, then the therapist is advised to elicit the client's views on the point. A client may fully understand a point but disagree with it or may misunderstand its implications. In such cases, the therapist is advised to discuss any matters arising and correct any misconceptions that the client may hold about the REBT principle enshrined in the didactic explanation.

Didactic explanations: the thinking and interventions of a trained therapist

In the following sequence, a trained REBT therapist has been working with Oscar, disputing his rigid demand Socratically using the empirical argument. Oscar's demand is as follows: 'Because I am good to my friend Peter, he absolutely has to be good to me'. After three attempts to help Oscar to see that this demand is false using Socratic questions, the therapist decides to make his point didactically. Here is his thinking and subsequent interventions.

[REBTer's thinking: I have made three attempts to help Oscar understand the idea that his rigid demand is false and I am no nearer achieving my goal. So let me make my point didactically and see if this makes a difference.]

REBTer: OK, Oscar let me put this another way. If it were true that Peter had to be good to you because you were good to him. He would have no choice but to do that. He would lose free will. Does he have free will?

Oscar: Yes he does.

REBTer: So it follows that he doesn't have to be good to you because he can choose not to and from what you have said he has chosen to exercise his free will not be good to you even though you have been good to him.

[REBTer's thinking: Now that I have made my point let me see if Oscar can put this in his own words.]

REBTer: Do you get my point?

Oscar: I think so.

REBTer: Can you put the point into your own words?

Oscar: Let me see. When I demand that Peter has to be good to me because I am good to him, that is untrue because if he had to reciprocate, he would lose free will. This is not the case because he can always choose to act according to his priorities and not in line with mine.

[REBTer's thinking; Oscar has summarised the point I was trying to make very well. Now let me see what he truly thinks of this idea.]

REBTer: That's a good summary. Do you agree with that idea?

Oscar: Actually I do. It's a hard idea to digest, but I can see that it is true.

Didactic explanations: the thinking and interventions of a trainee

Now let's see how a trainee might think and intervene in response to Oscar

[Trainee's thinking: I don't think that Oscar is responding well to Socratic questioning so I will use didactic explanation to make my point.]

Trainee: OK, Oscar, let me put this another way. If there was a law of nature that said that Peter had to

be good to you then he would have to be good
to you. As he wasn't good to you it follows that
no such law exists.

Didactic explanations: A comparison between the thinking and interventions of the trained therapist and those of the trainee

It is clear that both the trainee and the trained therapist are aware
that their use of Socratic questioning with Oscar was not bearing
fruit. This led them to decide to give a didactic explanation concerning why Oscar's rigid demand was false. Both their explanations were short and to the point. However, while the trained
therapist checked Oscar's understanding and opinion of his didactically presented point, the trainee did neither of these things. As a
result, there is no way for the trainee to gauge the level of Oscar's
understanding. In addition, even if Oscar does understand the
point that his rigid demand is false, the trainee also has no way of
ascertaining what he thinks of this idea. If Oscar has an objection
to this point based, for example, on a misconception, the trainee
would not know this and therefore cannot deal with it. As a result,
there is a real danger that the trainee will encounter 'resistance'
in Oscar in the disputing process, but will not respond to this
resistance productively because he will not know the source of this
resistance.

The conjoint use of Socratic questioning, didactic explanations and other disputing styles

While I have dealt with Socratic questioning and didactic explanations as if they are used separately, in actuality this is not the case.
During a disputing sequence an REBT therapist may use a variety
of different disputing styles. Thus, he might begin with Socratic
questioning, use a brief didactic explanation to clarify a point that
the trainee appears unclear about, provide a metaphor to underscore the point so that the client's understanding is deepened and
provide self-disclosure to show the client that he has been through
the same process of change.

It is beyond the scope of this book to cover all aspects of the
disputing process and in one important sense no book can teach

you to improve your disputing skills. In my experience, the best ways to hone these skills include the following:

1   View DVDs and listen to audio-recordings of skilled REBT therapists. For example, the Albert Ellis Institute has in its catalogue a number of DVDs of experienced therapists practising REBT with a variety of clients in their 'Master Therapists' series.
2   Read and learn from the transcripts of experienced REBT therapists practising therapy. For example I compiled and edited a number of live demonstration sessions conducted with Albert Ellis which contained much fine disputing work (Dryden and Ellis, 2003).
3   Record your disputing work and play these recordings to your supervisor for feedback.
4   Read articles and book chapters on disputing (e.g. Beal *et al.*, 1996; DiGiuseppe, 1991).

Albert Ellis's typical disputing strategy

I close this chapter on disputing with the master of this art – Dr Albert Ellis, the founder of REBT. One of his most typical disputing strategies involved him didactically stating a rational principle and then asking the client to articulate reasons in favour of the rational position.

Here are a few examples of this disputing strategy:

• OK, now, you are not worthless as a person. Why is that a true statement?
• It's not logical for you to conclude that because you really want to do well on your forthcoming test therefore you absolutely have to do so. Now why is that an illogical conclusion?
• As long as you believe that you have to sing that aria well, then that belief will lead to a variety of unhealthy consequences for you. What are they?

In the next chapter, I will consider the clinical thinking and interventions that are related to homework assignments and will again compare the thoughts and responses of a trained REBT therapist with those of a trainee.

Chapter 10

Thinking and intervening related to homework assignments

Homework assignments are generally those tasks that a client carries out in between therapy sessions. The term 'homework' is not intended to mean that the client has to carry out the assignments literally 'at home', although it can of course mean that. Rather, the idea is that the client does something outside therapy sessions in the service of her therapeutic goals.

Research has shown that there is a strong relationship between therapeutic outcome and the completion of homework assignments in CBT (e.g. Burns and Spangler, 2000). As such, the issue of homework assignments is an important one for REBT therapists to address effectively. The issue of homework assignments can be divided into two main areas:

- negotiating homework assignments
- reviewing homework assignments.

Raymond DiGiuseppe (personal communication) has often said in his professional workshops that the ideal structure for an REBT therapy session is as follows:

- Review the previous homework assignment
- Continue work on the client's target problem(s)
- Negotiate a new homework assignment.

This structure demonstrates the importance of homework assignments in REBT. As such, I regard this chapter as perhaps the most central one in the book. For a client will achieve minimal gains from this approach to therapy unless she consistently puts into practice in her own life what she learns within therapy sessions.

I will begin with a discussion of the issues that arise when negotiating homework assignments with clients and follow this with considering salient issues when reviewing these assignments in the following sessions. While I will not have the space to show the thinking and interventions of both trained REBT therapist and trainee on all these issues, I will present client work which shows how both think and intervene when some of these issues come to the fore. As before, I will then compare and contrast their work and the thinking that underpins it.

Negotiating homework assignments

In my long experience as an REBT trainer and supervisor, trained REBT therapists tend to be more proficient than trainees when it comes to the process of negotiating homework assignments with their clients. In particular, trained REBT therapists tend to:

1 regularly negotiate homework assignments with their clients;
2 give themselves sufficient time in therapy sessions to negotiate homework assignments with their clients;
3 negotiate homework assignments with their clients rather than unilaterally assign them;
4 ensure that homework assignments follow logically from the work done in therapy sessions;
5 communicate clearly with their clients so that the latter know exactly what they have agreed to do;
6 help their clients to see the purpose of the agreed homework assignments;
7 ensure that their clients have the necessary skills to carry out agreed homework assignments;
8 ensure that homework assignments are relevant to their clients' therapeutic goals;
9 negotiate homework assignments with their clients that are relevant to the stage reached on the problem being targeted for change;
10 help clients to specify where, when and how often they will carry out their homework assignments;
11 help their clients to identify and overcome any obstacles to homework completion;
12 encourage their clients to make a written note of negotiated homework assignments;

13   rehearse homework assignments in therapy sessions whenever possible.

By contrast, trainees tend to:

1   discuss homework assignments with their clients in an irregular fashion;
2   give themselves insufficient time in therapy sessions to discuss homework assignments with their clients;
3   unilaterally assign homework assignments to their clients rather than negotiate these assignments with them;
4   discuss homework assignments with their clients that do not always follow logically from the work done in therapy sessions;
5   communicate with their clients in such a way that the latter are often confused about what they have agreed to do;
6   often not help their clients see the purpose of the agreed homework assignments;
7   not systematically ensure that their clients have the necessary skills to carry out agreed homework assignments;
8   often not ensure that homework assignments are relevant to their clients' therapeutic goals;
9   often not take into account the stage reached on a problem when discussing homework assignments with their clients;
10   not be systematic in helping clients to specify where, when and how often they will carry out their homework assignments;
11   not be systematic in helping their clients to identify and overcome any obstacles to homework completion;
12   leave it up to clients whether or not they make a written note of agreed homework tasks;
13   not rehearse homework assignments in therapy sessions or do so intermittently.

Negotiating homework assignments: how a trained REBT therapist thinks and intervenes

Donald is a 23-year-old man with rejection anxiety. He has coped with this anxiety mainly by avoidance. Up to this point in therapy, his therapist has helped him to understand the irrational beliefs that underpin his anxiety and the alternative rational beliefs that he needs to develop if he is to approach women while being duly concerned, but not anxious about being rejected. After some negotiation his therapist has helped Donald to understand that being concerned, but not anxious about rejection is a realistic, viable goal and one to which he has made a commitment. Donald also understands the nature of belief change. In the session from which this excerpt is taken, the therapist has disputed the following rigid demand and alternative non-dogmatic preference:

- Rigid demand: 'If I go up to speak to a woman in a bar, she absolutely must not reject me'.
- Non-dogmatic preference: 'If I go up to speak to a woman in a bar, I would much prefer it if she does not reject me, but that does not mean that I have to be immune from rejection'.

At the end of the disputing sequence, Donald acknowledged that his rigid demand belief was false, illogical and harmful to him and that his non-dogmatic preference was true, logical and helpful to him. However, as Donald himself said, 'Knowing this does not make me feel it'.

About ten minutes from the end of the session from which the following exchange is taken, the trained therapist is aware that he needs to begin to negotiate a relevant homework assignment with Donald.

[REBTer's thinking: Right, it's about ten minutes before the end of the session and I need to negotiate a homework assignment with Donald.]

REBTer: So you understand that knowing that your rational belief is true, logical and useful to you does not on its own help you to feel it in the sense that it impacts on the way you subsequently act. We need to talk about ways you can put your understanding into action. Now what can you do between now and next week that will help you to strengthen your rational belief and weaken your irrational belief?

Donald: I'm not sure . . . Go out and get rejected?

[REBTer's thinking: Donald seems to be joking, but there is a serious point in there that I want to highlight.]

REBTer: Actually, yes! In the sense that you need to approach an agreed number of women and practise your rational belief at the same time. What do you think of that idea?

Donald: I can see the sense of it, but it seems a bit daunting.

[REBTer's thinking: I need to see if this sense of it being daunting will serve as an obstacle to Donald doing the homework that we are about to negotiate.]

REBTer: I can understand that the idea of approaching women when you have been used to avoiding them seems a bit daunting. Will that stop you from approaching women between now and our next session?

Donald: Depends on how many you want me to approach.

[REBTer's thinking: Donald talks in terms of how many women I want him to approach. I need to address this issue with him straight away.]

REBTer: How many women I want you to approach? I thought it was you who wanted a girlfriend?

Donald: I do!

REBTer: So how many women do you realistically want to approach between now and next week without it seeming overly daunting to you?

Donald: I would say two.

[REBTer's thinking: That's reasonable. I am going to encourage Donald to be specific about time and place.]

REBTer: Where and when are you going to approach these two women?

Donald: Well I am going to a quiz night on Wednesday and there is a woman there I have always wanted to talk to, but have always shied away from. And on Saturday, I am going to a pub with a few mates and I will try and chat with one other woman then.

[REBTer's thinking: I need to remind Donald that it is important for him to rehearse his rational belief while he approaches the women.]

REBTer: And what belief are you going to rehearse before during and after talking to them?

Donald: They don't have to accept me, although it would be nice if they did.

REBTer: Excellent!

[REBTer's thinking: I will see if Donald foresees any other obstacles to completing his homework.]

REBTer: Apart from approaching two women seeming daunting, can you think of other ways in which you might stop yourself from talking to two women on those occasions?

Donald: No, I'm pretty sure I will do that.

[REBTer's thinking: While I have no reason to disbelieve Donald, I want him to have a contingency plan if one or both of those social engagements fall through.]

REBTer: That's good to hear. But if one or both social engagements fall through, will you still commit to approaching and talking to two women before our next session?

Donald: (*laughing*) You like to cover all the bases don't you! OK, whatever happens, I will approach and talk two women before our session next week.

[REBTer's thinking: I am going to encourage Donald to make a written note of his homework.]

REBTer: I'll make a written note in my notes, can you do the same in your therapy notebook?

Donald: . . . (*writing*) . . . OK.

[REBTer's thinking: I want to check if what Donald has written corresponds to what we have agreed.]

REBTer: Can I check with you what you have written?

Donald: 'I will approach and talk to two women before our next session, one at the quiz night and the

REBTer: other at the pub. However, if one or both of these nights out don't work out, I will still talk to two women before the session.' How's that?

REBTer: That's great, although can I suggest you add the bit about rehearsing your rational belief and it's worthwhile being specific about it in your notes.

Donald: Good point. OK . . . (writing) . . . 'and I will rehearse the following belief while approaching the woman: "I want her to accept me, but she doesn't have to do so".'

REBTer: Great!

Negotiating homework assignments: how a trainee thinks and intervenes

In this case it is a trainee working with Donald on the same set of beliefs as above and has reached the same point as the trained therapist. However, with two minutes of the session remaining, the trainee suddenly realises that he hasn't negotiated a homework assignment with Donald and needs to do so.

[Trainee's thinking: Oh God! I'm not keeping track of time. I have got two minutes left and I need to set homework.]

Trainee: OK, Donald, we have to finish in a minute. What can you do between now and next week to put into practice what we have discussed today?

Donald: I'm not sure. I guess I can review my notes and you can give me some appropriate reading.

[Trainee's thinking: Donald wants to play it safe. But I think he is ready for a behavioural assignment.]

Trainee: I think you could stretch yourself. We have to finish now, but I want you to approach and talk to two women and rehearse your rational belief as you do so. Will you do that?

Donald: I'll try.

Negotiating homework assignments: comparing
the thinking and interventions of the trained
REBT therapist with those of the trainee

Perhaps the most crucial difference between the trained REBT
therapist and the trainee is that the former gave himself plenty of
time to negotiate a homework assignment while the latter was
always on the back foot because he gave himself so little time to
deal with the salient issues to do with homework negotiation.
Consequently, the major differences between them in their thinking
and in their interventions were as follows:

1   The trained therapist was aware of the need to negotiate a
    homework assignment and put this into practice while the
    trainee assigned a task unilaterally.
2   The trained therapist was very clear at various points (with
    himself and with Donald) in detailing the two major elements
    – i.e. behavioural and cognitive – of the agreed task. In con-
    trast, while the trainee was clear about the behavioural
    element, he was vague with respect to the cognitive element.
3   The trained therapist recognised the importance of eliciting
    specific times and specific places for homework execution and
    put this into practice, while the trainee did neither of these
    things nor did he think about doing them.
4   The trained therapist considered the need to elicit and deal
    with possible obstacles to homework completion and did this
    on several occasions. In addition, he helped Donald come up
    with a contingency plan if his two social engagements fell
    through. By stark contrast, the trainee did not address the
    issue of potential obstacles with Donald, nor did he think
    about doing so.
5   The trained therapist elicited a commitment from Donald that
    he would do the homework assignment, while the trainee did
    not do this. As a result, with the trainee Donald said that he
    would 'try' to do the assignment which, in my experience, is a
    good predictor for non-completion of homework.
6   Finally, the trained therapist recognised the importance of
    encouraging Donald to make a written note and translated this
    into practice. He even checked this note for accuracy, dis-
    covering that Donald had included the behavioural component
    of the task, but had omitted the cognitive component. On

discovering this, the trained therapist was able to rectify the situation. Again, by stark contrast, the trainee did not think of and therefore did not encourage Donald to make a written note of the homework assignment.

Reviewing homework assignments

Trained REBT therapists also tend to be more proficient than trainees when it comes to the process of reviewing homework assignments with their clients. In particular, trained REBT therapists tend to:

1   systematically review homework assignments;
2   check that clients have done all agreed assignments as negotiated and have not changed them;
3   ascertain the reasons why clients have modified homework tasks and intervene accordingly;
4   ascertain reasons why clients have failed to do any agreed assignments and intervene accordingly;
5   discover whether or not clients who have completed agreed homework assignments have brought about desired changes by challenging and changing their irrational beliefs and intervene accordingly if this is not the case;
6   systematically review what clients have learned from carrying out homework assignments;
7   capitalise on clients' success;
8   reinforce the clients' efforts without praising them as people.

By contrast, trainees tend to:

1   haphazardly review homework assignments;
2   check that clients have done some, but not all agreed assignments as negotiated and if they have done them, they tend not to check if they have changed them;
3   not ascertain the reasons why clients have modified homework tasks and intervene accordingly;
4   reiterate the importance of doing homework assignments when clients have not done them rather than ascertain reasons why clients have failed to do such assignments and intervene accordingly;

5   not assess how clients have brought about changes as a result of doing homework assignments;
6   not systematically review what clients have learned from carrying out homework assignments;
7   not capitalise on clients' success;
8   praise clients as people as well as reinforce their efforts. In doing so, they irrationally assign their clients a global positive evaluation and this, inadvertently, teach their clients that people can be rated globally.

Reviewing homework assignments: how a trained REBT therapist thinks and intervenes

Vanessa is a 33-year-old woman with anxiety about her hands shaking in public. Consequently, she avoids whenever possible doing anything publicly where her hands may shake, e.g. writing cheques, carrying a coffee cup in a café or holding a wine glass in a bar. She thus avoids going into banks or building societies, cafés and bars or pubs.

In her previous session with a trained REBT therapist, she had agreed to do the following: go into a wine bar with a friend who knew about and was sympathetic to her problem and hold a small glass of wine without putting it down for twenty minutes and without having first taken a beta-blocker. As she did this she agreed to rehearse the following rational beliefs:

'I would prefer not to shake, but that does not mean that I must not do so. I don't have to appear normal in public and I can accept myself if some people think I'm weird if I shake.'

We pick up the dialogue at the beginning of the next session after the usual pleasantries.

REBTer:	So, Vanessa, can we start by reviewing your homework assignment?
Vanessa:	OK. I went to the wine bar with Sylvia as we agreed and she bought me a small glass of wine, which I held.
REBTer:	For how long?

Vanessa:	For the agreed twenty minutes.
REBTer:	And did you rehearse the rational beliefs that we formulated the week before?
Vanessa:	I told myself that I don't have to be immune from shaking even though I'd rather not do it and if I do and others notice, I can accept myself even if they think I'm strange for shaking.
REBTer:	Excellent. What happened?
Vanessa:	Well I didn't shake. I felt quite relaxed in fact.

[REBTer's thinking: This sounds too good to be true and I'm reminded of what they say on the TV series, 'The Real Hustle': if something seems too good to be true, then it probably is.]

REBTer:	Gosh, it's difficult to believe that you had severe anxiety about your hands shaking.
Vanessa:	It does sound too good to be true, doesn't it.

[REBTer's thinking: Vanessa is looking very sheepish. I have to tread very carefully. Otherwise she will either retreat into herself, get defensive, feel ashamed or any combination of the above.]

Vanessa:	Well . . . and I feel really terrible saying this, but I did have a few drinks before I went to the wine bar with my friend.

[REBTer's thinking: I need Vanessa to be more precise about this.]

REBTer:	So what precisely did you drink before going out?
Vanessa:	I had two large gin and tonics to settle my nerves.
REBTer:	And if you had not had them, how would you have felt?
Vanessa:	Very anxious!
REBTer:	So, it seems like you did want to deal with your anxiety, but in a way which meant that you didn't deal with it in the longer term.
Vanessa:	Very true. I feel so ashamed now.

[REBTer's thinking: Vanessa is revealing a number of issues that we may have to tackle before we focus more directly on her anxiety about shaking. She seems to have a low tolerance for feeling anxious which means that she looks for ways to avoid the experience rather than face it. Second, she is ashamed about what she does to get rid of her anxiety quickly, like use alcohol. I will need to put this to her with care.]

REBTer: Can I check something out with you, Vanessa. It seems like the homework has taught us that we need to deal with your tendency to avoid anxiety rather than face it before we deal head on with your anxiety itself. What do you think of this idea?

Vanessa: I think that is very true.

REBTer: The homework has also taught us that when you drink to deal with your problems you feel ashamed. Do we need to deal with this emotion, as realistically, you may at times slip back?

Vanessa: I see what you mean.

[REBTer's thinking: It looks like I am going to rethink my assessment and redo my therapeutic plan.]

REBTer: So let's take stock and see where we are and what your experiences with this homework have taught us. OK?

Vanessa: OK.

Reviewing homework assignments: how a trainee thinks and intervenes

Now let's see how the trainee dealt with exactly the same event.

Trainee: So, Vanessa, can we start by reviewing your homework assignment.

Vanessa: OK. I went to the wine bar with Sylvia as we agreed and she bought me a small glass of wine, which I held.

Trainee: For how long?

Vanessa:	For the agreed twenty minutes.
Trainee:	And did you rehearse the rational beliefs that we formulated the week before?
Vanessa:	I told myself that I am not immune from shaking even though I'd rather not do it and if I do and others notice, I can accept myself even if they think I'm strange for shaking.
Trainee:	Excellent. What happened?
Vanessa:	Well I didn't shake. I felt quite relaxed in fact.
Trainee:	Fantastic. Let's capitalise on this and go to the next stage.

Reviewing homework assignments: comparing the thinking and interventions of the trained REBT therapist with those of the trainee

The main difference between the trained REBT therapist and the trainee in this excerpt is in their reading of the client's 'successful' completion of the negotiated homework assignment. It is clear that the trainee takes at face value the client's verbal report of 'success', while the trained therapist is sceptical that Vanessa could have made such a dramatic improvement. His sceptical thinking leads to him voicing his concerns, but in a very delicate way. This enables Vanessa to admit to drinking alcohol to calm her nerves and it is this alcohol rather than rational thinking that is responsible for her 'successful' completion of the assignment. By contrast, the trainee is oblivious to this and is about to capitalise on Vanessa's 'success', something which may lead Vanessa to continue to use alcohol as an anxiolytic. The trained therapist helps Vanessa to identify her shame issue and problem with experiencing anxiety, meta-emotional problems which if not dealt with will serve to prevent Vanessa from dealing effectively with her original problem. Since the trainee is unaware of the existence of these meta-emotional problems, he cannot help Vanessa deal with them.

In the next chapter, I will discuss how trained and trainee REBT therapists deal with a variety of obstacles to change.

Chapter 11

Thinking and intervening related to dealing with obstacles to change

The process of REBT like the path of true love rarely runs smoothly and the skilled REBT therapist needs to be able to identify and deal effectively with a variety of obstacles to change. A full discussion of how trained therapists and trainees think and intervene in the face of such obstacles merits a book and there are a number of such books in the literature (e.g. Neenan and Dryden, 1996; Ellis, 2002).

In this chapter, I will first briefly outline the most common obstacles to change that REBT therapists encounter. Then I will present, discuss and compare the thinking and interventions of both trained therapist and trainee in responding to two such obstacles.

Common obstacles to change in the working alliance

A good way of understanding common obstacles to change in REBT is by using the working alliance as a framework for such understanding (Bordin, 1979; Dryden, 2006). Working alliance theory states that the working alliance between therapist and client has four major components: bonds, views, goals and tasks. Here I will outline each component and list the major obstacles that occur in REBT under each heading.

Bonds

A bond refers to the interpersonal connectedness between therapist and client. There are many dimensions of the therapeutic bond to consider when trying to ascertain the reason for an obstacle to client change. Here are some of the most common obstacles in the bond domain:

- The client does not 'feel' understood by the therapist.
- The client does not 'feel' respected by the therapist.
- The client does not experience the therapist as genuine.
- The therapist's interpersonal style does not facilitate client learning (e.g. the therapist is overly active or works too quickly for the client).
- The client does not respect the therapist's expertise.
- The client does not experience the therapist as trustworthy.
- The therapist is under-involved with the client.
- The therapist is over-involved with the client.
- The therapist's style is informal and the client would benefit from a more formal style.
- The therapist's style is formal and the client would benefit from a more informal style.

Views

The views refer to the explicit and implicit understandings between therapist and client on a range of therapeutic and practical matters.

Here are some of the most common obstacles in the views domain:

- The therapist and client disagree on the conceptualisation of the client's problems.
- The therapist and client disagree on the treatment of the client's problems.
- The therapist and client disagree on a variety of practical issues to do with therapy (e.g. the therapist's cancellation policy).

Goals

REBT is a purposive activity and ideally therapist and client should agree with one another with respect to the client's goals for change. Here are some of the most common obstacles in the goals domain:

- The client and therapist disagree on the client's goals.
- The therapist and client are working on overcoming the client's dissatisfaction when the client is disturbed about the dissatisfaction.
- The therapist endeavours to help the client achieve a goal that is outside of her control to achieve.
- The therapist agrees to help the client achieve the elimination of a disturbed feeling, thought or impulse, which is, in reality, impossible to achieve.

Tasks

Tasks are activities carried out by both therapist and client ideally in the service of the client's goals. Tasks can be specific (e.g. disputing irrational beliefs) or more general in nature (e.g. free association in psychoanalysis or self-exploration in person-centred therapy). Here are some of the most common obstacles in the tasks domain:

- The client does not know what her tasks are in REBT and the therapist does not help her to understand these (e.g. she does not know that she has to dispute her irrational beliefs outside of therapy sessions).
- The client does not see that performing her tasks will help her to achieve her goals.
- The client does not understand that she has to work to change in REBT.
- The client does not have the capability to carry out the therapeutic tasks required of her in REBT.
- The client does not have the necessary skills to carry out the therapeutic tasks asked of her in REBT.
- The client does not have the confidence to execute the relevant tasks in REBT.
- The client carries out cognitive tasks alone to achieve goals that can only be achieved by cognitive and behavioural tasks used conjointly.
- The tasks that the client and/or the therapist execute unwittingly serve to perpetuate the client's problems.
- The client does not understand the nature of the REBT therapist's tasks and how these tasks relate to her own tasks and to her own goals.
- The client is too disturbed to carry out her own tasks in REBT.

A philosophy of low frustration tolerance

I discussed the philosophy of low frustration tolerance (LFT) in Chapter 5. If you recall, this philosophy stems from a demand about discomfort in all its forms and can be held by the REBT therapist, the client or both. While there are numerous forms of discomfort disturbance (Dryden, 1999b), they can all be divided into two main areas:

- Area 1: I must have good experiences.
- Area 2: I must get rid of bad experiences.

Here is a sample of common client and therapist LFT-based obstacles to change.

Client LFT

- The client believes that she absolutely should not have to work to change either inside or outside REBT therapy sessions.
- The client believes that any tasks that she is called upon to execute must not be difficult to perform. Thus, she will do easy homework such as reading, but not difficult homework like confronting fears.
- The client will only work on herself when she feels motivated to do so.
- The client believes that she has to get rid of disturbed experiences as quickly as possible.
- The client procrastinates on therapy tasks and waits until the last minute before doing them.
- The client terminates therapy when the going gets tough or when she does not make progress quickly enough when this expectation is unrealistic.

When client obstacles to change are due to client LFT, the task of the REBT therapist is to do the following:

1   Agree with the client that an obstacle to change exists.
2   Assess this obstacle and agree with the client that it is based on the client's LFT.
3   Identify the client's LFT belief and help her to develop an alternative high frustration tolerance (HFT) belief.

4 Engage the client in a process of questioning or disputing these beliefs until the client can acknowledge that her LFT belief is irrational and her HFT belief is rational. When this occurs the client has achieved the stage of intellectual insight (see p. 135).
5 Encourage the client to strengthen her HFT belief by rehearsing it and acting in ways that are consistent with this belief.
6 Repeat this process until the obstacle has been overcome.

Therapist LFT

A philosophy of LFT is not just the province of the client. The REBT therapist can also have LFT. Here are some instances of therapist LFT that may lead to or exacerbate a client's obstacles to change:

• The therapist gets impatient at the client's pace and/or rate of change and demonstrates this.
• The therapist avoids working rigorously because he finds doing so too hard (e.g. he negotiates homework with his client, but does not do so rigorously).
• The therapist wants an easy ride in therapy (e.g. he will allow the client to ramble on without helping the client to become and remain problem focused).
• The therapist is dogmatic in his use of REBT. For example, he thinks that because REBT has a good framework for understanding a client's problems and for helping a client address these problems effectively, therefore the client must make use of REBT and work assiduously in therapy. Holding this belief, the therapist may show anger and irritation when the client does not behave in the required manner.

The main approach to therapist LFT is for the therapist to be observant of his own feelings, thoughts and behaviour in therapy, identify instances of LFT and the irrational beliefs that underpin it. Then the therapist needs to challenge and change this LFT belief and encourage himself to act in ways that would reinforce his developing rational beliefs in this area. Recording therapy sessions and playing back the recordings is useful here in that the therapist may detect signs of LFT that he wasn't aware of during the therapy session. Playing and discussing such recordings in supervision can be especially useful in this process.

Dealing with doubts, reservations and objections

REBT can be seen as an educational approach to therapy in that the therapist explicitly teaches the client – using a variety of styles – the REBT perspective on psychological problems and how they can be addressed therapeutically. As I pointed out in the section on didactic explanations in Chapter 9, it is not only important for the therapist to check the client's understanding of REBT concepts and points of practice, it is also important for him to gauge the client's attitude towards these concepts and points. It sometimes happens that a client may hold a doubt, reservation or objection to an REBT concept or intervention and these are often based on misconceptions of these REBT-based ideas. If the client holds such an objection, for example, and the therapist does not know about it then he cannot deal with it. In this case, the unidentified objection may well serve as an obstacle to change as the client 'resists' accepting the REBT idea and holds on to the idea enshrined in the objection and perpetuates her problem as a result.

Consequently, it is important that the REBT therapist provides his client an opportunity to voice her doubts, reservations and objections as a prelude to addressing potential obstacles to change. Here are some example of such client doubts, reservations and objections:

- doubts about giving up a demand in favour of a non-dogmatic preference
- doubts about giving up an awfulising belief in favour of a non-awfulising belief
- doubts about giving up an LFT belief in favour of an HFT belief
- doubts about giving up a depreciation belief in favour of an acceptance belief
- doubts about feeling HNEs instead of UNEs (particularly concern rather than anxiety, remorse rather than guilt and healthy anger rather than unhealthy anger)
- doubts about overcoming procrastination
- doubts about asserting oneself instead of staying quiet.

I will show how a trained therapist differs from a trainee in his thinking and intervening in response to one such doubt later in this chapter. However, for more suggestions on how to deal with such doubts, reservations and objections see Dryden (2001) and Dryden and Branch (2008).

How a trained therapist and a trainee think and intervene in response to an obstacle to change based on client LFT

In this section, I will follow the now familiar structure by first considering how a trained REBT therapist thinks and intervenes when a client presents an obstacle to change based on her philosophy of LFT, then considering how a trainee might think and intervene in the same situation before comparing the two.

How a trained therapist thinks and intervenes in response to an obstacle to change based on client LFT

Tamsin has come to therapy because she is not fulfilling her potential in her job working for a PR firm. She was referred to a trained REBT therapist on the suggestion of her life coach who was becoming frustrated in working with Tamsin because she would not follow through on tasks that would advance her career. The life coach reasoned that Tamsin needed therapy rather than coaching at this point of her life.

On assessment the REBT therapist discovered that Tamsin had a dread of being evaluated in formal situations where she and her colleagues would have to make presentations to potential clients and would avoid such situations as much as possible. However, she was fantastic at these presentations in rehearsal when the clients were not present. The therapist helped Tamsin to identify and dispute both her irrational and alternative rational beliefs and the outcome of this work was that she committed herself to rehearsing her rational beliefs while joining her colleagues at the formal presentations. However, Tamsin continued to find excuses to miss these formal presentations. We pick up the interchange when the therapist begins to address the obstacle to change.

REBTer: So, Tamsin, we seem to have hit a block here. You keep committing yourself to rehearsing your rational belief in a formal situation, but you continue not to do so. What's your view on what is happening?

Tamsin: Well, I do have legitimate reasons.

[REBTer's thinking: I am pretty sure the reasons are not legitimate and I need to address this issue first before identifying the reason behind the obstacle.]

REBTer: If you were managing someone who had missed seven formal presentations in a row even though the person attended all seven run-throughs, what would you think was happening with the person?

Tamsin: I would think that she had a problem with presentations.

REBTer: She could have this problem and have legitimate reasons for missing them.

Tamsin: She could, but I would be highly sceptical. OK, I get your point, I am copping out.

REBTer: Why do you think you are doing that?

Tamsin: I am good at rehearsing my rational beliefs before I go and I even see myself in my mind's eye holding on to these beliefs when I am in the presentations. However, on the day, I get jittery and pull out.

[REBTer's thinking: I need to focus on her jitteriness since this is probably her 'A' to which she responds with avoidance.]

REBTer: So is it when you begin to feel jittery that you decide to pull out?

Tamsin: Now you come to mention it, yes, it is.

[REBTer's thinking: So 'A' is her feeling of jitteriness and 'C' in this case is her pulling out of the presentation. I am going to see if Tamsin can find and question her own irrational belief at 'B' since we have done a number of 'ABCs' and she can do the work for herself now.]

REBTer: So in this situation your behavioural 'C' is your pulling out of the presentation and this happens when you begin to feel jittery on the day. Is that right?

Tamsin: Yes.

REBTer: So your 'A' is your jittery feelings. Do you recall what we said about 'B'?

Tamsin: Yes, 'B' are my beliefs, in this case my irrational beliefs about my jitteriness and it is these beliefs not the jittery feelings alone that lead me to avoid the presentation.

REBTer: That's right. Now what are you demanding in this situation?

Tamsin: I must not feel jittery.

REBTer: And the alternative rational belief?

Tamsin: I'd much rather not feel jittery, but I don't have to be free of the jitters.

[REBTer's thinking: I'm not sure if Tamsin's demand is ego-related or LFT-related, so let me ask.]

REBTer: When you demand that you must not feel jittery are you saying that you are less worthy if you do or that you can't bear to feel the jitters?

Tamsin: Definitely that I can't bear the feeling.

[REBTer's thinking: So, Tamsin's obstacle is LFT-based.]

REBTer: What's the rational alternative to that belief?

Tamsin: I don't like feeling the jitters, but I can bear it.

REBTer: And is it worth bearing?

Tamsin: Yes.

REBTer: Because?

Tamsin: Because if I bear it, it will help me to deal with my ego fears about being evaluated.

[REBTer's thinking: I am going to suggest that Tamsin disputes these two sets of belief for homework. I will also encourage her to attend the next presentation and to rehearse her rational beliefs.]

REBTer: How about questioning those beliefs and if you come out in favour of your rational beliefs what do you think would be the next stage?

Tamsin: I guess do the actual presentation even though I'm jittery.

> *REBTer*:   While rehearsing what belief?
> *Tamsin*:   I can stand feeling jittery and although I'd like to be free of them, this isn't necessary.
> *REBTer*:   Excellent.

The REBT therapist then proceeded to negotiate the homework assignment more formally with Tamsin using the guidelines that I outlined in the previous chapter.

How a trainee might think and intervene in response to an obstacle to change based on client LFT

In the following segment, I will present how a trainee might deal with the same situation.

> *Trainee*:   So, Tamsin, we seem to have hit a block here. You keep committing yourself to rehearsing your rational belief in a formal situation, but you continue not to do so. What's your view on what is happening?
> *Tamsin*:   Well, I do have legitimate reasons.
>
> *[Trainee's thinking: I need to listen carefully to what Tamsin has to say here.]*
>
> *Trainee*:   What are they?
> *Tamsin*:   Well, there were two occasions when I was ill, then I had to take my aunt to a doctor's appointment. Then there was the time when I put the wrong date in my diary.
>
> *[Trainee's thinking: These are all excuses not good reasons. Albert Ellis would tell her that she is full of shit so I am going to do the same, but in my own way.]*
>
> *Trainee*:   I'm sorry, Tamsin, I don't buy any of these so-called reasons. I think they are excuses and you are deluding yourself.
> *Tamsin*:   I thought you were supposed to be on my side in counselling.

> *Trainee*:   I am on your side, but that doesn't mean that I
>   have to accept as true everything you say.
> *Tamsin*:   So are you calling me a liar?

Responding to an obstacle based on client LFT: comparing the thinking and interventions of a trained therapist with those of a trainee

Both the trained therapist and the trainee think that Tamsin's reasons for not addressing her evaluation anxiety by rehearsing her rational beliefs while actually attending PR presentation sessions are actually excuses rather than good reasons for non-attendance. However, while the trained therapist helps Tamsin to stand back and take an observer position while thinking about whether her reasons are really excuses, the trainee directly confronts Tamsin on this issue citing Albert Ellis to himself as a reason for this intervention.

It is clear from the two segments presented that these two interventions would have had different outcomes for Tamsin. The trained therapist's indirect approach enables Tamsin to admit to herself that her avoidance is an obstacle to change and not the result of good reasons for non-attendance at the presentations. By contrast, the trainee's direct approach and harsh manner leads to increased, not decreased client defensiveness and gets in the way of identifying Tamsin's avoidance as an obstacle.

Having helped Tamsin to admit to her avoidance being an obstacle, the trained therapist carefully and methodically works to help her to identify what she is avoiding and the irrational beliefs that underpin her avoidance. In doing this, the trained therapist ascertains that the client obstacle is LFT-based. Having done so he encourages Tamsin to question her irrational beliefs and their rational alternatives and from there to rehearse healthy HFT-based beliefs while confronting her issue with being evaluated rather than avoiding it.

How a trained therapist and a trainee think and intervene in response to an obstacle to change based on a client objection to a rational concept

In this final section, I will once again first consider how a trained REBT therapist thinks and intervenes this time when a client presents an obstacle to change based on her objection to a rational concept. Then, I will present how a trainee might think and intervene in the same situation before comparing the two.

How a trained therapist thinks and intervenes in response to an obstacle to change based on a client objection to a rational concept

In this example, Malcolm is a mature student who has come to therapy for help with his chronic procrastination. The therapist helps Malcolm to identify the following irrational belief that underpins his procrastination:

'I must be motivated to do the work before I start doing it and can't bear not having this motivation.'

The therapist helps Malcolm to see that his alternative rational belief is as follows:

'I'd like to be motivated to do the work before I start doing it, but I don't need this motivation. If I don't have the motivation, this is uncomfortable and I can bear it and it's worth doing so.'

The therapist has written these two beliefs on his whiteboard for future reference.

We pick up the dialogue at a point where the therapist is going to ask Malcolm what he honestly thinks about the rational belief.

[REBTer's thinking: Malcolm's seems to have understood the effect of his irrational belief on his behaviour so now I am going to enquire what he thinks about his irrational belief and its rational alternative.]

REBTer: When you stand back, which belief will help you overcome your procrastination?

Malcolm: Well, I know what you want me to say.

[REBTer's thinking: Malcolm's response indicates the presence of some kind of obstacle or doubt. Let me see if I can identify it.]

REBTer: I'm genuinely interested in what you think of the two beliefs that we are focusing on here, Malcolm.

Malcolm: Well, I think that I do need motivation. If I don't have it then I will definitely not do any work. With motivation at least I have the possibility of doing some work.

[REBTer's thinking: Malcolm is expressing a common misconception. He does not see that his demand is the problem here. He thinks it is lack of motivation. I need to address this straight away. But first, it's important that I convey empathic understanding of his position. If he 'feels' understood, he may be open to standing back and considering a different perspective.]

REBTer: So from your perspective the only way you can do work is if you are motivated to do it. If you are not motivated there is no way of doing it. That's why you are really reluctant to give up your demand for if you do so, you have no chance of doing the work. As you say, having the demand at least keeps alive the possibility of working because there is always the possibility of feeling motivated. Have I understood you correctly?

Malcolm: That's exactly how I feel.

REBTer: And I can see now exactly why you would be reluctant to surrender your demand in favour of your non-dogmatic preference.

[REBTer's thinking: Now I am going to invite Malcolm to stand back and consider a different view. If he says 'yes', he has made a commitment to at least considering this view. If he says 'no', we can explore his reluctance to do this. I am also going to add a touch of humour to lighten the discussion, since that will help Malcolm to be open-minded.]

REBTer: Malcolm, are you willing to stand back and consider a different viewpoint on this issue? I am not asking you to buy it, just consider it. No obligation!

Malcolm: (*laughing*) Put like that, what have I got to lose.

[REBTer's thinking: I have now got Malcolm's permission and his response to my humour is encouraging. I am going to begin my strategy by stressing what for Malcolm is his ideal state to do work, i.e. being motivated to do it.]

REBTer: OK, Malcolm, from what you are saying, the ideal position for you in respect to doing the work is being motivated to do it. Is that right?

Malcolm: That's right.

REBTer: When you feel motivated you do it.

Malcolm: I do.

[REBTer's thinking: I am now going to outline what I think is Malcolm's 'A' – not being motivated to work – and help him to see what his belief options are with respect to this 'A'.]

REBTer: The problem seems to start, if I understand you correctly, when you don't feel motivated to do the work. Is that right?

Malcolm: Yes, that's right.

REBTer: Now if we put that in the 'ABC' framework that we have been using in therapy, your 'A' then is 'Not being motivated to do the work'. Right?

Malcolm: Right.

[REBTer's thinking: Rather than help Malcolm choose between options I am going to introduce a third. I am doing this because I think that choosing from three options will be less pressurising for Malcolm than choosing from two. Considering this option will also give Malcolm the experience of agreeing with me as hopefully this will be the case and will strengthen our working alliance on this issue. This will help us to work together when we come to evaluate his demand and non-dogmatic preference.]

REBTer: Now let's see what your belief options are at 'B'. Although we have outlined two possible options which are up here on the board, there is a third option. Do you know what that is?

Malcolm: No.

REBTer: It is what I call the attitude of indifference. In this case it would be something like: 'I don't care

	if I am motivated to do the work or not'. What do you think of that belief?
Malcolm:	It's ridiculous.
REBTer:	Why?
Malcolm:	Because I do care.
REBTer:	That's right. An indifference belief involves you lying to yourself since it says that being motivated doesn't matter to you when the reality is that it does. Right?
Malcolm:	Right.
REBTer:	So is your indifference belief a viable option for you?
Malcolm:	No.

[REBTer's thinking: I need to lighten the mood a bit again.]

REBTer:	It was hardly worth me asking the question was it?
Malcolm:	(*smiling*) Not really.

[REBTer's thinking: I am now going to help Malcolm stand back and evaluate his demand. I will deliberately use the term stand back because I want Malcolm to get into an objective frame of mind. I want him to make a commitment to considering the demand objectively before proceeding and to help him do that, I will reiterate the 'no obligation' principle.]

REBTer:	Now let's consider your demand which is up on the board here. Before we do this, do you think you can stand back and look at it from an objective viewpoint or are you so attached to it that you can't do this? Remember you are under no obligation to purchase.
Malcolm:	No, I can be objective.

[REBTer's thinking: I will first look at the consequences of Malcolm's demand when he is facing his 'A'.]

REBTer:	Now when you are not feeling motivated to work and you believe that you must be motivated to work does that belief give you motivation?
Malcolm:	No, it doesn't.

REBTer:	Why not?
Malcolm:	Well I get depressed about not being motivated.
REBTer:	And when you aren't feeling motivated to work and believe that you have to work, does that belief help you work?
Malcolm:	Not at all. It leads me to procrastinate.

[REBTer's thinking: I am going to summarise what Malcolm has said to lay bare the dysfunctional aspects of his belief.]

REBTer:	So when you are not motivated to work, your demand that you must be motivated doesn't create motivation. Rather, it creates your feelings of depression. And it doesn't help you to work. Rather, it leads you to put off the work that it is important for you to do. So what's great about this belief, Malcolm?
Malcolm:	(*laughing*) Put like that, not much!

[REBTer's thinking: I am now ready to help Malcolm look at his non-dogmatic preference and evaluate this.]

REBTer:	Now when you are not in a motivated frame of mind, let's consider the third belief option, which is your non-dogmatic preference. This states that being motivated matters to you, but isn't crucial. Let's look at this. OK?
Malcolm:	OK.

[REBTer's thinking: Rather than directly ask Malcolm if being motivated is crucial to him, which there is still a good chance of him saying, I am going to take a slight detour and help him to see that motivation is not a crucial ingredient to starting work on something.]

REBTer:	Can you think of a time when you had work to do, but you weren't motivated to do it?
Malcolm:	That's an easy one. It was last night.
REBTer:	What happened?
Malcolm:	The usual. I did not do it.
REBTer:	Focus on the fact that you weren't motivated to do the work and bear with me while I ask you a strange question. OK?

Malcolm:	OK.
REBTer:	Would you have done the work if I had given you one million pounds to do it?
Malcolm:	Of course.
REBTer:	Even though you weren't motivated to do the work?
Malcolm:	That would have motivated me.

[REBTer's thinking: I need to help Malcolm see the difference between being motivated by the outcome and being motivated to work.]

REBTer:	Would you have done the work because you were motivated to do it or because you were motivated to have the million pounds?
Malcolm:	Motivated to have the million pounds.
REBTer:	So is it possible for you do something that you aren't motivated to do to get a result that you are motivated to have?
Malcolm:	Put like that, yes.

[REBTer's thinking: I am now going to elicit Malcolm's motivation to do the work and use this to help him see that he can work when he is motivated by an outcome even though he is not motivated to do the activity that leads to the outcome.]

REBTer:	Now let's come back to last night, but sorry, Malcolm there is no million pounds.
Malcolm:	Shame!
REBTer:	Was is it in your interests to do the work?
Malcolm:	Yes.
REBTer:	Why?
Malcolm:	Well, it is a course requirement and has to be done if I am to get my degree.
REBTer:	And you want to get your degree?
Malcolm:	I sure do.

[REBTer's thinking: It would be helpful to have Malcolm spell out the reasons why he wants his degree since these are the reasons that I want him to focus on when he is not motivated to do work. To this end I will write these reason on the whiteboard.]

REBTer:	Why?
Malcolm:	It will help to get me a better job and improve my future job prospects. It will make my aging parents proud of me. I would see it as a great achievement. I'll improve my financial prospects in the long run. And I may want to do post-graduate study in the future and having a degree will help me to do that.
REBTer:	So that's equivalent to the million pounds in a way isn't it?
Malcolm:	I guess so.

[REBTer's thinking: Now I am going to ask Malcolm an important question. If he answers 'yes' then I will use his response to drive home my point later.]

REBTer:	Now Malcolm, if you had kept these reasons to the front of your mind last night, is it possible that you would have begun the work even though you were not motivated to do the work itself?

The crucial component in the trained therapist's question here is the phrase 'is it possible'. If Malcolm agrees that it is possible, then he has already articulated a flexible position.

Malcolm:	Yes it's possible.

[REBTer's thinking: Now I am going to ask Malcolm to evaluate his demand and his non-dogmatic preference in this specific situation that we are using.]

REBTer:	So, it's possible. But what would have happened if you had demanded last night you had to be motivated to do the task?
Malcolm:	I would not have done it.
REBTer:	And what could have happened if you had honestly reminded yourself that such motivation was desirable but not necessary?
Malcolm:	I would have done the task because I would have allowed myself to be motivated by my wish

> to get a degree and the reason why getting it is so important to me. I get it! My demand makes the motivation of the moment the only thing that is important and if I am not motivated in the moment, I am stuffed.

The REBT therapist then went on to help Malcolm put his learning into his own words, after which the trained therapist helped Malcolm to revisit his doubt about surrendering his demand and asked him to re-evaluate it, as shown in the following dialogue.

> *REBTer*:   We did this piece of work because you had a big doubt about giving up your demand: 'I must be motivated to do the work before I start doing it and can't bear not having this motivation'. Your doubt was that the only way you could do work was if you were motivated to do it. If you were not motivated there was no way you could do it. That's why you were reluctant to give up your demand since if you did so you believed you had no chance of doing the work. Do you remember saying that?
>
> *Malcolm*:   I do.
>
> *REBTer*:   And what do you think of your doubt now?
>
> *Malcolm*:   It's unjustified.
>
> *REBTer*:   In what way?
>
> *Malcolm*:   Well, I was in effect saying that there was only one way I could work and that is if I am motivated in the moment to do the work. You helped me to see that this is not true and that I can work when I am not motivated by the task but when I am motivated by all the things that I am working for in my future. That's really important and I am going to let that be my guiding principle.

The REBT therapist then helped Malcolm operationalise his new 'guiding principle' and negotiated a specific homework assignment along the lines discussed in the previous chapter.

How a trainee might think and intervene in response to an obstacle to change based on a client objection to a rational concept

Now let's see how a trainee might think and intervene in response to the same situation. In this following sequence the trainee has identified Malcolm's demand and non-dogmatic preference (see pp. 197–199) and has written both on a whiteboard.

Trainee: When you look at these two beliefs which belief will help you overcome your procrastination?
Malcolm: Well, I know what you want me to say.
Trainee: Which is what?
Malcolm: You want me to say the non-dogmatic preference.

[Trainee's thinking: The way Malcolm is talking it is clear that he disagrees. I need to flush out his doubt as I have been taught to do.]

Trainee: And what do you think?
Malcolm: I think that if I believed the non-dogmatic preference I would never get any work done.
Trainee: Why?
Malcolm: Because my demand motivates me and the other belief lets me off the hook.

[Trainee's thinking: That's a misconception. I need to help Malcolm to see this.]

Trainee: Well, your demand isn't helping you to work at the moment, is it?
Malcolm: But it keeps work in my mind. If I held the other belief, I would not think about doing the work.
Trainee: That's not the case. You would think about the work because it's important for you to do it.
Malcolm: But you don't know how my mind works.

[Trainee's thinking: I am getting stuck here. I don't know what to do. I am going to change the subject and discuss the matter later with my supervisor.]

Responding to an obstacle based on a client objection to a rational concept: comparing the thinking and interventions of a trained therapist with those of a trainee

Both the trained therapist and the trainee showed that they were aware that Malcolm had a doubt about surrendering his demand about being motivated to do work before doing it in favour of his non-dogmatic preference. Apart from this, they differed in their approach to Malcolm's expressed doubt.

Thus, the trained therapist:

- Conveyed that he understood the reasons for Malcolm's doubt about giving up his demand in favour of his non-dogmatic preference.
- Invited Malcolm to stand back and consider a different viewpoint about his demand. He stressed humorously that Malcolm was not obliged to accept this different viewpoint.
- Worked with a specific example of Malcolm's procrastination to demonstrate this alternative viewpoint.
- Used the 'ABC' framework to help Malcolm to evaluate his three belief options towards his 'A' of not being motivated to start work.
- Began with the indifference belief to strengthen the alliance between him and Malcolm.
- Helped Malcolm to see that his demand led to depression and procrastination and did not lead to motivation.
- Used an indirect approach while evaluating Malcolm's non-dogmatic preference and in doing so helped him to see that being motivated was not a necessary condition for starting work. Instead, the therapist showed Malcolm that he could begin work because doing so would help him to achieve his longer-term goals and that he did not need to be motivated to do the task before starting it.
- Revisited Malcolm's original doubt with him, at which point Malcolm indicated that he no longer was doubtful about surrendering his demand in favour of his non-dogmatic preference.

By contrast, the trainee tried to deal head on with the misconceptions inherent in Malcolm's doubt. He showed no understanding of Malcolm's doubt and tried to convince him by general assertion rather than by specific evidence, which was the route chosen by the trained therapist. The trainee did not use a specific example of Malcolm's procrastination to help Malcolm to test his view that motivation was necessary to him. As a result, Malcolm quickly showed with irritation that he did not 'feel' understood by the trainee.

In the final chapter, I will consider how a trained therapist thinks and intervenes when opportunities arise to help a client maintain and generalise her gains. I will compare this with how a trainee might think and intervene in response to the same situations.

Chapter 12

Thinking and intervening related to maintaining change

In this final chapter of the book, I am going to consider how a trained REBT therapist and a trainee think and intervene when faced with opportunities to help clients to maintain the gains that they have made in therapy. In particular, I will consider two issues:

- encouraging the client to be her own therapist
- helping the client to prevent relapse.

Teaching the client to be her own therapist

One of the ultimate goals of REBT is to encourage a client to serve as her own therapist as soon as she can during therapy and after formal therapy has come to an end. Unless a client has internalised a set of self-helping strategies and techniques, she may well fail to deal with any new aversive activating events that she might encounter in therapy and once therapy has come to an end.

Thus, two central tasks that the REBT therapist has are to: (1) introduce the concept of self-help into therapy and (2) systematically help his client to acquire REBT self-help skills. He can best do this in a structured way. Thus, he can formally and deliberately teach his client such REBT skills as: (1) using a variety of self-help forms; (2) identifying 'As'; (3) discriminating keenly between her rational beliefs and her irrational beliefs; and (4) questioning beliefs. The therapist can also teach his client the large number of emotive and behavioural techniques which will help her to weaken her irrational beliefs and strengthen her rational beliefs.

Thorough coverage of this important topic lies outside the scope of this book. The reader is referred to Dryden (2001), which is an REBT workbook designed to teach clients such self-help skills.

Once the therapist has taught his client these skills in a structured and deliberate way, then he needs to encourage her to use the skills on her own. The therapist can serve as her consultant while she does this, providing her with useful feedback on any problems she may experience in doing this. It is important that the therapist gives his client an opportunity to serve as her own therapist as early in the therapeutic process as is clinically indicated.

What follows is a discussion of how a trained therapist thinks and intervenes when faced with an opportunity for a client to be her own therapist. I will contrast this with how a trainee thinks and intervenes in response to the same situation. Since trainees tend not to encourage clients to adopt a self-therapist role, the trainee's work in the segment to be presented will reflect this.

Frank has sought help for his anger problem. So far in therapy he has learned to assess specific examples of his anger using the 'ABCs' of REBT, to challenge his beliefs and to assert himself rather than to be aggressive. In the following exchanges he has lost his temper in the week and wants to discuss this episode with his therapist.

Helping a client to be his own therapist: the thinking and interventions of a trained therapist

REBTer: OK, Frank, what happened?
Frank: I lost my temper while driving my car when someone cut me up.
REBTer: What did you do?
Frank: I caught the guy up and verbally abused him.
REBTer: Did you use any of the skills you learned here to help yourself?
Frank: I didn't, I'm afraid.
REBTer: We'll consider why later. But first let's understand how you made yourself angry.

[*REBTer's thinking: Since Frank knows how to assess his own problems, I am going to ask him to take the lead in assessing this episode of anger. If he runs into difficulty, I will help him out.*]

REBTer: OK, Frank, why don't you take the lead and assess this episode.

Frank: So my emotional 'C' was unhealthy anger. I know it was anger because I wanted to beat the guy to a pulp. Now my 'A' was the guy taking the piss out of me by cutting me up and my 'B' was the guy must not take the piss out of me.

[REBTer: I want to see if this is an example of LFT anger or ego-defensive anger, so let me ask Frank.]

REBTer: And because the guy took the piss out of you when he absolutely should not have done so?

Frank: He makes me look like an idiot and I am an idiot if I don't get back at him.

[REBTer's thinking: So it's ego-defensive anger.]

REBTer: OK, you have assessed the episode. Now what?

Frank: I need to specify my rational belief.

REBTer: Which is?

Frank: I would prefer it if he did not take the piss out of me, but I am not immune from this. And I'm not an idiot even if he treats me like one and even if I don't get back at him.

REBTer: Now what?

Frank: Now I need to question these beliefs. My demand is unhealthy since it leads to my angry feelings and behaviour, while with my non-dogmatic preference I would have been pissed off, but would not have chased and verbally abused the guy. My non-dogmatic preference is true. Thus, it's true that I would prefer him not to take the piss out of me and it's also true that he doesn't have to do what I want. It's also true that I am not an idiot even if he treats me like one and even if I let the incident go.

REBTer: Very good. Now let's see why you didn't do any of this at the time.

Helping a client to be his own therapist: the thinking and interventions of a trainee

Trainee:	OK, Frank, what happened?
Frank:	I lost my temper while driving my car when someone cut me up.
Trainee:	What did you do?
Frank:	I caught the guy up and verbally abused him.

[Trainee's thinking: OK, let me use the 'ABC' framework to assess this episode.]

Trainee:	It sounds like your anger was unhealthy.
Frank:	Yes it was.
Trainee:	Now that is your 'C'. Now 'A' is the aspect of the situation that you were most angry about. What were you most angry about in this situation?
Frank:	I was most angry about the guy taking the piss out of me.
Trainee:	Now if you recall, 'A' doesn't cause 'C'. What largely determined your anger?
Frank:	(*getting exasperated*) You are talking as if I don't know these principles. You are treating me like a new client.

Helping a client to be his own therapist: the thinking and interventions of the trained therapist and the trainee compared

It is clear from these two excerpts that the trained therapist knows that Frank is knowledgeable about the 'ABCs' of REBT and uses the opportunity to have Frank take the lead in assessing and helping himself. The trainee, by contrast, does not use the opportunity to have Frank practise self-therapy. While the trainee is technically correct in his approach, he manages to antagonise Frank by going over the basics of REBT, treating him as if he knows little or nothing about the REBT framework. As a consequence, Frank becomes exasperated.

Helping a client to be his own therapist: a caution

The trained therapist knows that not all of his clients will be able to become their own therapist. Some of them may be so handicapped that they may not find it possible to serve as their own therapist for any extended period of time. If a therapist has unrealistic expectations of such clients and pushes them into a self-therapy mode, he may unwittingly discourage them from using the limited self-help abilities that they do possess.

Helping the client to prevent relapse

Relapse prevention is a term which originated in work with the addictions to highlight the fact that relapse often occurs and that a concerted effort to help clients prevent relapse is frequently necessary on the part of the therapist. A major part of relapse prevention involves helping a client to become aware of a variety of vulnerability factors. These client vulnerability factors can occur in the client's external and internal environment. Taking dealing with alcohol problems as an example, external vulnerability factors include the sight and smell of alcohol, other people drinking and TV adverts for drink, while internal vulnerability factors include clients' styles of thinking (thinking of all the positive aspects of drinking alcohol), behaviour patterns (deliberately walking past pubs and bars) and emotional responses (positive feelings associated with drink). All of these serve as invitations to drink.

I have already made the point that the course of therapy rarely runs smoothly and a client will frequently take two steps forward and one step back and even one step forward and two steps back! When these setbacks are small and when they occur in the context of general client progress, they are best described as lapses. However, when a client experiences a significant setback this is perhaps better described as a relapse. In REBT relapse prevention, the therapist asks his client to take each problem on her problem list and identify the set of internal and external circumstances in which she may experience a relapse. The therapist helps her as specifically as he can to identify relapse-triggering activating events, and the irrational beliefs she holds about such events. In particular, the therapist helps his client to identify any vulnerable feelings which may discourage her from using REBT techniques.

Then, the therapist encourages her to imagine that she is experiencing such a vulnerable feeling or is entering into a situation in which she may be vulnerable to relapse and asks her to use her rational thinking skills to prevent the situation leading to relapse. The client can do this by using imagery techniques or self-help forms. In fact, she can use any of the numerous REBT change techniques at this point. After she has successfully coped with her vulnerability factors in imagination, she is then encouraged to seek them out in reality so that she can gain experience at using her developing rational thinking skills in vivo (in real-life situations).

Helping a client to prevent relapse: the thinking and interventions of a trained therapist

Gemma is a 35-year-old woman who has come to therapy for help with giving up smoking. She has done well in therapy and when the following takes place she has not smoked a cigarette for two weeks, the longest period she has not smoked since she began to smoke at age 17. In the following dialogue she is working with a trained REBT therapist who has just explained the difference between a lapse and a relapse.

Gemma: OK, I see the difference between a lapse and a relapse, but I don't want to ever smoke again.

[REBTer's thinking: So it seems as if I may have to help Gemma deal with two sets of issues here: dealing effectively with her vulnerability factors that render her vulnerable to smoking and her feelings should she lapse and smoke again. My sense is because Gemma is so keen not to smoke again she would resist me if I push for starting with the meta-disturbance issue first, so I will put both issues to her and have her choose the order. As long we deal with both, that should be OK.]

REBTer: My sense is, Gemma, that we need to deal with two issues. I will outline them and if you agree, we can talk about the best order in which to tackle them. OK?

Gemma:	OK.
REBTer:	You have done very well to refrain from smoking for two weeks, but do you still have the sense that you are vulnerable to smoking.
Gemma:	Yes.
REBTer:	So do you think we should do some work helping you to deal with those times when you consider yourself to be at risk, as it were, of smoking again?
Gemma:	Definitely.
REBTer:	The other issue concerns dealing with your feelings should you lapse and smoke again. How would you feel if that happened?
Gemma:	Devastated.
REBTer:	And would that feeling make it more or less likely that you would smoke again?
Gemma:	More likely, definitely.
REBTer:	So do we need to work on this issue as well?
Gemma:	Well, to be honest with you I was hoping that you would help me get to the point that I wouldn't smoke again, but I'm beginning to see that this goal is a bit unrealistic. So, reluctantly, I agree that we need to work on that as well, But can we start with the other issue first, please?
REBTer:	I was just going to ask you that question and you've answered it for me.

The trained therapist then helped Gemma to list the situations in which she felt at risk of smoking. Having done this, the therapist suggested that Gemma pick one situation that she felt would be most relevant to start with.

| *Gemma:* | Well, I'm going to a wedding over the weekend and I will meet some mates who I haven't seen for some time, They are all smokers and I know there will be a time where we all go outside for a breather which means a ciggy! I guess I should avoid going out there with them. |

[REBTer's thinking: The point of relapse prevention is facing up to vulnerable situations and using skills so that, in Gemma's case, she does not smoke even though her mates are smoking. On the other hand, she may be so vulnerable to smoking in this situation that it might be best if she avoids the situation. I am going to suggest that we deal with this issue in the session and I will encourage her to use her skills in the 'at risk' situation. However, should she be so vulnerable that she will smoke I am going to suggest that she avoids going outside or leaves immediately rather than actually take a cigarette and smoke.]

REBTer:　What about if I help you to deal with this situation here in the session, but if you feel so vulnerable at the wedding you abandon your attempt to put these skills into practice and avoid going outside with your smoking mates or leave immediately rather than smoke?

Gemma:　OK, sounds like a good way forward.

REBTer:　OK, so imagine you are outside with your mates, what is likely to happen?

Gemma:　Well, we will be drinking and then one of them will take out a packet of cigarettes and offer them around.

[REBTer's thinking: I am going to see what Gemma is most vulnerable to and help her deal with that.]

REBTer:　At that point what might lead you to smoke?

Gemma:　The sense that I will be the odd one out if I don't. That's a real issue for me across the board.

[REBTer's thinking: I have an opportunity here to stress the importance of generalising the skills of dealing with being the odd one out.]

REBTer:　So, being the odd one out is something that is a general vulnerability factor for you not just in this situation. Is that right?

Gemma:　Yes, that's correct.

REBTer:　OK, so whatever you learn here about dealing with the sense of being the odd one out in this specific situation, you can learn to apply in every situation where you experience that sense. OK?

Gemma: That would be great.

[REBTer's thinking: I am now going to use Gemma's 'A' – being the odd one out – and use the 'ABC' framework to assess 'B' and 'C'. My hunch is that Gemma would smoke in this situation to get rid of a disturbed feeling about being the odd one out and to experience the sense that she is part of the crowd. Let's see.]

REBTer: Let's though start by focusing on this specific event. Imagine that everybody has taken a cigarette and you haven't. How do you feel about being the odd one out in this situation?

Gemma: Depressed.

[REBTer's thinking: Gemma knows about irrational beliefs and their rational alternative beliefs since we have gone over this a few times and she seems to have grasped the point so let me get straight to the point.]

REBTer: And what would your irrational belief be?

Gemma: I must be part of the group and I am unlikeable if I'm not.

REBTer: And what would your rational alternative belief be?

Gemma: I'd like to be part of the group, but I don't have to be. I can accept myself in this situation and it does not prove that I am unlikeable.

[REBTer's thinking: Before I do more work on this issue I first need to establish that if Gemma held this belief then she would not smoke.]

REBTer: If you rehearsed this belief at the time would you smoke or not?

Gemma: I wouldn't smoke, especially if I also reminded myself of the reason why I want to refrain from smoking that we discussed in the first session and that I wrote on my flash card.

[REBTer's thinking: Let me take Gemma through this situation using imagery, but I first need to help her to see that she will have a healthy negative emotion when she thinks rationally about being the odd one out.]

REBTer: That's great, but when you rehearse your rational belief about being the odd one out in this situation you will still feel bad won't you?

Gemma: Yes, I will feel sad, but I would not feel depressed.

REBTer: And what impact would your sadness have on your cigarette smoking?

Gemma: Oh I would not smoke. It's the depression that would be the clincher.

REBTer: OK, let's rehearse what we have covered. Close your eyes and imagine that you are at the wedding and are outside with your smoking mates. Can you get that image?

Gemma: Yes I can.

REBTer: OK, one of them brings out a pack of ciggies and offers them around. Everyone takes them apart from you and you begin to get a sense that you are the odd one out. You use that sense as a cue to rehearse your rational belief: I'd like to be part of the group, but I don't have to be. I can accept myself in this situation and it does not prove that I am unlikeable. Can you see yourself doing that?

Gemma: Yes.

REBTer: And how are you feeling?

Gemma: Sad about being the odd one out, but pleased that I am not smoking even though they tease me about being a goody-goody, which I know that they will.

[REBTer's thinking: I need to see if that pressure is another vulnerability factor that I need to help Gemma deal with.]

REBTer: Can you handle that pressure without smoking.

Gemma: Oh yes. In fact it's easier not to smoke when I am under that kind of pressure. It brings out the bolshy in me and I become even more determined not to smoke.

The trained therapist then negotiated homework which comprised the following:

- questioning her rational and irrational beliefs;
- rehearsing thinking rationally about being the odd one out at the wedding using daily imagery practice as demonstrated above;
- confronting the vulnerability situation in reality while thinking rationally about being the odd one out, but with the back-up plan of avoidance or withdrawal if the situation is too much for her.

Helping a client to prevent relapse: the thinking and interventions of a trainee

Gemma: OK, I see the difference between a lapse and a relapse, but I don't want to ever smoke again.

[Trainee's thinking: So it seems as if I have to help Gemma deal with two sets of issues here: dealing effectively with her vulnerability factors that render her vulnerable to smoking and her feelings should she lapse and smoke again. I will deal with the latter first because that is the meta-disturbance and in REBT we tend to deal with such issues first.]

Trainee: OK, Gemma, it seems as if I need to help you with two things: dealing with your vulnerability factors so that you don't smoke and dealing with your feelings when you lapse. Now, in REBT we deal with the second problem first. So let's imagine that you lapse and you smoke, how would you feel about that?

Gemma: I don't want to tempt fate like that, I want you to help me deal with what for me are vulnerable situations so that I don't smoke.

[Trainee's thinking: I need to make the rationale clearer for dealing with her meta-disturbance first.]

Trainee: But if you are disturbed about smoking then this will make it more likely that you will smoke.

Gemma: That's why we need to start with your feelings about smoking.

Gemma: I can't see that. I would have thought if you helped me to deal with my vulnerability factors, I wouldn't smoke and thus, I wouldn't have to deal with these feelings.

Trainee: But as a fallible human being, it's always possible to lapse and if you don't deal with that possibility in a healthy fashion, you will be more likely to relapse. Trust me on this one, let's work on this problem about lapsing and then I will get back to helping you with your vulnerability factors.

Gemma: It looks like I don't have much of a choice do I!

Helping a client to prevent relapse: the thinking and interventions of the trained therapist and the trainee compared

The main differences between the trained therapist and the trainee in working with Gemma lie in the degree of flexibility with which they apply REBT and the degree of attention that they give to the working alliance between them and the client. The trained therapist shows in his thinking and in his interventions that he attends closely to the working alliance between him and Gemma. He also shows a high degree of flexibility in using, in this case, the order of addressing Gemma's issues. He knows that as an REBT therapist he might prefer to deal with Gemma's meta-disturbance issue first, but also knows that doing so at the expense of the working alliance is counterproductive. Thus, he is happy to go with the order desired by his client.

The trainee, on the other hand, shows in his thinking and in his interventions that he is not concerned with the working alliance between him and Gemma. All he seems concerned with is doing the right thing and as such he is rigid in his determination to work with Gemma's meta-disturbance problem first. In doing so, he seems to antagonise her and she ends up by sensing that she has no choice but to go along with him. By being rigid, the trainee is a poor role model for REBT, which advocates flexibility!

When the trained therapist deals with Gemma's vulnerability factors he does so in the way advocated by REBT theory.

1   He helps her to develop a list of such factors.
2   He asks her to choose one factor to deal with at a time.
3   He encourages her to select a specific example of the target factor.
4   He assesses this factor using the 'ABC' framework.
5   Having ascertained that Gemma's rational belief will help her not to smoke in the chosen example, he uses imagery rehearsal to help her to see how she can handle the vulnerability factor in situ.
6   He helps her to see that she can avoid the situation or leave it if she finds dealing with the factor too difficult in the actual situation.
7   He negotiates appropriate homework on the basis of this session work.

By contrast, the trainee probably encounters resistance when attempting to help Gemma deal with her meta-disturbance issue at a time when she would rather be dealing with her vulnerability factors.

Helping a client to prevent relapse: a caution

It is particularly important for the therapist to encourage his client to accept herself if she fails to use her rational thinking skills in real-life vulnerable situations and experiences a relapse. Part of relapse prevention includes helping a client to think rationally about relapse and so get back on track having accepted herself for relapsing. When a client thinks rationally about relapse she can more easily learn from the experience than when she thinks irrationally about it. Thinking rationally in this area will enable a client to see that every setback is a useful learning experience if she can remain sufficiently open-minded rather than self-depreciating about these setbacks.

This brings us to the end of the book. I hope I have showed you how to think and intervene like an REBT therapist. I would appreciate feedback from you and would be pleased to hear your comments sent to me c/o the publisher.

References

Beal, D., Kopec, A.M., and DiGiuseppe, R. (1996). Disputing clients' irrational beliefs. *Journal of Rational-Emotive and Cognitive-Behavior Therapy, 14*(4), 215–229.

Beck, A.T. (1976). *Cognitive therapy and the emotional disorders.* New York: International Universities Press.

Beck, A.T., Rush, A.J., Shaw, B.F., and Emery, G. (1979). *Cognitive therapy of depression.* New York: Wiley.

Bordin, E.S. (1979). The generalizability of the psychoanalytic concept of the working alliance. *Psychotherapy: Theory, Research and Practice, 16*(3): 252–260.

Burns, D.D., and Spangler, D.L. (2000). Does psychotherapy homework lead to improvements in depression in cognitive–behavioral therapy or does improvement lead to increased homework compliance? *Journal of Consulting and Clinical Psychology, 68,* 46–56.

DiGiuseppe, R. (1991). Comprehensive cognitive disputing in RET. In M.E. Bernard (Ed.), *Using rational-emotive therapy effectively: A practitioner's guide.* New York: Plenum.

Dryden, W. (1986a). Vivid methods in rational-emotive therapy. In A. Ellis and R. Grieger (Eds.), *Handbook of rational-emotive therapy,* Volume 2. New York: Springer.

Dryden, W. (1986b). Language and meaning in RET. *Journal of Rational-Emotive Therapy, 4*(2), 131–142.

Dryden, W. (1987). *Current issues in rational-emotive therapy.* London: Croom Helm.

Dryden, W. (1999a). *Rational emotive behaviour therapy: A personal approach.* Bicester, Oxon: Winslow Press.

Dryden, W. (1999b). Beyond LFT and discomfort disturbance: The case for the term 'non-ego disturbance'. *Journal of Rational-Emotive and Cognitive-Behavior Therapy, 17*(3), 165–200.

Dryden, W. (2001). *Reason to change: A rational emotive behaviour therapy (REBT) workbook.* Hove, East Sussex: Brunner-Routledge.

Dryden, W. (Ed.). (2002). *Idiosyncratic rational emotive behaviour therapy.* Ross-on-Wye: PCCS Books.

Dryden, W. (2006). *Counselling in a nutshell.* London: Sage.

Dryden, W. (Ed.). (2007). *Dryden's handbook of individual therapy.* London: Sage.

Dryden, W. (2008). *Rational emotive behavour therapy: Distinctive features.* London: Routledge.

Dryden, W. (2009). *Understanding emotional problems: The REBT perspective.* London: Routledge.

Dryden, W., and Branch, R. (2008). *The fundamentals of rational emotive behaviour therapy: A training handbook,* 2nd edn. Chichester: Wiley.

Dryden, W., and Ellis, A. (2003). *Albert Ellis Live!* London: Sage.

Ellis, A. (1963). Toward a more precise definition of 'emotional' and 'intellectual' insight. *Psychological Reports, 13,* 125–126.

Ellis, A. (1994). *Reason and emotion in psychotherapy,* revised and updated edition. New York: Birch Lane Press.

Ellis, A. (2002). *Overcoming resistance: A rational emotive behavior therapy integrated approach,* 2nd edn. New York: Springer.

Garvin, C.D., and Seabury, B.A (1997). *Interpersonal practice in social work: Promoting competence and social competence,* 2nd edn. Boston, MA: Allyn & Bacon.

Neenan, M., and Dryden, W. (1996). *Dealing with difficulties in rational emotive behaviour therapy.* London: Whurr.

Neenan, M., and Dryden, W. (1999). *Rational emotive behaviour therapy: Advances in theory and practice.* London: Whurr.

Wampold, B.E. (2001). *The great psychotherapy debate: Models, methods and findings,* 2nd edn. Hillsdale, NJ: Lawrence Erlbaum Associates.

Woods, P. (1991). Orthodox RET taught effectively with graphics, feedback on irrational beliefs, a structured homework series and models of disputation. In M.E. Bernard (Ed.), *Using rational-emotive therapy effectively: A practitioner's guide.* New York: Plenum.

Index